THE ENCYCLOPEDIA OF

MEN'S REPRODUCTIVE CANCER

Carol Turkington
Charles R. Pound, M.D.

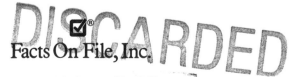

Facts On File, Inc.

The Encyclopedia of Men's Reproductive Cancer

Facts On File, Inc.
132 West 31st Street
New York NY 10001

Library of Congress Cataloging-in-Publication Data

Turkington, Carol.
The encyclopedia of men's reproductive cancer / Carol Turkington.
p. cm.
Includes bibliographical references and index.
ISBN 0-8160-5030-9 (hc : alk. paper)
1. Generative organs, Male—Cancer—Encyclopedias. I. Title.
RC280.G52T876 2004
616.99'46'003—dc222004010241

Text and cover design by Cathy Rincon

Printed in the United States of America

VB Hermitage 10 9 8 7 6 5 4 3 2 1

This book is printed on acid-free paper.

CONTENTS

FOREWORD

Cancers of the male reproductive tract can play a significant role in the lives of both young and older men. Prostate cancer is the most commonly diagnosed solid malignancy and the second leading cause of cancer death in American men. Although testicular and penile cancers occur much less often, they also are serious health issues.

Due to the fact that these problems often cause symptoms of a sensitive nature, many patients are reluctant to discuss signs and symptoms of these diseases with health care professionals. This can lead to a delay in both diagnosis and treatment that could have a dramatic effect on the patient's outcome.

The Encyclopedia of Men's Reproductive Cancer is an attempt to provide useful information to readers who do not have a thorough understanding of genitourinary cancers and potential treatments. We have made a specific effort to clarify issues pertaining to anatomy, medical terminology, and potential treatment options for persons without any medical background. Areas of groundbreaking research and possible future treatment modalities are also discussed.

Special emphasis is placed on lifestyle changes and dietary options that may affect one's likelihood of developing or fighting cancer. In an effort to provide as much concise information as possible, we have provided references to other sources of detailed information for those who may seek specialized information or support in a specific area of need.

Our hope is that through education and understanding, we may provide assistance to men at risk of, or affected by, cancer of the reproductive tract. Major advances have been made in recent decades in earlier and more effective treatments for both prostate and testicular cancer. For this to continue, we should strive to educate men about the importance of screening and early treatment of these diseases. Although penile cancer can be devastating in its later stages, it can be effectively treated without significant side effects if discovered in its early stages. There is also great potential for prevention of penile cancer altogether in men at risk if certain lifestyle canges can be implemented. The first step in this direction must be increased knowedge and understanding.

—Charles R. Pound, M.D.
Director Urologic Oncology
The University of Mississippi Medical Center

ACKNOWLEDGMENTS

The creation of a detailed encyclopedia involves the help and guidance of a wide range of experts. Without these, this book could not have been written.

First, thanks to the staff at Fox Chase Cancer Center in Philadelphia and to Dr. Charles Pound. Thanks also to the staffs of the National Institute of Mental Health, the American Medical Association, the National Institutes of Health, American Heart Association, American Psychiatric Association, American Psychological Association, American Society of Hematology, the Cancer Information Service, the Food and Drug Administration, the National Cancer Institute, and the American Board of Plastic and Reconstructive Surgeons.

I also thank the National Prostate Cancer Coalition (NPCC), Complementary and Alternative Medicine; Exceptional Cancer Patient, Inc.; Well Spouse Foundation; Chemotherapy Foundation; Cancer Liaison Program; Coalition of National Cancer Cooperative Groups; Widowed Persons Service; National Society of Genetic Counselors; Centers for Disease Control and Prevention Division of Cancer Prevention and Control; Fertile Hope; Klinefelter Syndrome and Associates; American Urological Association Alliance for Prostate Cancer Prevention; American Foundation for Urologic Disease; American Prostate Society; CaP CURE, National Prostate Cancer Coalition; Man to Man; Men's Cancer Resource Group; Patient Advocates for Advanced Cancer Treatments; Us Too International; American Brachytherapy Society; Cancer Hope Network; Cancer Information and Counseling Line; Cancer Information Service; Cancer Net; Cancer Research Institute; Cancer Survivors Network; CanSurmount; I Can Cope; International Union Against Cancer; CHEMOcare; Chemotherapy Foundation; National Association of Hospital Hospitality; Hereditary Cancer Institute; National Cancer Institute; Hospice Education Institute; HospiceLink; and the National Hospice and Palliative Care Organization.

Also, thanks to the National Hospice Foundation, Cancer Legal Resource Center, American College of Radiology, American Society of Clinical Oncology, Association of Community Cancer Centers, American College of Radiology, American Institute for Cancer Research, Cancer Research Foundation of America, Cancer Research Institute, and the European Organisation for Research and Treatment of Cancer.

Thanks also to the librarians at the Hershey Medical Center medical library, the National Library of Medicine, the Reading Public Library, and the Pennsylvania State Library.

Finally, thanks to my agent, Gene Brissie of James Peter Associates, to Bert Holtje, to my editor James Chambers, to Vanessa Nittoli at Facts On File, and to Kara and Michael.

INTRODUCTION

Each year, more than 300,000 American men are diagnosed with some type of reproductive cancer, including cancers of the prostate, penis, and testicles. Although most men diagnosed with these cancers will survive their diagnoses for years, others will not. Prostate cancer is the most common solid tumor among American men, striking about one out of every 11 white American men and one out of every nine African-American men: about 220,000 new cases occur each year. The incidence has been rising quickly in recent years, probably because of more screening and public awareness.

The early detection and appropriate treatment of reproductive cancers are key in lowering this death toll, because, when diagnosed at their earliest stages, these cancers offer excellent prognoses for long-term survival. Still, prostate cancer is the second-leading cause of cancer deaths in the United States.

Just as prostate cancer is essentially a cancer of old age (most men are over age 70 when they are diagnosed), testicular cancer is a disease of the young—and it is on the increase, especially among men in the 20 to 44 age group. About 7,400 American men are diagnosed with testicular cancer each year, accounting for just 1 percent of all cancers in men. In addition, testicular cancer is the most common form of cancer in young men between the ages of 15 and 35. The good news is that more than 95 percent of testicular cancer cases that are detected early can be successfully treated; more advanced stages (stage III and beyond) have about a 75 percent recovery rate.

Most rare of all the male reproductive cancers is penile cancer, diagnosed in just 1,400 American men each year, about 200 of whom will die of the disease. This type of cancer occurs in just one American man out of every 100,000—much more rare than in Africa, where it accounts for up to 10 percent of all cancers in men.

The Encyclopedia of Men's Reproductive Cancer is designed to answer questions about reproductive cancer and includes the most up-to-date information on cancers of the penis, testicles, and prostate that may affect a man during his lifetime. It has been designed as a guide and reference to a wide range of subjects important to the understanding of a man's reproductive health, and includes a wide variety of contact information for organization and governmental agencies affiliated with cancer issues, including current Web site addresses and phone numbers.

However, the book is not designed as a substitute for prompt assessment and treatment by oncologic experts in the diagnosis and treatment of men's reproductive and urologic cancer.

In this encyclopedia, we have tried to present the latest information in the field, based on the newest research. Although information in this book comes from the most up-to-date medical journals and research sources, readers should keep in mind that changes occur very quickly in reproductive oncology. A bibliography has been included for those who seek additional sources of information.

ENTRIES A–Z

abarelix A gonadotropin-releasing hormone (GNRH) antagonist currently being studied as a possible treatment for PROSTATE CANCER. Abarelix and other GnRH agonists work to decrease TESTOSTERONE level quickly. Abarelix is given as a monthly injection with a booster after about two weeks.

Side Effects
Reported side effects of this drug are similar to those of LUTEINIZING HORMONE–RELEASING HORMONE ANALOGS, which include HOT FLASHES, sleep problems, FATIGUE, and headache.

acid phosphatase An enzyme found in high levels in the normal prostate as well as in primary and metastatic PROSTATE CANCER. Acid phosphatase may also originate in other tissues.

A sensitive immunological test, such as radioimmunosorbent assay (RIA) or counterimmunoelectrophoresis for prostatic acid phosphatase, which are specific for the enzyme of prostate tissue, often has a positive result in the early stages of disease. Because acid phosphatase is very reliable as a marker in early disease, experts hoped the test could be used as a screening tool. However, acid phosphatase levels also may be high in up to 6 percent of cases of BENIGN PROSTATIC HYPERTROPHY and other conditions.

acupressure A noninvasive treatment for CHEMOTHERAPY-related nausea, based on the same principles as ACUPUNCTURE. In acupressure, a therapist presses on acupuncture points with the fingers instead of using needles. (Some therapists use electrical impulses, heat, laser beams, sound waves, friction, suction, or magnets instead of their fingers at the acupressure points, to the same purpose.)

Although acupressure cannot cure cancer, numerous studies have shown it is effective in relieving the nausea that follows CHEMOTHERAPY treatment or surgery. The technique can be used alone or as part of an entire system of manual healing such as in shiatsu massage.

See also ACUSTIMULATION.

acupuncture A technique in which very thin needles of varying lengths are inserted through the skin to treat a variety of conditions. Although there is no evidence that acupuncture is effective as a treatment for cancer, clinical studies have found it to be effective in treating nausea caused by chemotherapy drugs and surgical anesthesia. This finding was supported by a National Institutes of Health (NIH) expert panel consisting of scientists, researchers, and health care providers. There is also some evidence that acupuncture may lessen the need for conventional pain-relieving drugs.

Acupuncture has been practiced for the past 2,000 years and is an important component of current traditional Chinese medicine. Traditional Chinese practitioners believe that health depends on a vital energy called *qi* (pronounced "chee"), which they believe flows through pathways in the body called meridians. Practitioners believe that an obstruction along a meridian blocks the natural flow of energy, creating pain and disease. Also important to traditional Chinese physicians is the idea of the opposing forces of *yin* and *yang*, which, when balanced, are said to work together with *qi* to promote physical and mental wellness. The insertion of needles into precise points on the skin is believed to unblock energy flow, balance yin and yang, and restore health. Originally, 365 acupoints, corresponding to the number of days in a year, were identified; gradually, the number of acupoints grew to more than 2,000.

Some practitioners in the West reject the traditional philosophies of Chinese medicine and claim that acupuncture works by stimulating the production of natural painkiller substances in the body called endorphins. Because Western scientists have found the study of meridians (that do not exactly correspond to nerve or blood circulation pathways) difficult, some deny that meridians exist. Nevertheless, several studies have found that acupuncture used along with mainstream medicine can have real benefits, such as helping to relieve pain and reduce the nausea and vomiting of chemotherapy. There is no evidence that acupuncture used alone is effective in treating or preventing cancer.

Traditional acupuncture needles were made of bone, stone, or metal (including silver and gold), but modern disposable acupuncture needles are made of very thin stainless steel. In 1996 the U.S. Food and Drug Administration (FDA) approved the use of acupuncture needles by licensed practitioners; by law, needles must be labeled for one-time use only.

The procedure should cause little or no discomfort, because the needles are as thin as a strand of hair, and they usually are left in place for less than half an hour. Some acupuncturists twirl the needles or apply low-voltage electricity to them as a way to enhance the results. When conducted by a trained professional, acupuncture is generally considered safe. The number of complications reported has been relatively low, but there is a risk that a patient may be harmed by an acupuncturist who is not well trained.

There are more than 10,000 acupuncturists in the United States, and about 32 states have established training standards for licensing the practice of acupuncture. MEDICARE does not cover acupuncture, but it is covered by some private health insurance plans and health maintenance organizations (HMOs). Consumers should consult an experienced, qualified practitioner who is state licensed or board certified. The American Academy of Medical Acupuncture (http://www.medicalacupuncture.org) can refer patients to physicians (M.D.s or D.O.s) who practice acupuncture.

See also ACUPRESSURE; ACUSTIMULATION.

acustimulation   Mild electrical stimulation of ACUPUNCTURE points to control symptoms such as nausea and vomiting.

See also ACUPRESSURE.

adenocarcinoma   A type of cancerous gland cell that begins with a malignant change in the lining or inner area of an organ. Almost all PROSTATE CANCER is adenocarcinoma, which originates within the tiny glands of the prostate itself. As with every other type of cancer, an adenocarcinoma begins as one mutant abnormal cell that multiplies and grows into a larger tumor.

If untreated, the cancer cells eventually spread through the capsule of the gland and out into nearby lymph nodes, bones, or other tissues. This may occur early in the life of the tumor or may not occur for many years. Even before the tumor is big enough to penetrate the area outside the capsule, sometimes a few cancer cells may escape from the prostate into blood or lymph nodes.

adenomatoid tumor   A very rare, benign tumor of the epididymis (one of a pair of long coiled tubes that carry sperm from the testicles to the vas deferens). The vas deferens then empties into the ejaculatory duct within the prostate. From there, the sperm enters the penis. On ultrasound, this tumor appears as a well-defined mass separate from the testicle.

adjuvant treatment   Treatment for cancer that is used after (in addition to) primary treatment to increase the effectiveness of the primary surgical treatment. It usually entails the use of CHEMOTHERAPY, HORMONAL THERAPY, or RADIATION THERAPY after surgery, to increase the likelihood of killing all cancer cells.

A secondary form of treatment begun prior to the primary therapy is called neo-adjuvant treatment.

adrenal glands   Gland located on the top of each kidney that produces male sex hormones (ANDROGEN) and some female sex hormones (estrogen and progesterone). They also produce other hormones, such as aldosterone and hydrocortisone, which help control the body's metabolism, and epinephrine and norepinephrine, which help regulate heart rate, breathing, and digestion.

Adriamycin (doxorubicin) An anthracycline antibiotic used in combination with other CHEMOTHERAPY drugs to treat PROSTATE CANCER, and many other types of cancer. Doxorubicin disrupts the growth of cancer cells, destroying them. Side effects include loss of appetite, nausea and vomiting, HAIR LOSS, and decreased white blood cell and platelet counts. Less common side effects include mouth or lip sores, radiation recall, and irregular heartbeat. Rarely, Adriamycin may cause heart damage, leading to congestive heart failure.

Adrucil See FLUOROURACIL.

advance directives A written document, completed and signed when a person is legally competent, that explains what the person would or would not want if he or she were unable to make decisions about medical care. Common advance directives include the following:

- HEALTH CARE PROXY (or health care power of attorney), which gives another person the authority to make decisions for a patient when the person is unable to do so
- LIVING WILL, which directs a doctor to use, not start, or stop treatment that is keeping a dying patient alive when the patient cannot make his or her preferences known
- Nonhospital DO NOT RESUSCITATE ORDER (DNR order), which directs emergency staff not to resuscitate a person in a life-threatening situation who is not in a hospital or other health care facility

Advance directives are an important part of any patient's financial affairs, since such documents allow someone else to make treatment decisions on a patient's behalf when the person is no longer capable of making those decisions.

Patients should prepare and sign advance directives that comply with state law and give copies to family, friends, and doctors. The document should reflect the patient's wishes and appoint someone who is willing to carry out those wishes to make decisions.

African Americans The incidence of male reproductive cancers varies strikingly for African Americans and Caucasian Americans. In most cases, African-American men have higher rates of these cancers than do Caucasian men. Overall cancer rates have been inching down for African Americans in the last decade, but the disparity between races continues.

Members of minorities receive substandard medical care because of racial discrimination in health care settings, time pressures on health care workers, and low-end health insurance plans, according to a recent landmark report (*Unequal Treatment: Confronting Racial and Ethnic Disparities in Health Care* 2003). As a result, more African Americans and members of other minority groups die of cancer than do Caucasians. Lower-quality medical care was found even when minority patients' income, age, medical condition, and insurance coverage were similar to those of Caucasian patients.

Early detection could lower the high cancer death rates among African Americans, since regular checkups and other tests detect cancer early, when treatment is more successful. About half of all cancers can now be discovered early by such screening methods. But African Americans are not getting this preventive care. Some cancers detectable by screening are diagnosed in African Americans at a later stage.

Prostate Cancer

The PROSTATE CANCER rate among African Americans is the most dramatic evidence of the cancer gap between races. African-American men have the highest rates of prostate cancer and death of cancer in the world—more than twice the rates for Caucasian men in the United States. Moreover, some studies have shown that African Americans who have cancer have shorter survival time than Caucasians at all stages of diagnosis. Other studies of African-American men with equal access to health care (such as in the military) have shown that they have similar survival rates to Caucasians when diagnosed at the same stage.

PROSTATE CANCER is about 66 percent more common in African-American men than in Caucasian men. In fact, African-American men may have the highest rate of prostate cancer in the world. In addition, the risk that an African-American man will die of prostate cancer is twice as high as the risk of Caucasians. Death rates also are increasing much more rapidly among African-American men.

Because they are at higher risk, African Americans should begin screening for prostate cancer by age 40—10 years earlier than Caucasian men, according to the AMERICAN UROLOGIC ASSOCIATION and the American College of Surgeons. On the other hand, Africans in Africa have one of the lowest rates of prostate cancer in the world.

In addition to these race-related causes, studies have also found an increased risk of prostate cancer associated with a DIET high in saturated fat among African Americans. Other factors such as genetically determined HORMONE levels and diet during adolescence may account for differences in incidence among the ethnic groups studied.

The AMERICAN CANCER SOCIETY (ACS) has developed a prostate education program for African Americans called Let's Talk About It cosponsored by the 100 Black Men of America, Inc. The ACS Man to Man program enlists survivors and others concerned about prostate cancer to help people newly diagnosed with the disease and to develop local support groups, screenings, and educational events.

Testicular Cancer

Caucasian-American men have about five times the risk of TESTICULAR CANCER of African-American men. Whereas the risk for testicular cancer has doubled among Caucasian Americans in the past 40 years, it has remained the same for African Americans. The reasons for these differences are not known.

age The incidence of male reproductive tract cancers generally increases with age, generally occurring in men older than age 50 (except for TESTICULAR CANCER). Even if cancer incidence rates remain steady, the number of people diagnosed with cancer in the next 50 years is expected to double, barring any major breakthroughs in prevention. The aging of the population alone will increase the number of people who are diagnosed

and treated for cancer but who also survive longer at increasingly older ages. Advances in cancer prevention, detection, and treatment should continue to reduce cancer death rates.

Prostate Cancer

For example, in the United States, PROSTATE CANCER is found mainly in men older than age 50; the median age is 69. In fact, more than 70 percent of all prostate cancers are diagnosed in men older than 65 years old. It is unclear why this increase with age occurs for this type of cancer; the average age of patients at the time of diagnosis is 70. In fact, the increase in the prevalence of prostate cancer with age is greater for prostate cancer than for any other cancer. For every 10 years after the age of 40, the incidence of a significant prostate cancer nearly doubles. Men in their 50s have a risk of 10 percent, which increases to 70 percent for men in their 80s. (However, in most older men the prostate cancer is not fatal; many die of other causes and are never diagnosed with prostate cancer).

Alarmingly, the rates of prostate cancer are on the rise: Incidence rates have increased both for men younger than age 50 and for men aged 50 to 64.

Penile Cancer

Age is also a risk factor for PENILE CANCER. Most cases of the disease are diagnosed in men older than age 50, although about 20 percent occur in men younger than 40 years of age.

Testicular Cancer

Although advanced age is a critical factor in other types of male reproductive cancers, the exception is testicular cancer, which is the most common form of cancer in men 15 to 40 years old. It may also occur in young boys; about 3 percent of all testicular cancer is found in this group.

Agent Orange A toxic herbicide containing dioxin used by U.S. soldiers during the Vietnam War that has been linked to a number of cancers, including PROSTATE CANCER, according to the U.S. Veterans Administration. Shortly after their military service in Vietnam, some veterans reported a variety of health problems (including cancer) that many attributed to exposure to Agent Orange or other herbicides.

Agent Orange was the code name for a herbicide developed in the 1940s for military use in tropical climates; extensive testing for military applications did not begin until the early 1960s. The purpose of the product was to destroy enemy cover in dense terrain by defoliating trees and shrubbery. Agent Orange (the name refers to the orange band that was used to mark the drums in which it was stored) was tested in Vietnam in the early 1960s and used more extensively during the height of the war (1967–68). It was eventually phased out and its use discontinued in 1971. Agent Orange was a mixture of two chemicals—2,4,D (2,4-dichlorophenoxyacetic acid) and 2,4,5,-T (2,4,5-trichlorophenoxyacetic acid)—that was then combined with kerosene or diesel fuel and dispersed by aircraft, vehicle, and hand spraying. An estimated 19 million gallons of Agent Orange were used in South Vietnam during the war.

The earliest health concerns about Agent Orange focused on the product's contamination with chlorinated dioxin 2,3,7,8-tetrachlorodibenzo-p-dioxin (TCDD) (dioxin). TCDD is one of a family of dioxins that are cousins of cancer-causing polychlorinated biphenyls (PCBs). The TCDD found in Agent Orange is believed to be harmful to humans; in animal tests, TCDD has caused a wide variety of fatal diseases. TCDD is a synthetic, always unwanted byproduct of the chemical manufacturing process. The Agent Orange used in Vietnam was later found to be extensively contaminated with TCDD.

The Agent Orange Settlement Fund was created as a result of class action lawsuits by Vietnam veterans and their families about injuries allegedly incurred as a result of their exposure to chemical herbicides used during the Vietnam War. The suit, brought against the major manufacturers of these herbicides, was settled out of court in 1984 for $180 million—reportedly the largest settlement of its kind at that time. The Settlement Fund was given to class members according to a distribution plan established by the courts. Because the class involved an estimated 10 million people, the fund was distributed to class members in the United States through two separate programs designed to provide most benefits to Vietnam vets and their families most in need of assistance.

A payment program provided cash to totally disabled veterans and survivors of deceased veterans, and an assistance program provided money for social services organizations to establish programs to benefit all the affected veterans. The payment program distributed a total of $197 million to about 52,000 veterans between 1988 and 1994. The assistance program functioned as a foundation, distributing $74 million to 83 organizations between 1989 and 1996. These agencies, which ranged from disability and veterans service organizations to community-based not-for-profits, provided counseling, advocacy, and medical and case-management services. During this period, these organizations helped more than 239,000 Vietnam veterans and their families.

The Department of Veterans Affairs has developed a comprehensive program to respond to veterans' medical problems, including health-care services, disability compensation for veterans who have service-connected illnesses, scientific research, and outreach and education.

Air Care Alliance A national league of humanitarian flying organizations dedicated to providing air travel for severely ill patients (such as cancer patients) who cannot afford air transportation. The alliance has member groups whose activities include health-care, patient transport, and other kinds of public-benefit flying. For contact information, see Appendix I.

AirLifeLine The oldest and largest national volunteer pilot organization in the United States, dedicated to providing transportation to and from medical destinations for patients in financial need. For a quarter-century, AirLifeLine has helped to ensure equal access to health care and improve the quality of life for thousands of people throughout the United States. Flights are staffed with volunteer pilots who donate their time and all of the flight costs.

AirLifeLine is a charitable nonprofit organization funded by donations from individuals, foundations, corporations, and volunteer pilots. For contact information, see Appendix I.

alcohol Moderate to heavy alcohol intake (three or more drinks per day) increases a man's risk of developing PROSTATE CANCER. Alcohol increases production of TESTOSTERONE, which may stimulate the growth of prostate cells. Testosterone is a hormone that stimulates growth in both normal and cancerous prostate cells, and may play a role in the development of prostate cancer.

Although the increased risk related to alcohol appears to be relatively slight in some studies, prostate cancer is so prevalent that even a small association could translate into a significant number of prostate cancers. The risk of prostate cancer appears to be higher for both African-Americans and Caucasians according to the amount of alcohol they consume. The increased risk of prostate cancer associated with alcohol consumption in general was found to be only slight for both groups, but there was a significant increase in risk for those considered to be heavy or very heavy drinkers, whether younger or older than age 65.

No difference was found between men who had stopped drinking alcohol and men who still drank, leading researchers to suspect that alcohol use is related to the early stages of the disease. Alcohol may cause prostate cancer either indirectly, through its effect on the body's ability to absorb nutrients, or directly, through its possible carcinogenic properties.

alendronate sodium A drug that affects bone metabolism that is being studied as a possible treatment for bone pain caused by cancer. Alendronate sodium belongs to the family of drugs called BISPHOSPHONATES.

alkaline phosphatase An enzyme made by cells in the bones and liver. Levels of alkaline phosphatase in the blood often rise in men whose PROSTATE CANCER has spread to the bones or liver.

See also ALKALINE PHOSPHATASE TEST.

alkaline phosphatase test (ALP test) A test measures the level of an enzyme called ALKALINE PHOSPHATASE (ALP) in the blood. This enzyme is found in all tissues, especially in the liver, bile ducts, and bone. Since damaged or diseased tissue releases enzymes into the blood, ALP level measurements can be abnormal in many conditions, including cancer. (Serum ALP level is also high in some normal conditions, such as during normal bone growth or in response to a variety of drugs.) The ALP test is one of several that may be used to help diagnose cancers that typically spread to the bone, including PROSTATE CANCER. The normal range is 44 to 147 IU/l. Higher-than-normal levels may indicate leukemia or bone cancer.

alkylating agents Drugs that cause a chemical process to disrupt cell division, especially in fast-growing cells. Types of alkylating agents include alkyl sulfonates, ethyleneamines, nitrogen mustards, nitrosoureas, and triagenes. Alkylating agents carry a very high risk of infertility. They are often used as a form of CHEMOTHERAPY to treat various cancers.

Alliance for Prostate Cancer Patients An organization whose aim is to recruit public and private business leaders, legislators, health providers and administrators, researchers, and federal, state, and local health officials into a coordinated cohesive forum to enhance and promote prostate cancer awareness, education, research, and primary and secondary prevention programs. The goal of this diversified stakeholder group is to implement and evaluate ambitious plans that are designed to eliminate PROSTATE CANCER as a health threat in the United States by 2010. For contact information, see Appendix I.

allicin A phytochemical found in onions and GARLIC that experts suspect may help protect against cancer. Allicin is most widely recognized for its action as an antiviral, antifungal, and antibacterial agent with the ability to block the toxins produced by bacteria and viruses. It is also an ANTIOXIDANT and helps to eliminate toxins from the body.

alopecia See HAIR LOSS.

alpha-fetoprotein (AFP) A protein found in the bloodstream of some men who have TESTICULAR CANCER. The alpha-fetoprotein (AFP) level rises when the cancer is growing and falls when the cancer is shrinking or has been surgically removed, so a blood test can potentially measure the progress of the disease and success of treatment. Because of its action, AFP is considered to be a TUMOR MARKER.

Higher levels of AFP occur in 75 percent of TERATOCARCINOMA, EMBRYONAL CELL CARCINOMA, and YOLK SAC CARCINOMA patients. (However, increased levels of AFP are also found in people who have liver diseases, such as cirrhosis, acute and chronic hepatitis, and hepatic necrosis.) The half-life of AFP in the blood is five to seven days; therefore, high levels of AFP should fall by one-half of the initial level per week and should probably return to normal within 25 to 35 days after surgery if all of the tumor has been removed. The higher the level, however, the longer the interval before it returns to normal.

AFP level is normally less than about 5 ng/ml, but presence of cancer cannot be assumed until the level is above 25 ng/ml. A very small number of people have a naturally high level of this protein in their blood (less than 25 ng/ml) though they do not have cancer.

American Association for Cancer Education (AACE) A professional organization of educators in many disciplines who are working to improve the quality of education in the field of cancer. The association provides a forum for those concerned with the education of health professionals working to advance the prevention of cancer, expedite early cancer detection, promote individualized therapy, and develop rehabilitation programs for cancer patients.

American Association for Cancer Education (AACE) efforts include the faculties of schools of medicine, dentistry, osteopathy, education, pharmacy, nursing, public health, and social work. The association encourages projects for the training of paramedical personnel and educational programs for the general public, populations at risk, and cancer patients.

The group was founded in 1947 as the Cancer Coordinators, an association of cancer educators in U.S. medical and dental schools who met annually to discuss issues in the field. The mission of the association today is to foster cancer education by individuals throughout the world involved in cancer education. It provides a forum for health-related professionals concerned with the study and improvement of cancer education at the undergraduate, graduate, continuing professional, and paraprofessional levels.

Active members include physicians, dentists, nurses, health educators, social workers, occupational therapists, and other professionals interested in cancer education. Cancer education efforts are related to prevention, early detection, treatment, and rehabilitation.

Other interests of the association include educational programs for the general public, for populations at special risk, and for cancer patients. Such efforts involve developing and evaluating new educational strategies and methods, including the examination of objectives, courses, and evaluation instruments; expanding public education; fostering international cooperative efforts in cancer education; and furthering education in cancer prevention. For contact information, see Appendix I.

American Association of Tissue Banks (AATB) A scientific nonprofit organization founded in 1976 that sets guidelines to ensure the safety and availability of high-quality transplantable human tissue. Organizations such as sperm banks attain American Association of Tissue Banks (AATB) membership through a process of inspection and accreditation by adhering to the published standards of the group. The AATB further promotes the quality and safety of tissues and cells for transplantation through its program of voluntary inspection and accreditation of tissue banks. The association also maintains a registry of U.S. sperm banks.

Some men who are interested in fathering children consider sperm banking before surgery, RADIATION THERAPY, or CHEMOTHERAPY treatments that may render them infertile. Sperm banks are facilities at a limited number of health care institutions where sperm are frozen and stored in liquid nitrogen–cooled refrigerators.

Before treatment, patients are usually advised to collect specimens over at least two weeks. Specimens can be stored because the capacity of sperm to fertilize eggs does not change for an extended period.

Sperm banks charge fees for freezing, storing, and retrieving sperm for the donor. Costs vary among institutions, and some portions are covered by some insurance companies. Since most physicians want patients to start cancer treatment shortly after diagnosis, it is important to locate a sperm bank as soon as possible to begin storing sperm.

See also INFERTILITY; SPERM BANKING.

American Brachytherapy Society (ABS) A nonprofit, professional organization founded in 1978 that seeks to provide insight and research into the use of BRACHYTHERAPY in malignant and benign conditions. Members include physicists, physicians, and other health care providers interested in brachytherapy. The mission of the American Brachytherapy Society (ABS) is to provide information directly to the consumer, promote the highest standards of practice of brachytherapy, and help health-care professionals by encouraging improved and continuing education for radiation ONCOLOGISTS and other professionals involved in the treatment of cancer. In addition, the ABS promotes clinical and laboratory research into the practice of brachytherapy. For contact information, see Appendix I.

American Cancer Society (ACS) A nationwide community-based organization dedicated to eliminating cancer as a major health problem by preventing cancer, saving lives, and easing suffering through research, education, advocacy, and service. It is one of the oldest and largest voluntary health agencies in the United States: more than two million Americans are involved in programs of research, education, patient service, advocacy, and rehabilitation. Headquartered in Atlanta, Georgia, the American Cancer Society (ACS) has state divisions throughout the country and more than 3,400 local offices.

To ease the impact of cancer on patients and their families, the American Cancer Society provides service and rehabilitation programs, as well as patient and family education and support programs. The ACS provides printed materials and conducts educational programs. Society staff members also accept calls and distribute publications in Spanish and sponsor a number of related support groups, including CANCER SURVIVORS NETWORK, I

Can Cope, Look Good . . . Feel Better, and Reach To Recovery. A local ACS group may be listed in the white pages of the telephone directory.

The society has invested more than $2.4 billion in cancer research and has provided grant support to 32 Nobel Prize winners early in their career. The society's overall annual expenditure in research grew steadily from $1 million in 1946 to more than $125 million in 2002. The research program focuses primarily on peer-reviewed projects initiated by beginning investigators working in leading medical and scientific institutions across the country. The research program consists of three components: extramural grants, intramural epidemiology and surveillance research, and the intramural behavioral research center. The society's prevention programs focus primarily on tobacco control, the relationship between diet and physical activity and cancer, promotion of comprehensive school health education, and reduction of the risk of skin cancer.

The society also gives patients and professionals information via its early detection guidelines and its detection education and advocacy programs, in order to ensure that all cancers are detected at the earliest possible stage, when there is the greatest chance of successful treatment. The society sponsors national conferences and workshops, audiovisual and print publications, the American Cancer Society Web site, and the National Call Center, as well as clinical awards, professorships, and scholarships. For contact information, see Appendix I.

American Cancer Society Web site This Web site (at www.cancer.org) is sponsored by the AMERICAN CANCER SOCIETY to provide lifesaving information to the public. The site includes an interactive cancer resource center containing in-depth information on every major cancer type. Through the resource center, visitors can order American Cancer Society publications, gain access to recent news articles, and find additional on- and off-line resources. Other sections on the Web site include a directory of medical resources, links to other sites organized by cancer type or topic, resources for media representatives, and information on the society's research grants program, advocacy efforts, and special events. For contact information see Appendix I.

American Chronic Pain Association (ACPA) A nonprofit tax-exempt organization that has more than 400 chapters in the United States, Canada, Australia, New Zealand, Mexico, England, Ireland, Wales, Scotland, India, Jordan, and Russia. Since 1980 the association has provided a support system for people with chronic pain through education in pain management skills and self-help group activities. Groups are open to anyone who has chronic pain, regardless of race, creed, sexual orientation, or source of the pain.

The American Chronic Pain Association (ACPA) facilitates peer support and education for individuals who have chronic pain and their families so that these individuals may live more fully in spite of their pain. The association also works to raise awareness among the health care community, policy makers, and the public about issues related to living with chronic pain. For contact information, see Appendix I.

American College of Radiology (ACR) A medical specialty society of more than 31,000 members established in 1923 that promotes high-quality medical imaging. A leader in radiation oncology for the past 25 years, the American College of Radiology (ACR) recently created the American College of Radiology Imaging Network (ACRIN), a multicenter network that conducts diagnostic imaging studies comparing current techniques and equipment with new technology.

The members of the American College of Radiology include radiologists, radiation ONCOLOGISTS, and medical physicists. For more than three-quarters of a century the ACR has devoted its resources to making imaging safe, effective, and accessible to those who need it.

The ACR supports a number of accreditation programs, including programs in ultrasound, magnetic resonance imaging, nuclear medicine, radiation oncology, radiography/fluoroscopy, and computed tomography. Patients can search for accredited facilities at the ACR Web site. For contact information, see Appendix I.

American Foundation for Urologic Disease (AFUD) A nonprofit agency interested in the prevention and cure of urologic disease through the expansion of patient education, public awareness, research, and advocacy. The agency, founded in 1987, has earmarked more than $2.4 million for research and public education initiatives. *Family Urology,* the official magazine of the foundation, reaches more than 100,000 readers each quarter.

The foundation offers a membership program to help support its mission and to keep medical professionals, patients, family members, and friends informed about urologic disease and dysfunctions, including PROSTATE CANCER treatment options and sexual function. They also offer prostate cancer support groups, such as Prostate Cancer Network. Some Spanish-language publications are available.

The foundation's education councils have distributed more than 6 million brochures nationwide to patients, grassroots organizations, physicians, medical specialty groups, allied health-care workers, and corporations. For contact information, see Appendix I.

American Institute for Cancer Research (AICR) A nonprofit group that provides information about cancer prevention, particularly through DIET and nutrition, and supports research at sites throughout the country. The institute also offers a toll-free nutrition hotline, a pen pal support network, and a wide array of consumer and health professional brochures, plus health aids related to diet and nutrition and their link to cancer and cancer prevention.

The American Institute for Cancer Research (AICR) also supports CancerResource, an information and resource program for cancer patients. A limited selection of Spanish-language publications is available.

Since its founding in 1982 the American Institute for Cancer Research has grown into the nation's leading charity in the field of diet, nutrition, and cancer. AICR also offers a wide range of cancer prevention education programs and publications for health professionals and the public. Through these pioneering efforts, AICR has helped focus attention on the link between cancer and lifestyle choices. Over the past several years, the institute has spent 66 percent to 72 percent of its funds on research and education. For contact information, see Appendix I.

American Joint Committee on Cancer (AJCC)
An organization established in 1959 to publish systems of classification of cancer, including staging and end results reporting, for doctors. This information is used to help select the most effective treatment, determine prognosis, and continue evaluation of cancer control measures.

The organization is comprised of six founding organizations, four sponsoring organizations, and seven liaison organizations. Membership is reserved for those organizations whose missions or goals are consistent with or complementary to those of the American Joint Committee on Cancer (AJCC).

These organizations generally demonstrate involvement or activity in one or more of the following areas: cancer epidemiology, patient care, cancer control, cancer registration, professional education, research, and biostatistics.

Sponsoring organizations include the AMERICAN CANCER SOCIETY, the American College of Surgeons, the AMERICAN SOCIETY OF CLINICAL ONCOLOGY, and the Centers for Disease Control and Prevention. For contact information, see Appendix I.

American Pain Society   A multidisciplinary organization of basic and clinical scientists, practicing clinicians, policy analysts, and others interested in advancing pain-related research, education, treatment, and professional practice. The American Pain Society was founded on March 6, 1977, in Chicago. In its *Pain Facilities Directory*, the society offers information on more than 500 specialized pain treatment centers across the country. It also offers counseling for pain, referrals, and education programs. For contact information, see Appendix I.

American Prostate Society (APS)   A nonprofit organization that provides information on the most up-to-date treatments for PROSTATE CANCER, PROSTATITIS, prostate growth, and impotence. In addition to a Web site featuring frequently asked questions (FAQs) and other information, the American Prostate Society (APS) offers a free newsletter on request. For contact information, see Appendix I.

American Society of Clinical Oncology (ASCO)
A nonprofit organization dedicated to supporting all types of cancer research, but especially patient-oriented clinical research. The American Society of Clinical Oncology (ASCO) mission is to facilitate the delivery of high-quality health care, foster the exchange of information, further the training of researchers, and encourage communication among the various cancer specialties.

ASCO has more than 16,000 professional members worldwide, including clinical ONCOLOGISTS in medical oncology, therapeutic radiology, surgical oncology, pediatric oncology, gynecologic oncology, urologic oncology, and hematology; students; oncology nurses; and other health-care practitioners. International members make up 20 percent of the total membership and represent 75 countries worldwide. For contact information, see Appendix I.

Americans with Disabilities Act   A law that protects American employees (in companies that have more than 15 workers) from employment discrimination. Cancer patients are included under this law, which requires employers to make accommodations for those who have temporary or permanent disabilities. Men who have REPRODUCTIVE CANCERS who think they may have been discriminated against at work can contact their company's human resources office for information or consider filing a complaint with the U.S. Justice Department.

American Urological Association (AVA)   The world's preeminent urological association, which conducts a wide range of activities to ensure that more than 13,000 members remain current on the most recent research and best practices in the field of urology.

An educational nonprofit organization, the American Urological Association (AUA) fosters the highest standards of urologic care by providing a wide range of services, including publications, an annual meeting, continuing medical education, and health policy advocacy. For contact information, see Appendix I.

analgesic pump   A device containing narcotic medication that can be operated by a patient as a way of controlling pain, first made available in 1974. The pump is hooked up to an intravenous feed (IV) so that patients can obtain immediate pain relief by pressing a button to self-administer a preset dose of medication as often as needed. A control protects against excessive doses. The analgesic pump offers the psychological advantage of allowing the patient to exercise some control over pain, not to have to wait for a nurse to administer an injection.

These are generally used on a short-term basis after surgery, but in patients with advanced cancer it can be implanted under the skin for longer periods.

androgen A type of male hormone that stimulates the development of male sexual characteristics, such as beard growth, testicular enlargement, and voice deepening. TESTOSTERONE and ANDROSTERONE are two androgens that are also used to treat cancer. Androgens appear to change the hormonal environment in the cancer cell, removing the stimulus to grow so that it does not divide. The exact mechanism is unknown.

Androgens are produced by the testicles and, to a limited degree, by the adrenal glands.

Androgen medications should not be used by people who have PROSTATE CANCER, because most prostate cancer cells require testosterone to grow.

Patients who take androgens may retain salt and water; after using androgens for more than three months they may experience decreased sexual interest, increased body hair, and acne.

Androgen medications include the following:

- Calusterone (Methosarb)
- Dromostanolone propionate (Drolban, Masteril, Macleron, Permastril)
- Fluoxymesteron (Halotestin, Ora-Testryl)
- Nandrolone decanoate (Deca-Durabolin)
- Testosterone propionate (Neohombreol, Oraton)

androsterone A type of steroid hormone (an ANDROGEN) that is synthesized and released by the testes, and is responsible for stimulating the development of male sexual characteristics.

anemia A decrease in red blood cells. Anemia is common in cancer patients and may cause debilitating FATIGUE, often as a result of a decline in the level of hemoglobin, the part of blood that carries oxygen to the body's tissues. About three in four cancer patients experience fatigue caused by anemia or by cancer treatment.

In some cases, anemia occurs when the body's red blood cells are being destroyed at a faster than normal rate because of the side effects of radiation or chemotherapy. Anemia also can be caused by bleeding from a tumor or by insufficient production of red blood cells by BONE MARROW.

Several forms of anemia may occur in cancer patients. *Hemolytic anemia* occurs when red blood cells are destroyed, possibly as a result of chemotherapy. *Aplastic anemia* occurs when the bone marrow makes too few red blood cells as a result of either chemotherapy or radiation. Levels of white blood cells and platelets also decline. *Iron-deficiency anemia* occurs when the level of iron in the blood is too low; the low level leads to a lack of hemoglobin, which in turn causes anemia. In those who have cancer, iron deficiency may be a result of bleeding (such as from a tumor in the colon). *Pernicious anemia* occurs when there is a lack of vitamin B_{12} in the diet. Many cancer patients often have a poor appetite and may not eat enough foods that contain vitamin B_{12}. Anemia also may occur if cancer has spread to the bone or may be a response to hormone therapy.

Symptoms

If blood counts drop slowly, initial symptoms may not be readily apparent. Once anemia becomes significant, it may cause lowering of blood pressure when a person stands up quickly, weakness, dizziness, pallor, shortness of breath, heart palpitations, feeling of cold, or fatigue. A sudden (or large amount of) bleeding from a tumor may cause the rapid onset of these symptoms.

Treatment

Anemia that results from CHEMOTHERAPY may be treated by iron and vitamin supplements, bone marrow stimulants such as ERYTHROPOIETIN (a medication that stimulates the production of blood cells), or transfusion therapy.

aneuploid Having either too few or too many chromosomes in a cell. In humans, an aneuploid cell would be considered abnormal.

Normally, each cell should have two copies of each chromosome, one inherited from the mother and one from the father. A cell with the normal number of each chromosome (two) is called a "diploid" cell. A triploid cell has three copies of each chromosome, and is abnormal.

An "aneuploid" cell has a chromosome number that is not an exact multiple of the normal diploid number (two), with either fewer or more than the normal number of chromosomes in the cell. A triploid cell would be an example of aneuploidy in humans.

Most cancerous cells are aneuploid cells—and the more aneuploid they are (that is, the more chromosomes they have in each cell), the more aggressive the cancer. FLOW CYTOMETRY can measure the amount of cellular chromosomes and determine whether the cell has the correct number of chromosomes.

angiogenesis The formation of a network of blood vessels that penetrates cancerous growths, supplying nutrients and oxygen and removing waste products. This process helps cancer to spread.

Tumor angiogenesis actually starts when cancerous tumor cells release molecules that send signals to surrounding normal host tissue; the signals activate certain genes that in turn make proteins to encourage growth of new blood vessels. Other chemicals, called ANGIOGENESIS INHIBITORS, cause the process to stop.

The walls of blood vessels are formed by cells that divide only about once every three years. However, when required, angiogenesis can stimulate them to divide.

Angiogenesis is regulated by both activator and inhibitor molecules. Normally, the inhibitors predominate, blocking growth. Should a need for new blood vessels arise (such as to repair a wound), angiogenesis activators increase in number and inhibitors decrease. This process prompts the formation of new blood vessels.

Because cancer cannot grow or spread without the formation of new blood vessels, scientists are trying to find ways to stop angiogenesis. They are studying natural and synthetic angiogenesis inhibitors, also called antiangiogenesis agents, for the potential of these chemicals to prevent the growth of cancer by blocking the formation of new blood vessels. In animal studies, angiogenesis inhibitors have stopped the formation of new blood vessels, causing cancerous cells to shrink and die.

When researchers realized that cancer cells can release molecules to activate the process of angiogenesis, the challenge became to find and study these angiogenesis-stimulating molecules in animal and human tumors. From such studies more than a dozen different proteins, as well as several smaller molecules, have been identified as angiogenic, meaning that they are released by tumors as signals for angiogenesis. Among these molecules, two proteins appear to be the most important for sustaining tumor growth: vascular endothelial growth factor (VEGF) and basic fibroblast growth factor (bFGF). VEGF and bFGF are produced by many kinds of cancer cells and by certain types of normal cells, too.

Although many tumors produce angiogenic molecules such as VEGF and bFGF, presence of the molecules is not sufficient to begin blood vessel growth. For angiogenesis to begin, these activator molecules must overcome a variety of angiogenesis inhibitors that normally restrain blood vessel growth. Almost a dozen naturally occurring proteins, including the proteins angiostatin, endostatin, and thrombospondin, can inhibit angiogenesis. A finely tuned balance between the concentration of angiogenesis inhibitors and the concentration of activators such as VEGF and bFGF determines whether a tumor can induce the growth of new blood vessels. Angiogenesis is triggered when the production of activators increases as the production of inhibitors decreases.

The discovery that angiogenesis inhibitors such as endostatin can restrain the growth of primary tumors raises the possibility that such inhibitors may also be able to slow tumor spread.

It has been known for many years that cancer cells originating in a primary tumor can spread to another organ and form tiny, microscopic tumor masses that can remain dormant for years. A likely explanation for this tumor dormancy is that no angiogenesis occurred, so the small tumor lacked the new blood vessels needed for continued growth. One possible reason for tumor dormancy may be that some primary tumors secrete the inhibitor angiostatin into the bloodstream; angiostatin then circulates throughout the body and inhibits blood vessel growth at other sites. This process could prevent microscopic cancer cells from growing into visible tumors.

Researchers are now studying whether interfering with angiogenesis can slow or prevent the growth and spread of cancer cells in humans. To answer this question, almost two dozen angiogenesis inhibitors are currently being tested in patients who have cancers of the breast. If the results of clinical trials show that angiogenesis inhibitors are both safe and effective in treating cancer in humans, these agents may be approved by the U.S. Food and Drug Administration (FDA) and made available for widespread use. The process of producing and testing angiogenesis inhibitors is likely to take several years.

angiogenesis inhibitor   Substance (also called an antiangiogenesis agent) that may prevent the growth of blood vessels from surrounding tissue to a solid tumor.

See also ANGIOGENESIS.

anorexia   See APPETITE LOSS.

anthocyanins   A group of plant chemicals within the larger category of PHYTOCHEMICALS called PHENOLICS that give intense color to certain red and blue fruits and vegetables (especially blueberries). These plant pigments are very powerful ANTIOXIDANTS that have been studied extensively for their ability to fight cancer and to delay several diseases associated with the aging process.

antiandrogen   A medication that blocks or interferes with the body's ability to use androgens by preventing these HORMONES from reaching malignant PROSTATE CANCER cells. An ANDROGEN is a steroid hormone that stimulates the development of male sexual characteristics, such as beard growth, deepening voice, and muscle development. TESTOSTERONE and ANDROSTERONE are two examples of androgens. These hormones are principally produced in the testis, although they are also secreted by the adrenal cortex.

Because antiandrogens do not actually affect the production of testosterone, testosterone levels remain normal during treatment. This means that libido and erectile function are not affected by use of antiandrogens.

The antiandrogen BICALUTAMIDE (Casodex) has been shown to be effective in treating prostate cancer; it has not yet been approved by the U.S. Food and Drug Administration (FDA). Other antiandrogens include FLUTAMIDE (Eulexin) and NILUTAMIDE (Nilandron).

Antiandrogens used together with LUTEINIZING HORMONE–RELEASING HORMONE (LHRH) ANALOGS are considered to cause a total androgen blockade. Such a treatment method is used for men whose PROSTATE-SPECIFIC ANTIGEN (PSA) level increases greatly during the use of an LHRH analog.

Side Effects

Antiandrogens can cause nausea, vomiting, diarrhea, or breast growth or tenderness. If used a long time, KETOCONAZOLE may cause liver problems, and aminoglutethimide can cause skin rashes. Men who receive total androgen blockade may experience more side effects than men who receive a single method of hormonal therapy. Any method of hormonal therapy that lowers androgen levels can contribute to weakening of the bones in older men.

antiemetics   See ANTINAUSEA MEDICATION.

antigen   A substance that is foreign to the body. Several different studies are investigating the use of VACCINES against cancer which would trigger a natural response to an injected antigen. Depending on the specific antigen used, this natural response could also kill cancer cells in the process.

anti-inflammatory drugs and prostate cancer
Anti-inflammatory drugs that do not contain steroids are often used as nonprescription pain relievers. Regular use of aspirin, ibuprofen, and other nonsteroidal anti-inflammatory drugs (NSAIDs) may help protect against PROSTATE CANCER, according to researchers at the Mayo Clinic. In one 2002 study, men age 60 and older who used NSAIDs daily had a reduced risk of prostate cancer

of as much as 60 percent. The study also suggested that the beneficial effect may increase with age. The findings of this research were published in March 2002 in *Mayo Clinic Proceedings.*

In the study, 1,362 Caucasian men were followed for an average of five and a half years. Of the 569 men who reported using NSAIDs daily, 23 had prostate cancer, compared with 68 of 793 men in the same study who did not use NSAIDs daily and contracted the disease.

The association between NSAID use and prostate cancer appears to be stronger in older men: The risk of prostate cancer among NSAID users was 12 percent lower in men age 50 to 59 years, 60 percent lower in men 60 to 69 years, and 83 percent lower in men 70 to 79 years when compared to that in men in those same age groups who did not use NSAIDs daily.

Although the study findings provide important information that NSAIDs may protect against prostate cancer, they are not conclusive. More research is needed to show that the results in the study could be confirmed in other similar studies. Since the study included only Caucasian men in southeastern Minnesota, it is not known whether the findings apply to men of all races.

Researchers cautioned that although their findings complement those of previous studies that NSAIDs help protect against breast and colon cancers, and possibly against prostate cancer, there are also negative side effects of use of NSAIDs that must be considered and monitored for people who use NSAIDs on a daily basis.

antimetabolites   Anticancer drugs that closely resemble substances needed by cells for normal growth and that interfere with the normal metabolic processes within cells.

The CHEMOTHERAPY drugs FLUOROURACIL, methotrexate, and mercaptopurine are all antimetabolites that prevent cell growth at a short, specific period in the reproduction cycle of the cell by interfering with important enzyme reactions within the cell.

Antimetabolites sometimes must be administered over hours, days, or weeks. Side effects of use of antimetabolites can be severe, including blood cell disorders or stomach problems; sometimes, cancer cells can become resistant to specific metabolites.

antinausea medication   A type of drug that can prevent or reduce nausea and vomiting, common side effects of CHEMOTHERAPY and RADIATION THERAPY. Popular antinausea drugs include dexamethasone (DECADRON), prochlorperazine (COMPAZINE), thiethylperazine (Torecan), chlorpromazine (Thorazine), metoclopramide, lorazepam (ATIVAN), diazepam (Valium), dronabinol (MARINOL), granisetron (KYTRIL), dolasetron (Anzemet), and ondansetron (ZOFRAN). Often a combination of these drugs is prescribed; if the first combination does not work, others may work better. Antinausea medications are often administered along with chemotherapy drugs to prevent nausea. Typically, it is much easier to prevent nausea and vomiting than to treat them.

antioxidants   Compounds that fight cell damage caused by FREE RADICALS, rogue oxygen molecules that can attack cells throughout the body. Although free radicals serve important functions, such as helping the immune system fight off disease, at excessive levels they can cause problems.

These highly reactive oxygen radicals are formed both during normal metabolism and in response to infection and some chemicals. They cause damage to fatty acids in cell membranes, and the products of this damage can then damage proteins and DNA. The most widely accepted theory of the biochemical basis of many types of cancer is that they are triggered by free radical damage of tissues.

A number of different mechanisms are involved in protection against, or repair after, free radical damage, including a number of nutrients—especially vitamin E, beta-carotene, vitamin C, and selenium. Collectively known as antioxidant nutrients, they limit the cell and tissue damage caused by toxins and pollutants.

Because high dosages of antioxidant supplements can cause side effects, consumption of antioxidants as part of a healthy diet is safer than use of supplements. Antioxidants are found in

• Fruits and vegetables (especially blueberries and yellow fruits and vegetables)
• Brown rice
• Whole grains

- Meats
- Eggs
- Dairy products

Side Effects

Supplements that contain high levels of antioxidants can cause severe side effects, including internal bleeding, and may be toxic to patients who are taking anticoagulant medication. No one should use these or any supplements without consulting a doctor. In addition, high dosages of vitamin E are potentially harmful if combined with blood-thinning drugs.

antisperm antibodies   Antibodies that can attach to sperm and inhibit their ability to fertilize an egg. Normally, antibodies prevent infection, but when they attack the sperm, they cause infertility. Men produce antisperm antibodies only when their sperm are in contact with their blood, such as after surgery or an injury to the testicles. Testicular BIOPSY and TESTICULAR CANCER can both lead to production of antisperm antibodies.

Under normal circumstances, sperm are separated from the immune system by a natural mechanism called the blood–testes barrier, which maintains close connections between the cells lining the male reproductive tract so that immune cells cannot reach the sperm within. Normally, sperm develop in the testicles and are not exposed to blood. If accidental contact occurs, such as when an injury breaks down this barrier, the immune system has access to sperm. When this happens, the body responds to the sperm as intruders and develops antibodies against them.

Antisperm antibodies are produced by the immune system; once formed, they interfere with the sperm movement and ability to penetrate a woman's cervical mucus or directly affect the sperms' ability to penetrate and fertilize an egg, depending on where on the sperm the antibodies attach themselves. Antibodies may also cause the sperm to clump together, as is sometimes seen in a routine semen analysis.

The likelihood of production of antibodies rises dramatically in men who have had surgery on the reproductive tract: Nearly 70 percent of men who have had a VASECTOMY reversal have antibodies on their sperm.

Risks

Anything that interferes with the normal barrier between blood and testes can lead to the formation of antisperm antibodies, including the following conditions:

- CRYPTORCHIDISM (undescended testicles)
- Infection (orchitis, prostatitis)
- Inguinal hernia repair before puberty
- Testicular biopsy
- Testicular cancer
- Testicular torsion (twisting of the testicle)
- VARICOCELE (dilatation of the veins around the spermatic cord)
- Congenital absence of the vas deferens
- Vasectomy reversal

Diagnosis

Over the years many tests have been developed to detect antisperm antibodies. In women, blood testing for antisperm antibodies may be more practical than an attempt to measure antibodies in the cervical mucus, which is the primary location where the immune system interacts with sperm. The postcoital test, a standard part of the infertility evaluation, may suggest the presence of antisperm antibodies. Examination of the cervical mucus after intercourse near the time of ovulation can detect antisperm antibodies that may cause either a lack of sperm or sperm that do not swim but simply shake in place.

Direct examination of sperm for attached antibodies is more reliable than blood testing. Two common tests are the immunobead assay and the mixed agglutination reaction (MAR). Both tests use antibodies bound to a small marker, such as plastic beads or red blood cells, which attaches to sperm that have antibodies on the surface. The results are read as a percentage of sperm bound by antibodies.

Treatment

Suppressing the immune system with corticosteroids may decrease the production of antibodies but can also cause serious side effects. Current approaches to the treatment of antisperm antibodies include methods of sperm processing to remove surface antibodies, such as rapid washing, freeze-thawing, and enzyme cleavage. However, these methods have only a modest (if any) success rate.

antitumor antibiotics   Drugs used as a form of CHEMOTHERAPY that attack microbes and are also toxic to cells, interfering with DNA. They are widely used to treat cancer. Examples of antitumor antibiotics include bleomycin and doxorubicin (ADRIAMYCIN).

aorta   The large artery originating from the left ventricle of the heart whose branches carry blood to all parts of the body. The lymph nodes most often affected by TESTICULAR CANCER are located around the aorta and below the kidneys in the retroperitoneum.

apoptosis   Programmed cell death that occurs naturally during the development of a person's tissues and organs. During fetal development, apoptosis plays a vital role in determining the final size and form of tissues and organs. As more cells are produced than are required to produce tissues and organs, unwanted cells are programmed to die, either because the chemical signals that direct them to go on living are suppressed or because they receive a specific signal to die. Experts believe that the suppression of apoptosis is associated with the uncontrolled cell growth in leukemia and other cancers. Apoptosis also occurs when viruses infect cells. Apoptosis differs from cell necrosis, in which cell death may be triggered by a toxic substance.

appetite loss   Lack of interest in eating is a frequent problem experienced by cancer patients as a direct result of advancing disease and as a side effect of treatment. Most types of CHEMOTHERAPY drugs cause some degree of appetite loss. People may lose their appetite while struggling with cancer because chemotherapy-related nausea or mouth or stomach pain alters appetite—or because pain itself can trigger appetite loss.

Appetite loss is a serious problem among cancer patients because it can lead to poor nutrition, which can interfere with recovery. Loss of appetite and weight loss can lead to CACHEXIA, a form of malnutrition.

Because good nutrition is essential to recovery, maintaining a healthy diet during treatment is important.

Treatment

Drugs such as megestrol (Megace) or dronabinol (MARINOL, MARIJUANA) may be used to improve appetite. Patients also should eat:

• Small, frequent meals
• Nutritious snacks
• White, cold food, such as dairy products or poultry
• Skim milk or butter with food
• High-calorie, high-protein food
• Attractive, appetizing meals

In addition, patients should eat during the times when they feel most comfortable, stimulate appetite with light exercise, take medications with high-calorie drinks, and eat at a friend's home or a good restaurant. Patients should also try lemon-flavored drinks, rinse the mouth before eating, and try cold white food (ice cream, milk shakes, boiled chicken). Many patients find that eating meat becomes unpleasant; they should try to substitute other high-protein meals they find more palatable. Appetite usually returns after chemotherapy ends, although several weeks may elapse before it completely returns to normal.

arsenic   An element found throughout the Earth's crust that has been used for centuries both as a drug and as a poison. New research now suggests that men who have PROSTATE CANCER who do not respond to standard therapies may someday find hope in arsenic trioxide treatment, according to a Phase II clinical trial conducted by researchers at Montefiore Medical Center.

In the study, two of the 15 prostate cancer patients for whom at least two hormonal treatments had failed responded to the arsenic trioxide. One patient (who was also receiving radiation therapy) experienced a significant drop in his PROSTATE-SPECIFIC ANTIGEN (PSA) level. Expanded studies are needed to determine the effectiveness of the arsenic treatment in larger populations.

Arsenic has already proved to have remarkable clinical effectiveness in patients who have had relapsed acute promyelocitic leukemia.

Asian men Reproductive cancers are generally less common in American men of Asian descent than in white American men.

For example, American men of Asian descent living in the United States have lower rates of PROSTATE CANCER than do Caucasian-American men, but higher rates than Asian men living in Asia. Japan has the lowest rate of prostate cancer in the world.

Likewise, TESTICULAR CANCER is twice as common in Caucasians as in Asian-American men.

See also RACE.

aspiration Removal of fluid or cells from tissue by inserting a needle into an area and drawing the fluid into the syringe.

aspirin and prostate cancer See ANTI-INFLAMMATORY DRUGS AND PROSTATE CANCER.

Association for the Cure of Cancer of the Prostate (CaP CURE) A nonprofit organization dedicated to finding a cure for PROSTATE CANCER through support of research, education, and prevention. The group's activities include advocacy, research, referrals, and information on clinical trials. The Association for the Cure of Cancer of the Prostate (CaP CURE) is the largest private source of funding for prostate cancer research in the world. Since its inception in 1993 CaP CURE has awarded more than $104 million to fund 1,000 medical research projects worldwide. Its advocacy efforts likewise have had significant impact, resulting in an overall increase in U.S. government support for prostate cancer research from $60 million to $430 million annually, organization of the first National Cancer Summit and March on Washington, and sponsorship of more than 80 clinical trials. For contact information, see Appendix I.

Association of Cancer Online Resources (ACOR) A group of online communities designed to provide timely and accurate information about cancer in a supportive environment. The Association of Cancer Online Resources (ACOR) offers access to mailing lists that provide support, information, and community to everyone affected by cancer and related disorders. In addition to mailing lists, ACOR aims to provide patients with access to varied and credible information sources through Internet resource development and partnership with trusted content providers and to improve communication between patients and health-care professionals through advocacy in a variety of public forums, including professional journals and other media.

Association of Community Cancer Centers (ACCC) The leading U.S. oncology policy organization for the cancer care team, dedicated to helping cancer professionals adapt to the complex challenges of program management, reimbursement, legislation, and regulations. In the 1970s the Association of Community Cancer Centers (ACCC) presented the first U.S. meeting on hospital oncology units and HOSPICE care; throughout the 1990s, association support resulted in passage of ACCC's off-label drug legislation in 39 states. The association focuses on helping to assure that cancer programs are adequately funded. ACCC priorities also include cancer patient advocacy and long-term plans for the joint development of guidelines for standard patient care.

ACCC members include medical and radiation oncologists, surgeons, cancer program administrators, hospital executives, practice managers, oncology nurses and social workers, and cancer program data managers. ACCC Institution/Group Practice members include more than 650 medical centers, hospitals, oncology practices, and cancer programs across the United States. For contact information, see Appendix I.

atypical cells Abnormal cells. This term is generally used to describe cells that are not normal, but yet are not abnormal enough to be called a cancer. Cancer is the result of the division of atypical cells.

balanoposthitis   Also known as balanitis, this refers to a generalized inflammation of the fore-skin and head of an uncircumsized penis commonly caused by a yeast or bacterial infection below the foreskin. The inflammation causes pain, itching, redness, and swelling, which eventually can cause a narrowing of the urethra. Men who have balanoposthitis may later have chronic inflammation of the penis tip (balanitis xerotica obliterans), tightening of the foreskin (phimosis), inability of the foreskin to be pulled over the penis into the natural position (paraphimosis), and cancer.

B cells   White blood cells produced in the BONE MARROW, one of the two types of white blood cells that play an important part in the immune system.

benign prostatic hyperplasia (BPH)   This term most correctly describes what one would see under the microscope in a man with benign (nonmalignant) growth of the prostate. In the past, it was commonly used to refer to an enlarged prostate gland. The abnormal growth of benign prostate cells is not cancer but can cause many of the same symptoms as PROSTATE CANCER. Benign prostatic hyperplasia (BPH) does not usually affect sexual function; it causes problems when as the prostate enlarges, it presses against the bladder and the ure-thra, blocking the flow of urine.

Once the prostate begins to enlarge, it can grow in one of two ways. Cells can multiply around the urine passageway through the prostate, squeezing it closed. The second type of growth more likely to cause symptoms, and involves enlargement of the middle lobe; cells grow into the urine tube and even up and into the bladder. This type of growth more often needs to be treated with surgery.

Cause

BPH is the result of small noncancerous growths inside the prostate that may be related to hormone changes that occur with aging. By age 60, more than half of all American men have microscopic signs of BPH, and by age 70, more than 40 percent have enlargement that can be felt on physical examination.

The prostate normally starts out about the size of a walnut and begins to enlarge in all men by the time they reach 40, growing to the size of an apricot; by age 60, it may be as big as a lemon. Prostate growth generally continues throughout a man's lifetime. Effects of this growth vary from minor annoyance to almost unbearable discomfort. By age 60, one in four men is so severely affected by symptoms that he needs treatment.

Symptoms

This condition is normally diagnosed by its symptoms. A man who has BPH may find urinating or maintaining more than a dribble of urine difficult. He also may need to urinate frequently or may have sudden powerful urges to urinate. Many men are forced to get up several times a night; others have an annoying feeling that the bladder is never completely empty. Straining to empty the bladder can make the condition worse: The bladder stretches, the bladder wall thickens and loses its elasticity, and the bladder muscles become less efficient.

The pool of urine that collects in the bladder can foster urinary tract infections, and trying to force a urine stream can produce pressure that eventually damages the kidneys.

Complications

BPH can lead to a number of problems. For instance, a completely blocked urethra is a medical emergency that requires immediate catheterization, a procedure in which a tube called a catheter is inserted through the penis into the bladder to allow urine to escape. Other serious potential complications of BPH include bladder stones, bleeding, urinary infection, and kidney damage.

Self-Test

The AMERICAN UROLOGICAL ASSOCIATION has developed a seven-question self-test to help patients assess the severity of BPH symptoms. The test asks men to rate how often over the past month they have:

- Had a sensation of not emptying the bladder completely after urinating
- Had to urinate again less than two hours after urinating
- Stopped and started again several times during urination
- Found it difficult to postpone urination
- Had a weak urinary stream
- Had to push or strain to begin urination
- Had to get up several times at night to urinate (how many times)

Scoring for the first six questions:

- One point for having problems less than one time in five
- Two points for having problems less than half the time
- Three points for having problems about half the time
- Four points for having problems more than half the time
- Five points for having problems almost all the time

Scoring for the seventh question:

- One point for each time had to get up in the night
- Five points for getting up five times or more

Mild: one to seven points
Moderate: eight to 19 points
Severe: 20 to 35 points

Diagnosis

BPH is diagnosed with a detailed medical history focusing on the urinary tract—the kidneys, the ureters (the pair of tubes that carry urine from the kidneys to the bladder), the bladder, and the urethra.

The initial medical evaluation typically includes a physical exam called a DIGITAL RECTAL EXAMINATION (DRE), a URINALYSIS to check for infection or bleeding, and a blood test to measure kidney function. Some physicians may also check the level of PROSTATE-SPECIFIC ANTIGEN (PSA), using a PSA test to help rule out the likelihood of cancer. PSA is a protein that is produced by the cells of the prostate gland.

In addition, other tests may help a urologist determine whether BPH has affected the bladder or kidneys. These include tests that measure the speed of urine flow, pressure in the bladder during urination, and the quantity of urine that remains in the bladder after urination.

Some other tests that are widely used are expensive, sometimes risky, and unnecessary for most men, according to an expert panel sponsored by the U.S. Public Health Service (USPHS) Clinical Practice Guidelines. These include the following:

- CYSTOSCOPY, in which the doctor inserts a viewing tube into the urethra to get a direct look at the bladder
- UROGRAM, an X-ray to visualize the kidneys, ureter, and bladder in which urine is made visible after dye is injected into a vein
- ULTRASOUND, a test that obtains images of the kidneys and bladder after a probe is placed on the abdomen

Treatment

There is no cure for prostate growth, but there is no connection between BPH and prostate cancer. Although BPH may not be a threat to life, if not properly treated it can lead to extremely serious consequences, including kidney damage and failure. Some men may require treatment with medicine or surgery to relieve symptoms. Although BPH cannot be cured, its symptoms often can be relieved by surgery or by drugs. According to some experts, mild to moderate symptoms worsened in only about 20 percent of cases, improved (without any specific treatment) in another 20 percent, and remained about the same in the rest.

If a man has no serious complications such as inability to urinate, kidney damage, frequent urinary tract infections, major bleeding through the urethra, or bladder stones, the best approach for treating BPH is not clear. The USPHS guidelines advise doctors to leave treatment decisions to the patient after discussing the benefits and side effects of each treatment option.

The options selected by an individual are tied to his own preferences. For instance, some men with significant symptoms or complications want immediate relief and are willing to have surgery or begin a drug regimen. Others are reluctant or unwilling to have surgery or to take pills daily for an extended period.

Watchful waiting Men whose symptoms are mild often opt for WATCHFUL WAITING: they have regular checkups and have further treatment only if symptoms become very bothersome. The USPHS Clinical Practice Guidelines call watchful waiting "an appropriate treatment strategy for the majority of patients." Men who choose watchful waiting should have regular, perhaps annual, checkups, including DREs and laboratory tests.

For those who choose watchful waiting, a number of simple steps may help to reduce bothersome symptoms. These include limiting intake of fluid in the evening, especially of beverages that contain alcohol or caffeine, which can trigger the urge to urinate and can interfere with sleep; taking time to empty the bladder completely; and not allowing long intervals to pass without urinating. Men monitoring prostate conditions should also be aware that certain medications prescribed for other conditions may make their symptoms worse. These include some over-the-counter cough and cold remedies, prescribed tranquilizers, antidepressants, and drugs that control high blood pressure. Switching to a different prescription may help. Watchful waiting, of course, is not always enough for BPH, and surgery or drug therapy may be required. Both options are discussed in the following.

Surgery Several types of surgery can relieve the symptoms of an enlarged prostate, including the following:

- *Transurethral resection of the prostate (TURP):* TRANSURETHRAL RESECTION OF THE PROSTATE, which is considered to be the best way to treat prostate enlargement, accounts for a majority of all prostate surgery. However, its use is beginning to decline as alternatives have become more widely available. This procedure relieves symptoms quickly, generally improving the urinary flow within weeks. By inserting a slim fiberoptic scope through the penis and up the urethra as far as the prostate, the surgeon pares away the lining of the prostate and excess prostate tissue, expanding the passageway for flow of urine. The TURP procedure ordinarily does not cause incontinence or impotence.

- *Transurethral incision of the prostate (TUIP):* This procedure is used on small prostate glands and is far less common than TURP. As is TURP, TUIP is performed by passing an instrument through the penis to reach the prostate; however, the surgeon makes only one or two small incisions to relieve pressure in the prostate rather than trimming away tissue. As TURP does, the procedure considerably increases the urine flow. TUIP is an outpatient procedure with a low risk of side effects. Men interested in having children may want to consider this procedure, because it usually does not affect ejaculation or fertility.

- *Laser surgery:* Using a laser, a doctor can vaporize prostate tissue directly. In laser-induced and laser-assisted surgery, high-energy instruments heat prostate tissue to the boiling point, thereby killing the tissue.

- *Indigo laser:* In this minimally invasive procedure, a urologist threads a special indigo fiber into a tube through the urethra and into the prostate. The fiberoptic tip is carefully placed in the area targeted for treatment; laser energy through the fiberoptic tip is then used to precisely destroy the enlarged part of the prostate.

The destroyed prostate tissue is then absorbed naturally by the body. As the prostate shrinks over a few weeks, pressure on the bladder and the urethra eases, decreasing the symptoms of BPH. Symptoms continue to improve over several months.

The treatment is typically an outpatient procedure and can be completed in less than 30 minutes. There are several anesthesia options, including general, spinal (no feeling below a certain point), and local (only the immediate area being treated is numbed). Choice of anesthesia depends on the patient and the size of his prostate. Patients must use a catheter until the swelling subsides; this is usually removed within a week.

This is a relatively recent therapy, which some have compared favorably to the "gold-standard" TURP.

- *Transurethral needle ablation (TUNA):* This recently approved technique can be done with local anesthesia as an outpatient procedure. An instrument is inserted through the penis into the prostate's urine tube. Heat is applied to prostate tissues through needles, which removes excess tissue as that tissue later dies. Some clinical studies have reported that TUNA improves the urine flow with minimal side effects when compared with other procedures. TUNA is similar to use of lasers and other noninvasive techniques. TUNA works best on moderately enlarged prostates and is not very effective on very large prostates or those that have a median lobe.

- *Targis:* This type of microwave treatment was approved by the U.S. Food and Drug Administration in late 1997. As other new therapies have, this has appeared to be effective in the short term but has yet to demonstrate long-term benefits.

- *Prostatectomy:* This generalized term is used to describe any procedure that surgically removes prostate tissue. A radical prostatectomy is performed for cancer and involves removal of the entire prostate. Only the inner part of the prostate is removed during an open prostatectomy (also called suprapubic prostatectomy), which is done for men with BPH with very large prostates (about 5 percent of all cases) that are too big to remove using a scope.

Drug Therapy

Millions of American men have chosen drugs rather than surgery since drug therapy for BPH was first tried in the early 1990s. Although regarded as less effective than surgery, drug therapy is also less inva-

sive and usually free of major side effects. Drug types include alpha-adrenergic blockers and 5-alpha reductase inhibitors (finasteride).

Alpha adrenergic blockers   These originally were used to treat high blood pressure by relaxing smooth muscles in blood vessel walls. In BPH, they relax the muscular portion of the prostate and the bladder neck, allowing urine to flow more freely. For the average patient, these drugs increase the rate of urine flow and reduce symptoms, often within days. Side effects include dizziness, fatigue, and headache.

Finasteride   This shrinks the prostate by blocking an enzyme that converts the male hormone TESTOSTERONE into a stronger, growth-stimulating form. It may take finasteride at least six months to increase urinary flow rate and reduce symptoms, however. It seems to work best for men who have a greatly enlarged prostate.

In a small percentage of men, the drug can affect sexual activity, decreasing interest in sex, diminishing ability to have an erection, and causing problems with ejaculation. It sometimes also causes tenderness or swelling of the breasts, and causes a drop in PSA level. These side effects can be reversed by stopping use of the drug.

Some studies suggest combining the two types of drugs may produce better results. This is most often done in men with large prostates.

Other Treatments

Researchers are working to develop BPH treatments that are more effective and produce fewer side effects. These include using laser surgery, powerful electric currents, and microwaves. Doctors have also tried to enlarge the urethra by inserting a balloon into it and inflating it with fluid, and by inserting a stent (a small metal coil) into the urethra to hold it open. This treatment has a significant risk of long-term complications and is generally done only in patients when other treatments are not an option.

benign prostatic hypertrophy (BPH)   An alternate name for BENIGN PROSTATIC HYPERPLASIA.

BEP   The abbreviation for a common combination of chemotherapeutic drugs (CISPLATIN [Platinol],

BLEOMYCIN, and ETOPOSIDE) used in treatment of GERM CELL TUMORS.

beta-carotene A common plant chemical within a group of more than 600 called carotenoids. Beta-carotene is converted by the body into vitamin A, which has many vital functions, including the growth and repair of body tissues, formation of bones and teeth, resistance of the body to infection, and development of healthy eye tissues. Whereas vitamin A supplements can be toxic, excess beta-carotene is safely stored away and converted to vitamin A only when the body needs it. Epidemiologic studies have linked high intake of foods rich in beta-carotene and high blood levels of the micronutrient to a lower risk of cancer.

Beta-carotene acts as an ANTIOXIDANT and immune system booster; it is found in bright orange–colored fruits and vegetables such as carrots, pumpkins, peaches, and sweet potatoes. Some experts suspect it may be possible to shield the body's immune system from the risk of cancer by supplementing the diet with beta-carotene.

Most, but not all beta-carotene in supplements is synthetic, consisting of only one molecule (natural beta-carotene in food is made of two molecules). Researchers originally saw no meaningful difference between natural and synthetic beta-carotene, but this view was questioned when the link found between beta-carotene-containing foods and lung cancer prevention was not duplicated in studies using synthetic pills. The most common beta-carotene supplement is 25,000 IU (15 mg) per day; some people take as much as 100,000 IU (60 mg) per day. Excessive beta-carotene (more than 100,000 IU, or 60 mg per day) sometimes tints the skin yellow-orange. Individuals who take beta-carotene for long periods should also supplement with vitamin E, as beta-carotene may reduce vitamin E level.

bicalutamide (Casodex) An anticancer drug used to treat PROSTATE CANCER that belongs to the family of drugs called ANTIANDROGENS. Antiandrogens block the action of ANDROGENS (HORMONES that can help malignant cells grow).

Bicalutamide is most often used together with luteinizing hormone–releasing hormone (LHRH) to treat advanced prostate cancer. The most common side effects of these drugs include HOT FLASHES, FATIGUE, mood swings, and bone loss.

bioflavonoids See FLAVONOIDS.

biological response modifier (BRM) Substance developed by researchers to strengthen the ability of the IMMUNE SYSTEM to find and destroy cancer. Treatment with a BRM alters the body's natural antitumor response by stimulating the BONE MARROW to make specific tumor-killing blood cells. These substances may serve directly as tumor-killing agents or chemical messengers, decrease the body's normal methods of suppressing the immune response, or change tumor cells so that they are more likely to trigger an immune response to or be damaged by the immune system. Biological response modifiers also may improve the body's tolerance to RADIATION THERAPY or to CHEMOTHERAPY.

There are many types of these modifiers, some produced by the body and others created in the lab. Many ongoing studies are investigating the use of these substances in BIOLOGICAL THERAPY to treat a wide variety of cancers.

The primary biological response modifiers include antibodies, COLONY-STIMULATING FACTORS, CYTOKINES (including interferons and INTERLEUKINS), MONOCLONAL ANTIBODIES, and VACCINES. Interferon is the best known and most widely used biological response modifier. Although most human cells produce interferon, interferon also can be made by using recombinant (gene splicing) biologic techniques. Although experts are not sure exactly how interferon works, it can play a role in the treatment of several cancers.

Researchers continue to discover new BRMs, learn more about how they function, and develop ways to use them in cancer therapy. All of these substances alter the interaction between cancer cells and the body's immune defenses, restoring the body's ability to fight cancer. Biological therapies may be used to stop or control processes that allow cancer cells to grow, make cancer cells more recognizable to the immune system, boost the killing power of immune system cells, and alter the malignant growth patterns to make them more like those of healthy cells. BRMs also block or reverse the process that triggers the overgrowth of abnormal cells, and can prevent cancer cells from spreading to other parts of the body.

Some BRMs are a standard part of treatment for certain types of cancer; others are being studied as new types of treatments, either alone or in combination with each other. They are also being used with other treatments, such as radiation therapy and chemotherapy.

biological therapy A relatively new type of cancer treatment, sometimes called immunotherapy, biotherapy, or BIOLOGICAL RESPONSE MODIFIER therapy, that is designed to enhance the body's natural defenses against cancer. Biological therapies may be used to stop or suppress processes that allow cancer growth and to make cancer cells more recognizable and therefore more susceptible to destruction by the immune system. Biological therapies also boost the killing power of immune system cells and alter cancer cell growth patterns to promote healthy patterns. They can be used to block or reverse the process that triggers the malignant process, and to enhance the body's ability to repair normal cells damaged by other forms of cancer treatment, such as chemotherapy or radiation therapy. Biological therapy also can help prevent cancer cells from spreading to other parts of the body.

Biological Response Modifiers

Antibodies, CYTOKINES, and other immune system substances produced in the lab for use in cancer treatment alter the interaction between the body's immune defenses and cancer cells to boost the body's ability to fight the disease. BRMs include interferons, INTERLEUKINS, COLONY-STIMULATING FACTORS, MONOCLONAL ANTIBODIES, and VACCINES.

Interferons

There are three major types of interferon, a type of naturally occurring cytokine: interferon alfa, interferon beta, and interferon gamma. Interferon alfa is the type most widely used in cancer treatment.

Interferons can improve the capacity of a cancer patient's immune system to fight cancer cells and may slow the growth of cancer cells or promote their transformation into cells that behave more

normally. Researchers believe that some interferons may also stimulate natural killer (NK) cells, T cells, and macrophages, boosting the immune system's anticancer function.

Interleukins

Interleukins are also cytokines that occur naturally in the body and can be produced synthetically. There are many different kinds of interleukins; interleukin-2 (IL-2 or aldesleukin) has been the most widely studied in cancer treatment. IL-2 stimulates the growth and action of cancer-killing immune cells such as lymphocytes.

Colony-Stimulating Factors (CSFs)

CSFs (sometimes called hematopoietic growth factors) usually do not directly affect tumor cells; rather, they encourage BONE MARROW STEM CELLS to divide and develop into white blood cells, platelets, and red blood cells. Bone marrow is critical to the body's immune system because it is the source of all blood cells. The CSFs' stimulation of the immune system may benefit patients who are having cancer treatment. Because anticancer drugs can damage the body's ability to make white blood cells, red blood cells, and platelets, patients who receive anticancer drugs have an increased risk of development of infections, anemia, and ready bleeding.

By using CSFs to stimulate blood cell production, doctors can increase dosages of anticancer drugs without increasing the risk of infection or the need for transfusion with blood products. As a result, researchers have found CSFs particularly useful when combined with high-dose chemotherapy.

CSFs include the following:

- *Granulocyte colony-stimulating factor (G-CSF, filgrastim) and granulocyte-macrophage colony-stimulating factor (GM-CSF, sargramostim)* can increase the number of white blood cells, thereby reducing the risk of infection in patients who are receiving chemotherapy. G-CSF and GM-CSF can also stimulate the production of stem cells in preparation for stem cell or bone marrow transplants.

- *Erythropoietin* can increase the number of red blood cells and reduce the need for red blood cell transfusions of patients who receive chemotherapy.

- *Oprelvekin* can reduce the need for platelet transfusions of patients who are receiving chemotherapy.

Researchers are studying CSFs in clinical trials to treat some types of leukemia, metastatic colorectal cancer, melanoma, lung cancer, and other types of cancer.

Monoclonal Antibodies (MOABs)

MOABs are antibodies made in the laboratory that are produced by a single type of cell and are specific to a specific antigen. Researchers are trying to figure out how to create MOABs specific to the antigens found on the surface of the cancer cell being treated. MOABs that react with specific types of cancer may enhance a patient's immune response to the cancer. MOABs can be programmed to interfere with the growth of cancer cells; in addition, they may be linked to CHEMOTHERAPY drugs, radioactive substances, other biological response modifiers, or other toxins so that when the antibodies latch onto cancer cells, they deliver these poisons directly to the tumor, helping to destroy it.

MOABs may help destroy cancer cells in bone marrow that has been removed from a patient in preparation for a bone marrow transplant. MOABs carrying radioisotopes may also prove useful in diagnosing certain cancers, including PROSTATE CANCER.

Cancer Vaccines

Researchers are developing vaccines for cancer treatments that may encourage the immune system to recognize and reject cancer cells, preventing cancer recurrence. In contrast to vaccines against infectious diseases, cancer vaccines are designed to be injected after the disease is diagnosed, rather than before it develops.

Cancer vaccines given when the tumor is small may be able to cure the cancer. Early cancer vaccine studies focused on melanoma, but today vaccines are also being studied in the treatment of many other types of cancer, including lymphomas and cancers of the breast. Researchers are also investigating ways that cancer vaccines can be used in combination with other BRMs.

Side Effects

Biological therapies can cause a number of side effects, including rashes or swelling at the site where they are injected. Several biological response modifiers, including interferons and interleukins, may cause flulike symptoms such as fever, chills, nausea, vomiting, and appetite loss. Fatigue is another common side effect, and blood pressure may be affected. The side effects of IL-2 can often be severe, depending on the dosage given. Patients need to be closely monitored during treatment. Side effects of CSFs may include bone pain, fatigue, fever, and appetite loss. The side effects of MOABs vary, and severe allergic reactions may occur. Cancer vaccines can cause muscle aches and fever.

biomarkers Substances that may indicate the presence of cancer when they occur at high levels in blood, other body fluids, or tissues.

biopsy The surgical removal of a small piece of tissue or a small tumor for microscopic examination to determine whether cancer cells are present. If an open or incisional biopsy is required, a small incision is made to get to the tissue, which is removed. In a traditional needle biopsy, a large hollow needle removes a core or plug of the tissue. In a FINE NEEDLE ASPIRATION, the tissue is sucked out of the suspected area.

biotherapy Treatment to stimulate or restore the ability of the immune system to fight infection and disease, and to lessen side effects caused by some cancer treatments. Biotherapy is also known as immunotherapy, biological therapy, or BIOLOGICAL RESPONSE MODIFIER (BRM) therapy.

bisphosphonates Chemicals that block bone breakdown, and which are typically used to treat osteoporosis. They also can be used to treat bone pain that occurs when PROSTATE CANCER spreads to the bones. Although bisphosphonates appear to improve bone symptoms in men with prostate cancer, their use is still experimental.

bladder infection A bacterial infection in the bladder can mimic symptoms of BENIGN PROSTATIC HYPERPLASIA or PROSTATE CANCER. Symptoms of bladder infection include soreness of the urethra and bladder, pain with urination, difficulty with urination, frequent and urgent urination, bloody urine, back pain, and low to moderate fever.

A bladder infection can be diagnosed by a simple urinalysis that can be done in a doctor's office and/or a urine culture that must be sent to a lab for results within two days. Although the culture takes longer, it may reveal an infection that does not show up in a urinalysis.

Bladder infections are generally treated with antibiotics and drinking large amounts of water.

Blenoxane See BLEOMYCIN.

bleomycin (Blenoxane) A type of CHEMOTHERAPY drug used in the treatment of TESTICULAR CANCER (in combination with VP-16 and CISPLATIN given every three weeks). Bleomycin is a mixture of glycoprotein antibiotics derived from *Streptomyces verticillus*.

blood count, complete A test to measure the number of red blood cells, white blood cells, and platelets in a blood sample. Other factors also included in a complete blood count (CBC) are hemoglobin (the level of oxygen-carrying protein) and hematocrit (percentage of red blood cells). A separate count of young red cells (called a reticulocyte count or "retic") can be performed on the same blood sample, although it must be separately requested.

CBC results can reveal ANEMIA, a blood clotting problem, or an infection. A CBC is usually performed before each episode of CHEMOTHERAPY to measure the blood cell count, since chemotherapy often causes a drop in these levels. If the blood count is too low, the oncologist may postpone chemotherapy treatment until it begins to rise.

blood tests Tests that are sometimes helpful in diagnosing reproductive cancers, such as TESTICULAR CANCER or PROSTATE CANCER, because they can detect certain proteins, such as ALPHA-FETOPROTEIN (AFP), HUMAN CHORIONIC GONADOTROPIN (hCG), or PLACENTAL ALKALINE PHOSPHATASE (PLAP), that are secreted at high levels by some testicle and prostate cancers. The tumors may also increase the levels of enzymes such as LACTATE DEHYDROGENASE (LDH). NONSEMINOMAS often raise AFP level, whereas SEMINOMAS do not. LDH, hCG, and PLAP levels are increased in some seminomas and nonseminoma GERM CELL testicle cancers. These substances are not produced by Sertoli's cell or Leydig's cell tumors. Tests can measure the levels of these substances present in the fluid portion of blood.

Because levels of these proteins are not usually elevated in the plasma if the tumor is small, these tests are also useful in estimating the extent of cancer present, predicting a patient's prognosis, and evaluating the response to therapy to make sure the tumor has not recurred.

bone marrow The soft, fatty substance filling the cavities of the bones that contains immature cells called STEM CELLS. These cells produce all of the body's red blood cells and platelets and most of the white blood cells. Stem cells produce:

- White blood cells (leukocytes), which fight infection
- Red blood cells (erythrocytes), which carry oxygen to and remove waste products from organs and tissues
- Platelets (thrombocytes), which enable the blood to clot

CHEMOTHERAPY can affect the bone marrow, producing a temporary decrease in the number of cells in the blood (bone marrow depression).

bone marrow aspiration A procedure in which a needle is inserted into the center of a bone (usually the hip) to remove a small amount of BONE MARROW for microscopic examination. Bone marrow is the spongy substance on the inside of the bone in which blood cells are manufactured.

After the test, there may be some pain or soreness at the site. The sample is analyzed for iron stores, red blood cell and white blood cell production and maturation, and number of megakaryocytes (cells that produce platelets).

A bone marrow aspiration is used to determine the cause of an abnormal blood test result; to confirm the diagnosis of ANEMIA, an increase or drop in white blood cells, or a reduction of platelets in the blood; or to evaluate response to cancer treatments.

bone marrow biopsy See BONE MARROW ASPIRATION.

bone marrow depression See BONE MARROW.

Bone Marrow Foundation A nonprofit organization dedicated to improving the quality of life for BONE MARROW TRANSPLANT patients and their families by providing financial aid, education, and emotional support. The foundation was created in 1992 to respond to the critical gap in financial coverage for patient support services.

Its Patient Aid Program has assisted hundreds of patients with the cost of donor searches, compatibility testing, bone marrow harvesting, medications, home and child care services, medical equipment, transportation, cord blood banking, and housing expenses associated with the transplant.

The foundation currently accepts applications for aid from more than 70 bone marrow transplant centers throughout the United States. To fulfill the growing need for information and support to patients and their families, the foundation established the Marie M. Reynolds Resource and Educational Center to provide immediate information in a convenient format to patients, their families, and the clinicians who provide for their care. The center also seeks to provide support and encouragement to patients and families who are dealing with the challenge of a life-threatening disease. For contact information, see Appendix I.

bone marrow transplant A procedure to replace bone marrow that has been destroyed by high dosages of CHEMOTHERAPY drugs or RADIATION THERAPY. Transplants may be autologous (an individual's own marrow is saved before treatment), allogeneic (marrow is donated by someone else), or syngeneic (marrow is donated by an identical twin).

Bone marrow transplant is used as part of chemotherapy or radiation therapy treatments; in this procedure, a patient's marrow is removed and stored so that a much higher dosage of drugs or radiation, which would otherwise damage bone marrow, can be used. After the treatment is finished, the patient's healthy marrow is then returned.

Bone Marrow Transplant Family Support Network A national telephone support network for transplant patients and their families that provides referrals, information, counseling, and health insurance information. For contact information, see Appendix I.

Bone & Marrow Transplant Information Network A nonprofit organization dedicated exclusively to serving the needs of people facing a bone marrow, blood stem cell, or umbilical cord blood transplant. Founded in 1990 by BONE MARROW TRANSPLANT survivor Susan Stewart, BMT InfoNet strives to provide high-quality medical information in easy-to-understand language, so that patients can be active, knowledgeable participants in their healthcare planning and treatment.

In addition to publications, BMT InfoNet offers patients and survivors emotional support. Its volunteer network of more than 200 transplant survivors is available to help newly diagnosed patients and their loved ones cope with the stress of a life-threatening diagnosis, and the prospect of a bone marrow, stem cell, or cord blood transplant. For contact information, see Appendix I.

bone metastasis The spread of cancerous cells to the bone, where they can cause severe pain. Prostate, testicular, and PENILE CANCER all can spread to the bones.

Symptoms

Pain is the most common symptom of bone cancer, but symptoms may vary with the location and size of the cancer. Tumors that occur in or near joints may cause swelling or tenderness in the affected area. Some men may experience continuous pain, whereas others may only have occasional discomfort, at least at first. If there is pain, it may be restricted to one area or may appear in different spots.

Bone cancer can interfere with normal movements and can weaken the bones, occasionally leading to a fracture. Bone pain may change at different times of the day or in response to rest or activity.

The most common sites of bone metastasis are the back, ribs, shoulder, and hips. If the cancerous cells spread to the spine, the patient may be paralyzed if the nerves are compressed as the tumor grows into the spine.

Other symptoms may include FATIGUE, fever, weight loss, and ANEMIA.

Diagnosis

In addition to a complete medical exam, the doctor may suggest a blood test to determine the level of an enzyme called ALKALINE PHOSPHATASE. A high level of alkaline phosphatase can be found in the blood when the cells that form bone tissue are very active—such as when a broken bone is mending or when a tumor triggers the production of abnormal bone tissue.

X-rays can show the location, size, and shape of a bone tumor. If X-ray results suggest that a tumor may be cancer, the doctor may recommend special imaging tests such as a BONE SCAN, a computed tomography (CT) scan, magnetic resonance imaging (MRI) scan, or an angiogram.

Either a needle or an incisional BIOPSY can detect bone cancer. During a needle biopsy, the surgeon makes a small hole in the bone and removes a sample of tissue from the tumor with a needlelike instrument. In an incisional biopsy, the surgeon cuts into the tumor and removes a sample of tissue.

Treatment

Treatment options depend on the type, size, location, and stage of the original cancer, as well as the person's age and general health. Surgery is often the primary treatment; although amputation is sometimes necessary, pre- or postoperative chemotherapy has often made it possible to spare the limb. When possible, surgeons avoid amputation by removing only the cancerous section of the bone and replacing it with a prosthesis. CHEMOTHERAPY and RADIATION THERAPY may also be used alone or in combination.

Bone pain and progression of the disease may be treated by irradiation, BISPHOSPHONATES (clodronate or pamidronate), atrasentan, steroids such as oral prednisone, chemotherapy (MITOXANTRONE or a combination of taxotere and estramustine), or painkillers such as narcotics or nonsteroidal anti-inflammatory drugs.

bone scan   A specialized test that detects areas of altered bone metabolism by determining how much of a radioactive isotope collects in the bones. During the test, a small amount of radioactive chemical is injected through a vein into the blood and circulates throughout the body; it is absorbed by areas of fast bone growth that may be associated with bone healing or cancer.

As it decays, the chemical emits radiation, which is detected by a camera. When the tracer has collected in the bones a few hours after the injection, the scan is performed. Information from the camera is recorded in a computer, which then processes the data and creates an image. Although the chemical used in the study is radioactive, it is not considered to be harmful.

Normal distribution areas appear uniform and gray. "Hot spots" are areas where there is increased accumulation in the bone; these appear black. "Cold spots" are areas where there is less uptake of the radiotracer. These appear light or white.

The bone scan is the most sensitive way to identify PROSTATE CANCER that has spread to the bone. Although the scan is quite sensitive, it can still miss small numbers of malignant cells in the bone. In about 8 percent of cases the scan may miss bone cancer. On the other hand, certain other bone problems (such as a history of broken bones, Paget's disease, or arthritis) can cause an increase in the uptake of the radioactive substance.

Prostate cancer that has spread to the bone alters the appearance of bone in a different way than other cancers do. Prostate cancer that has spread to the bone tends to create the appearance that more bone is present on an X-ray, whereas other cancers cause what appears to be a loss of bone.

A bone scan is often performed as part of the staging evaluation of men newly diagnosed with prostate cancer who have a PROSTATE-SPECIFIC ANTIGEN (PSA) level above 10 ng/ml. A bone scan is not usually performed for men who have lower PSA levels because the risk of cancer spread to the bone is very low in this group.

BPH See BENIGN PROSTATIC HYPERPLASIA.

brachytherapy A procedure in which radioactive material sealed in needles, seeds, wires, or catheters is placed directly into or near a malignant tumor. The procedure is also called internal radiation, implant radiation, or interstitial RADIATION THERAPY. Another form of this treatment is called high-dose-rate remote brachytherapy (or high-dose-rate remote radiation therapy or remote brachytherapy), which is a type of internal radiation treatment in which the radioactive source is removed between treatments.

The term *brachytherapy* is derived from the ancient Greek words for "short distance" or "near to" and has been used for more than a century to treat a number of cancers. Henri Becquerel discovered natural radioactivity in 1896 when he realized that uranium produced a black spot on photographic plates that had not been exposed to sunlight. Two years later, Marie Curie and Pierre Curie, working in Becquerel's laboratory, extracted polonium from a ton of uranium ore and later in the same year, extracted radium. In 1901 Pierre Curie had the idea of inserting a small radium tube into a tumor. Two years later, Alexander Graham Bell made a similar suggestion (completely independently). With these early experiences, scientists found that inserting radioactive materials into tumors caused cancers to shrink.

In the early 20th century major brachytherapy research was carried out at the Curie Institute in Paris and at Memorial Hospital in New York. The advent of high-voltage teletherapy for deeper tumors and the problems associated with radiation exposure from high-energy radionuclides led to a decline in the use of brachytherapy toward the middle of the 20th century. However, over the past 30 years, scientists have again become interested in the use of brachytherapy, with newer types of imaging scans—computed tomography (CT) scan, MAGNETIC RESONANCE IMAGING (MRI), and ultrasound—and sophisticated computers, which improved positioning of the radiation for most effective dosage. TRANSRECTAL ULTRASOUND, C-arm fluoroscopy, and three-dimensional computerized treatment planning and postoperative CT-based dosimetry all have made the use of brachytherapy

more precise. The discovery of artificial radioisotopes and remote afterloading techniques also have reduced radiation exposure hazards.

There are several different types of seed implants that are used in brachytherapy:

- Palladium 103 (Pd 103) seeds produce radiation more rapidly and over a shorter period. Some researchers think that palladium seeds are best suited to treat faster growing, more aggressive tumors. These are used for permanent seed placement.
- Iodine (I 125) seeds are usually recommended for use in the treatment of slow-growing tumors.
- Echogenic seeds have a specific feature that helps the doctor place the seeds within the cancerous tissue.
- Iridium 192 is used for temporary placement; it is removed after 24 to 72 hours.

Palladium, which provides a higher initial dose of radiation, is preferred by some experts for fast-growing, high-grade tumors and for those tumors that have a Gleason score of at least seven. Iodine is preferred for tumors scored at six or lower.

Radioactive Risk

Though very sensitive Geiger counters could detect radiation in the body of someone who has received radioactive seeds, the person would not be considered radioactive. Intimate contact does not pass on the radiation.

In spite the very low risk, some doctors recommend that close contact with pregnant women and small children be avoided for two months after the initial procedure.

Side Effects

After surgery, there may be some swelling, bruising, or slight bleeding from the area under the scrotum and in front of the rectum. This is related to needle placement and usually fades after a few days. Presence of blood in the urine as a result of urethral irritation and of blood in the ejaculate may occur briefly but stop within a few days.

The most common side effects of brachytherapy for PROSTATE CANCER include urination problems such as urinary frequency, painful urination, or serious urinary incontinence. Rectal ulcers, bleeding or fistulas are possible but uncommon. A few patients may experience a harmless increase in PSA. Urinary symptoms usually appear earlier when palladium is used as opposed to iodine, because of the initial higher dose of radiation.

If urinary symptoms are not linked to urinary retention, they can be treated with nonsteroidal anti-inflammatory drugs (NSAIDs) or an alpha blocker such as doxazosin, terazosin, or tamsulosin. Symptoms usually fade after one to four months but may persist for more than a year in some cases.

Between 7 percent and 25 percent of prostate cancer patients who have interstitial seed placement may experience an obstruction of the bladder outlet as a result of blood clots in the bladder or prostate swelling. Blood clots can be removed by washing out the bladder. A swollen prostate may be treated with a catheter and medications.

Candidates

Because interstitial therapy is considered to be a way to cure prostate cancer, candidates who have a life expectancy of at least seven to 10 years and no underlying illness should be chosen. Men who have symptoms of significant obstructive voiding or size and weight of the prostate above 50 ml are at higher risk for development of urinary problems after the procedure.

Combination Therapy

Some doctors recommend a combination of brachytherapy and radiation therapy for prostate cancer patients, because the internal radiation may not be able to reach tissue outside the prostate.

See also the AMERICAN BRACHYTHERAPY SOCIETY.

BRCA1/BRCA2 Two genes (*breast cancer 1* and *breast cancer 2*) that normally help to suppress cell growth. A woman who inherits either gene in an altered form has a higher risk of breast or ovarian cancer. Men who have inherited a mutant form of BRCA1 may have as much as a threefold higher risk of development of PROSTATE CANCER than other men. Men who have an altered BRCA1 or BRCA2 gene also have an increased risk of breast cancer (primarily if the alteration is in BRCA2).

Genes are small pieces of DNA, the material that acts as a master blueprint for all the cells in the body. A person's genes determine such characteristics as hair or eye color, height, and skin color. Any mistake in a gene that interferes with its function can lead to disease.

The BRCA1 and BRCA2 genes produce a chemical substance that helps the body prevent cancer. Most men have two normal copies of the BRCA1 and BRCA2 genes, both of which produce this cancer-preventing substance. However, some men have a genetic defect in one copy of their two BRCA1 and BRCA2 genes; as a result, they do not produce a normal amount of this cancer-preventing substance. These men are at higher risk of prostate cancer.

People inherit one copy of each of their genes from their mother and a second copy of each gene from their father. If one parent has a defective BRCA1 or BRCA2 gene, there is a 50 percent chance the child may inherit the defective copy and a 50 percent chance the child may inherit the normal copy. If a person inherits a defective BRCA1 or BRCA2 gene, then each of that person's children likewise has a 50 percent chance of inheriting it. Because family members share a proportion of their genes and, often, their environment, it is possible that the large number of cancer cases seen in these families may be partly due to other genetic or environmental factors. Therefore, risk estimates that are based on families with many affected members may not accurately reflect the levels of risk in the general population.

Specific gene alterations have been identified in different ethnic groups. In Ashkenazi Jewish families, about 2.3 percent (23 of 1,000 persons) have an altered BRCA1 or BRCA2 gene—about five times higher than the percentage in the general population. Among people who have alterations in BRCA1 or BRCA2, three particular alterations have been found to be most common in the Ashkenazi Jewish population. Other ethnic and geographic populations, such as Norwegian, Dutch, and Icelandic people, also have a higher rate of certain genetic alterations in BRCA1 and BRCA2. This information about genetic differences between ethnic groups may help health-care providers determine the most appropriate genetic test to select.

Genetic Testing

A simple blood test can determine alterations in a person's *BRCA1* or *BRCA2* gene. However, the cost of genetic testing can range from several hundred to several thousand dollars, and not all insurance policies cover the test. Some people may choose to pay for the test even when their insurer would be willing to cover the cost, as a way of protecting their privacy. From the date that blood is drawn, several weeks or months may pass before test results become available. It may be possible to have the genetic test performed as part of a clinical study at a comprehensive cancer center for no charge.

In a family with a history of prostate cancer, it may be most informative first to test a family member who has the disease. If that person is found to have an altered *BRCA1* or *BRCA2* gene, the specific change is referred to as a known mutation. Other family members can then be tested to see whether they also carry that specific alteration. In this scenario, a positive test result indicates that a person has inherited a known mutation in *BRCA1* or *BRCA2* and has an increased risk of development of certain cancers. However, a positive result provides information only about a person's risk of development of cancer—it cannot predict whether cancer will actually develop.

If the Test Result Is Positive

If a patient tests positive for altered *BRCA1* or *BRCA2* genes, there are several possible responses. Careful monitoring for symptoms of cancer may allow the disease, if it occurs, to be diagnosed at an earlier stage, when treatment is more effective.

breakthrough pain   Intense increases in pain that occur with rapid onset even when painkillers are being used. Breakthrough pain can occur spontaneously or be related to a specific activity.

Brief Pain Inventory   A questionnaire used to measure pain.

buserelin   An anticancer drug that belongs to the family of drugs called gonadotropin-releasing hormone agonists. In prostate cancer therapy, buserelin prevents the production of testosterone in the testicles.

cachexia A loss of body weight and muscle mass that is common among cancer patients.

calcium and prostate cancer A diet rich in calcium may help reduce the risk of some types of colon cancer and is essential for strong bones. However, some scientists suggest that an excess of calcium intake may be linked to PROSTATE CANCER.

In a 2000 Harvard University study, scientists observed a moderate increase in the risk of prostate cancer associated with higher intake of dairy foods and dairy calcium. This increase could be related to the capacity of calcium to reduce the body's level of vitamin D, which has been shown to protect the prostate. Vitamin D is one of the HORMONES that slow the growth of many types of cells and can prevent the progression of cancer to a more advanced stage.

Researchers emphasized that their study suggests only a possible link between calcium and prostate cancer, and they are not recommending dietary changes. Not all studies see a link between calcium and prostate cancer, and most men never have too much calcium—which would be above 1,000 mg a day for men 50 or younger and 1,200 mg a day for those older than 50. Calcium may really be a concern only for men who consume more than 2,000 milligrams a day. Calcium-rich foods include the following:

- One cup of milk—300 mg
- One-half cup of broccoli—35 mg
- One-half cup of spinach—120 mg
- One and one-half ounces of cheddar cheese—300 mg
- Eight ounces of low-fat yogurt—300–415 mg
- One cup of calcium-fortified orange juice—300 mg

cancer A general term used to describe more than 100 different uncontrolled growths of abnormal cells in the body. A cancer cell divides and reproduces abnormally, continuing to grow, invade, and destroy surrounding tissue. It may spread from the original site and travel via lymph or blood systems to other parts of the body, where these cells can create new cancerous tumors. A new tumor that has arisen as a result of spread from a primary tumor is called a metastatic tumor.

Cancer Care A national nonprofit agency that offers free support, information, financial assistance, and practical help to people who have cancer and their loved ones. Services are provided by oncology social workers and are available in person, over the telephone, and through the agency's Web site.

Established in 1944, Cancer Care is the oldest and largest national nonprofit agency devoted to offering professional services. It has helped more than 2 million people nationwide through its toll-free counseling line and teleconference programs, its office-based services, and its Internet support. All services are provided free and are available to people of all ages, with all types of cancer, at any stage of the disease. Cancer Care's reach, including its cancer awareness initiatives, also extends to family members, caregivers, and professionals, providing vital information and assistance.

A section of the Cancer Care Web site and some publications are available in Spanish, and staff can respond to calls and e-mails in Spanish. For contact information, see Appendix I.

cancer centers Institutions dedicated to treating and researching cancer, as designated by the NATIONAL CANCER INSTITUTE. "Cancer center" refers to a cancer center that has a scientific agenda other than that of a "comprehensive" or "clinical" cancer center. Such centers may have a narrow research focus such as in basic science, population research, epidemiology, diagnosis, immunology or other areas.

A CLINICAL CANCER CENTER has reasonable research activities in clinical oncology, with or without research encompassing basic and prevention research. A COMPREHENSIVE CANCER CENTER has a wide range of research in basic research, clinical research, and prevention, control, behavioral and population-based research.

The Cancer Centers Program of the NCI supports cancer research programs in about 60 institutions across the United States through Cancer Center Support Grants.

CancerFax A service sponsored by the NATIONAL CANCER INSTITUTE (NCI) that provides summaries of cancer information (in English or Spanish) via fax machine. NCI fact sheets on various cancer topics, as well as other NCI information, are also available through CancerFax. CancerFax does not provide listings of clinical trials.

CancerFax can be accessed 24 hours a day, seven days a week, by anyone in the United States, by dialing (800) 624-2511 toll-free from a touch-tone phone or from the telephone on a fax machine (the machine must be set to touch-tone dialing) and following the recorded instructions. Anyone calling from outside the United States may use the local number, (301) 402-5874. For a fact sheet that explains how to use CancerFax, consumers may call the CANCER INFORMATION SERVICE at (800) 4-CANCER.

Cancer Fund of America (CFA) A national non-profit agency dedicated to helping cancer patients who are having financial difficulty. Its priority is patient care rather than research. Cancer Fund of America (CFA) provides supplies, such as food, crutches, lotions and ointments, dressings, seasonal gift boxes, adult diapers, and bed pads, through its patient assistance programs.

Cancer Fund of America's mission differs greatly from that of many of the more than 200 U.S. charities that offer cancer-related services, because its principal mission is to provide aid to the ill and needy rather than to conduct research. CFA gives support and services to financially indigent patients, disseminates information about early detection and prevention of cancer, provides commodities and gifts in kind to hospices and other health-care providers, and distributes donated merchandise to various nonprofit community service organizations that aid the ill, needy, and infants. For contact information, see Appendix I.

Cancer Genetics Network A national network of eight centers specializing in the study of inherited predisposition to cancer, together with the Informatics Technology Group, which provides supporting information. The network supports collaborative investigations on the genetic basis of cancer susceptibility, methods to integrate new knowledge into medical practice, and techniques to address the psychosocial, ethical, legal, and public health issues.

The network includes the following:

- Carolina–Georgia Cancer Genetics Network Center (Duke University Medical Center, Emory University, and the University of North Carolina/Chapel Hill)
- Georgetown University Medical Center's Cancer Genetics Network Center (Georgetown University Lombardi Cancer Center, Washington, D.C.)
- Mid-Atlantic Cancer Genetics Network Center (Johns Hopkins University and Greater Baltimore Medical Center)
- Northwest Cancer Genetics Network (Fred Hutchinson Cancer Research Center in Seattle and University of Washington School of Medicine in Seattle)
- Rocky Mountain Cancer Genetics Coalition (University of Utah, University of New Mexico, and University of Colorado)
- Texas Cancer Genetics Consortium (M. D. Anderson Cancer Center, Health Science Center at San Antonio, Southwestern Medical Center at Dallas, and Baylor College of Medicine)
- University of Pennsylvania Cancer Genetics Network

- UCI-UCSD Cancer Genetics Network Center (University of California Irvine and University of California San Diego)
- Informatics Technology Group

Cancer Hope Network A nonprofit organization that provides individual support to cancer patients and their families by matching them with trained volunteers who have undergone and recovered from a similar cancer experience. Matches are based on the type and stage of cancer, treatments used, side effects experienced, and other factors. Through this matching process, the network tries to provide support and hope, to help patients and family members look beyond the diagnosis and cope with treatment.

This unique program was built on the belief that matching a cancer patient with someone who has recovered from a similar experience could make a real difference in the patient's own fight. It is available to all cancer patients and their loved ones anywhere in the United States at no cost. After the office is contacted and the person's situation discussed, the office matches the patient with a volunteer who has recovered from the same cancer experience. The staff make a match based on characteristics of the cancer and treatment and on overall demographic similarities, such as age or gender.

Patients may contact the group at any point; ideally they recommend a match before the beginning of treatment, to give patients a chance to discuss any fears and questions about that treatment. However, the program benefits patients at all stages of their cancer experience.

Volunteers are former patients who have survived a cancer experience and who want to help others as they deal with the disease; they have been off treatment for at least one year and have had extensive training before their first patient visit. For contact information, see Appendix I.

Cancer Information and Counseling Line A toll-free telephone service that is part of the psychosocial program of the American Medical Center (AMC) Cancer Research Center. Professional counselors provide up-to-date medical information, emotional support through short-term counseling, and resource referrals to callers nationwide between the hours of 8:30 A.M. and 5:00 P.M. Mountain Standard Time (MST). Individuals may also submit questions about cancer and request resources via e-mail. For contact information, see Appendix I.

Cancer Information Service (CIS) A service sponsored by the NATIONAL CANCER INSTITUTE (NCI) to interpret research findings for the public and to provide personalized responses to specific questions about cancer. As a resource for information and education about cancer, the Cancer Information Service (CIS) helps people become active participants in their health care by providing the latest information on cancer in understandable language.

Through its network of regional offices, the CIS serves the United States, Puerto Rico, the U.S. Virgin Islands, and the Pacific Islands. For 25 years the CIS has provided the most accurate and up-to-date cancer information to patients and families, the public, and health professionals by interacting with individuals, working with organizations through its Partnership Program, participating in research efforts to find the best ways to help people adopt healthier behavior, and providing access to NCI information over the Internet.

Through the CIS toll-free telephone service, callers can speak with knowledgeable, caring staff who are experienced in explaining medical information in easy-to-understand terms. CIS information specialists answer calls in English and Spanish and provide cancer information to deaf and hearing-impaired callers through the service's toll-free TTY number, (800) 332-8615.

CIS staff have access to comprehensive, accurate information from the NCI on a range of cancer topics, including the most recent advances in cancer treatment. They take as much time as each caller needs, provide thorough and personal attention, and treat all calls as confidential.

The CIS also provides live online assistance to users of NCI Web sites through LiveHelp, an instant messaging service that is available from 9 A.M. to 10 P.M. Eastern Standard Time (EST), Monday through Friday. Through LiveHelp, information specialists answer questions about cancer and help people navigate Cancer.gov, the NCI's Web site.

CIS staffers can answer questions about cancer (including ways to prevent cancer, symptoms and risks, diagnosis, current treatments, and research studies), provide written materials from the NCI, and make referrals to clinical trials and cancer-related services such as treatment centers, mammography facilities, or other cancer organizations.

Through its Partnership Program, the CIS collaborates with established national, state, and regional organizations to reach minority and medically underserved groups with cancer information. Partnership Program staff provide assistance to organizations developing programs that focus on breast and cervical cancer, clinical trials, tobacco control, and cancer awareness for special populations. To reach those in need, the CIS helps give cancer information to people who do not traditionally seek health information or who may have trouble doing so as a result of educational, financial, cultural, or language barriers.

The CIS plays an important role in research by studying the most effective ways to communicate with people about healthy lifestyles, health risks, and options for preventing, diagnosing, and treating cancer. The capacity to conduct health communication research is a unique aspect of the CIS. Results of these research studies can be applied to improving CIS communication about cancer and can help other programs communicate more effectively. For contact information, see Appendix I.

Cancer Legal Resource Center   A legal organization that provides information and educational outreach on cancer-related legal issues to people who have cancer and others impacted by the disease. The center, a joint program of Loyola Law School and the Western Law Center for Disability Rights, provides outreach to cancer support groups, cancer survivors, and caregivers. It also provides speakers for outreach programs at hospitals, community centers, cancer organizations, and work places.

The center provides information about its services and, when necessary, matches patients with volunteer attorneys and other professionals for additional legal information. The center is presently working with major cancer centers in Los Angeles but accepts calls from the Greater Los Angeles area, Orange County, and outside California.

The center also trains law students to understand the legal needs of people battling cancer and of cancer survivors. For contact information, see Appendix I.

Cancer Liaison Program   A division of the U.S. Food and Drug Administration (FDA) that works directly with cancer patients and advocacy programs to provide information and education on the FDA drug approval process, cancer clinical trails, and access to investigational drugs when it is not possible for them to join a clinical trial. For contact information, see Appendix I.

CancerMail   A service of the NATIONAL CANCER INSTITUTE that provides comprehensive cancer information summaries and other related information via e-mail. To obtain a content list, consumers can send an e-mail to cancermail@cips.nci.nih.gov with the word *help* in the body of the message. CancerMail responds by sending a content list via e-mail. Instructions for ordering documents through e-mail are also provided.

CancerNet   A Web site that provides a wide range of cancer information from the NATIONAL CANCER INSTITUTE, including details on treatment options, clinical trials, reduction of cancer risk, and methods of coping with cancer. Resources on support groups, financial assistance, and educational materials are also available. The Web site address is http://cancernet.nci.nih.gov.

Cancer Research Foundation of America (CRFA)   A nonprofit group that seeks to prevent cancer by funding research and providing educational materials on early detection and nutrition. The group focuses on cancers that can be prevented through lifestyle changes or early detection followed by prompt treatment, including cancers of the prostate and testicles.

When Cancer Research Foundation of America (CRFA) began its work in 1987, cancer prevention was not regarded as a major strategy in the war against cancer. Scientists primarily focused on discovering new cancer treatments rather than ways to prevent the disease.

Today prevention research is recognized as essential to the fight against cancer. Now that scientists better understand how tumors develop, they are learning ways that people can reduce their cancer risks. Since its inception, the foundation has provided funding to more than 200 scientists at more than 100 leading academic institutions across the country. For contact information, see Appendix I.

Cancer Research Institute (CRI)   A nonprofit organization that funds research projects and scientists across the United States. The institute was founded in 1953 to foster the science of cancer immunology, which is based on the idea that the body's immune system can be mobilized against cancer. CRI helped develop this field. For nearly five decades the institute has been a sustaining force in cancer and immunology research, supporting more than 2,500 scientists and clinicians at leading universities and research centers worldwide. All such funding decisions are made by its Scientific Advisory Council, consisting of 63 of the world's leading immunologists, including four Nobel laureates, 24 members of the National Academy of Sciences, and 23 members of the Academy of Cancer Immunology. For contact information, see Appendix I.

Cancer Survivors Network   A telephone- and Internet-based service for cancer survivors, their families, caregivers, and friends. The telephone component, (877) 333-HOPE, gives survivors and families access to prerecorded discussions. The Web-based component offers live online chat sessions, virtual support groups, prerecorded talk shows, and personal stories. Cancer Survivors Network is supported by the AMERICAN CANCER SOCIETY. For contact information, see Appendix I.

cancerTrials   A Web site sponsored by the NATIONAL CANCER INSTITUTE that provides information and news about cancer research studies. The primary mission of cancerTrials is to help people consider clinical trials as an option when making cancer care decisions. Consumers can access cancerTrials at http://cancertrials.nci.nih.gov.

Cancervive   A Los Angeles nonprofit organization founded in 1985 by a childhood cancer survivor, Susan Nessium. The organization is dedicated to providing support, public education, and advocacy to those who have experienced cancer and to helping survivors reclaim their life after cancer. For contact information, see Appendix I.

capsule   A fibrous outer layer that surrounds many body organs. The tissue around the prostate is generally compressed and acts as a prostate capsule.

carboplatin (Paraplatin)   A platinum-based anticancer drug similar to CISPLATIN, but somewhat less toxic. Carboplatin is less effective than cisplatin in treatment of TESTICULAR CANCER.

carcinoma   Cancer that begins in the skin or in tissues that line or cover internal organs.

carcinoma in situ   A precancer that is confined to its original position, usually considered to be the earliest stage of cancer (or stage 0). Surgical removal of carcinoma in situ is often a cure (but not in the case of bladder cancer).

In TESTICULAR CANCER, carcinoma in situ does not produce a mass or cause any symptoms, but it does mean that the man is likely to develop testicular cancer. In some cases, it is detected in men who have a testicular biopsy in a medical evaluation of infertility.

carotenoid   A substance found in yellow and orange fruits and vegetables and in dark green, leafy vegetables that may reduce the risk of development of cancer. The most widespread pigments in the natural world, carotenoids are an important component of the colorful appearance of many plants and animals, including red peppers, tomatoes, paprika, flamingos, canaries, ladybugs, and salmon.

One study has found a link between consumption of LYCOPENE (a carotenoid found in tomato-based foods) and a reduced risk of PROSTATE CANCER.

The color-producing properties of carotenoids are so powerful that many manufactured products, such as soft drinks, use them as coloring (although in such low concentrations that they do not yield much nutritional benefit). The most common natural carotenoid is BETA-CAROTENE, a yellow-orange pigment that lends its color to carrots, sweet potatoes, and other fruits and vegetables. Beta-carotene is a provitamin A carotenoid: a type of carotenoid that the body readily converts into vitamin A.

In recent years studies have linked a variety of carotenoids with the prevention of several different kinds of cancer.

Beta-carotene pills, lutein pills, and other supplements can now be found at health food stores and supermarkets alongside such familiar products as vitamin C, echinacea, and folic acid.

However, experts caution that scientists still do not wholly understand how carotenoids work as preventative agents. Although studies reinforce the finding that a diet rich in fruits and vegetables may help prevent a wide variety of cancers, scientists still do not know precisely how carotenoids reduce cancer risk and how they may interact with other agents. In addition, the need for caution is reinforced by ambiguous results of other studies of the effects of carotenoids, especially studies of beta-carotene.

See also DIET.

Casodex   See BICALUTAMIDE.

castration   The surgical removal of both TESTICLES is called surgical castration. When medications are used to stop production of testosterone in the testicles, this is commonly referred to as "chemical castration."

cathepsin B (CB)   An enzyme that destroys proteins in the connective tissue that holds cells in place. It is produced in high amounts by malignant cells, which can then invade surrounding tissue and escape to blood vessels.

Cells also produce natural inhibitors of CB called stefins. By measuring the ratio of CB to stefins in a simple test, researchers have been able to identify patients who have the most aggressive prostate cancers, even among patients whose tumors are at the same stage.

The degree to which prostate cancers have progressed is determined by the GLEASON GRADING SYSTEM, which is based on the shape and microscopic

appearance of tumors. Patients who have higher grades of tumor are usually diagnosed with more advanced stages of the disease. The Gleason grading system assigns tumors a score between 2 and 10, in which 10 is the most aggressive cancer. People who have a Gleason score from 7 to 10 have a higher risk of dying of prostate cancer than those who have lower scores, but some patients who have higher scores can still be cured. Even among tumors that have a similar Gleason score, there are biologically aggressive and less aggressive forms of cancer. This variation makes prediction of outcomes for individual patients more difficult.

Researchers reasoned that a prostate tumor that had a stefin level that was equal to or higher than the CB level would be less aggressive; however, if the CB level were higher, the tumor would be more likely to spread.

In one recent study, Minnesota scientists found that the ratio of CB to stefin A was significantly higher in patients whose cancer had spread to one or more pelvic lymph nodes than in patients whose nodes were clear.

The ratio of CB to stefin A reveals differences in tumors that are not visible under the microscope. If this test were done on tumors of newly diagnosed patients, it would indicate which cancers were most aggressive, and those individuals could then have aggressive treatment. Patients whose tumor has a ratio of 1 or less than 1 may require less aggressive treatment.

Centers for Disease Control and Prevention, Division of Cancer Prevention and Control (CDC/DCPC)   A department of the U.S. federal government that conducts, supports, and promotes efforts to prevent cancer and to increase early detection of cancer. The Division of Cancer Prevention and Control (DCPC) works with partners in the government, private, and nonprofit sectors to develop, implement, and promote effective cancer prevention and control practices nationwide.

In addition to the Centers for Disease Control's (CDC) activities in monitoring cancer risk factors and use of cancer preventive services, DCPC specifically supports systems for monitoring cancer incidence and mortality rates through funding and technical assistance. Data from these systems serve a critical role in identifying and monitoring cancer trends, gaps, disparities, barriers, and successes; developing, guiding, and evaluating cancer prevention and control activities; and prioritizing allocation of resources.

In addition, DCPC helps translate basic research into public health practices, interventions, and health delivery services and then promotes, implements, and evaluates their use. DCPC conducts and funds studies to identify problems, needs, and opportunities related to modifiable behavioral and other risk factors for cancer and to evaluate the feasibility and effectiveness of cancer prevention and control strategies. Results are used to plan or improve cancer prevention and control activities.

DCPC also develops health communication campaigns, prepares and provides cancer prevention educational materials, and recommends priorities for health promotion, health education, and cancer risk reduction activities both for health professionals and for the public.

DCPC provides cancer-related Web sites; a public inquiries e-mail service (cancerinfo@cdc.gov); a toll-free phone number, (888) 842-6355, and a Web-based information system for selected cancer legislative issues. The division also provides support and technical assistance to improve education, training, and skills in the prevention, detection, and control of selected cancers. For contact information, see Appendix I.

CHEMOcare   A program and Web site sponsored by the Scott Hamilton initiative Cancer Alliance for Research Education and Survivorship (CARES) designed to provide the most up-to-date information about CHEMOTHERAPY to patients and their families.

The site contains information about having chemotherapy, managing side effects, and living well during treatment. For contact information, see Appendix I.

chemotherapy   The use of toxic drugs to control cancer by interfering with the growth or production of malignant cells. In general, chemotherapy is not usually used in the treatment of PROSTATE CANCER, a type of cancer that is characterized by slow growth, except when other treatments have failed.

However, scientists are studying possible uses of chemotherapy for men who do not respond, or who stop responding, to HORMONAL THERAPY. Researchers are also beginning to look into the possibility of using chemotherapy earlier in the treatment of prostate cancer to see if it will be more effective if used sooner.

History

The first drugs used as chemotherapy agents were not used to treat cancer, but to attack armies in chemical warfare. During mustard gas experiments after World War I and during World War II, a large number of soldiers were unintentionally exposed to the gas. They were subsequently discovered to have unusually low white blood counts. Scientists soon realized that a drug that damaged rapidly growing white blood cells might also damage rapidly growing malignant cells. Several individuals who had lymphoma during the 1940s were then injected with mustard gas and experienced a remarkable (albeit temporary) improvement.

How It Works

Chemotherapy drugs interfere with the ability of cancer cells throughout the body to divide and reproduce themselves. Whereas normal cells typically divide in very controlled ways, malignant cells grow and reproduce in a rapid, haphazard way. Chemotherapy drugs are taken up by rapidly dividing cells—which include cancerous cells and also some healthy cells that normally divide quickly, in the lining of the mouth, the bone marrow, the hair follicles, and the digestive system. However, whereas healthy cells can repair the damage caused by chemotherapy, cancer cells cannot, and so they eventually die.

Chemotherapy drugs damage cancer cells in different ways. If a combination of drugs is used, each drug is chosen because for its specific effects. Chemotherapy must be carefully planned so that it destroys more and more of the cancer cells during the course of treatment but does not destroy the normal cells and tissues. In some types of cancer, chemotherapy can destroy all the cancer cells and cure the disease.

Chemotherapy and Prostate Cancer

Chemotherapy cannot cure PROSTATE CANCER, and it is not the primary therapy for prostate cancer patients, but it may be used when prostate cancer has spread outside the prostate gland or in combination with other therapies. The AMERICAN CANCER SOCIETY does not consider chemotherapy effective against early prostate cancer. Although it may slow tumor growth and reduce pain, it has had limited success in the treatment of advanced disease.

However, several different drugs have been shown to improve symptoms and decrease the PROSTATE-SPECIFIC ANTIGEN (PSA) level or the size of a tumor. No drug has been shown to kill all prostate cancer cells. As a result, chemotherapy is often used when hormone therapy fails.

Drugs that have been used to treat prostate cancer include estramustine, vinblastine, taxanes, mitoxantrone, and suramin.

Chemotherapy and Testicular Cancer

The main drugs used to treat testicle cancer are cisplatin, vinblastine, bleomycin, cyclophosphamide, etoposide, and ifosfamide. These drugs are used in various combinations. Some of the drugs used to treat testicular cancer can cause long-term side effects, including kidney damage, heart damage, damage to small blood vessels that causes sensitivity to cold, nerve damage that causes numbness and abnormal tingling, hearing loss, and lung damage that causes shortness of breath and reduced capacity for physical activity. Development of a second cancer (usually leukemia) is a very serious but rare side effect that occurs in less than 1 percent of testicular cancer patients treated with chemotherapy.

Chemotherapy and Penile Cancer

Chemotherapy may be used in addition to surgical excision (cutting out and removing) of the penile tumor. Bleomycin is usually the chemotherapy drug of choice for treating penile cancer. Patients are usually hospitalized for the first few doses of chemotherapy to monitor them for possible side effects. Most people receive subsequent chemotherapy (after the initial dose) on an outpatient basis. FLUOROURACIL cream (a chemotherapy drug put on the skin of the penis) is sometimes used for very small surface cancers of the penis.

Adjuvant therapy   To reduce the chance of cancer recurrence, chemotherapy may be given after surgery, when all the visible cancer has been removed, or after RADIATION THERAPY, so that if any cancer cells remain that are too small to see, they can be destroyed. Chemotherapy is designed to kill any tiny cancer cells that may have been left behind. In advanced cancer, if a cure is not possible, chemotherapy is used to shrink and control the cancer, to extend life and improve its quality.

Neoadjuvant therapy   Chemotherapy also can be given before surgery to shrink a tumor and make removal easier. This is usually given to people whose cancer cannot be removed easily during an operation. Chemotherapy can also be used in this way before radiation therapy.

Types of Chemotherapy

Chemotherapy drugs are divided into different types, depending on the way they work and the parts of the cells they affect. (For a list of chemotherapy drugs for use in prostate, testicular, or PENILE CANCER, see Appendix III.)

How It Is Given

Chemotherapy may be given in different ways depending on the type of cancer and the specific chemotherapy drugs used. They can be given in pill or liquid form by mouth, on the skin as a lotion, intravenously, intra-muscularly, subcutaneously (under the skin), intra-arterially (into the artery), intrathecally (into the central nervous system through the cerebrospinal fluid), intrapleurally (into the chest cavity), intraperitoneally (into the abdomen), intravesically (into the bladder), or intralesionally (into the tumor itself).

Chemotherapy administered intravenously is given through catheters, ports, and pumps. A catheter is a soft, thin, flexible tube that is placed into a large vein in the body, where it remains throughout treatment. Patients who need many IV treatments often have a catheter to eliminate the need for frequent injections. Drugs can be given and blood samples can be drawn through the same catheter. Central venous catheters are usually placed into a large vein, usually in the chest.

A peripherally inserted central catheter (PICC) is inserted into a vein in the arm. Catheters can also be placed in an artery or other locations in the body; intrathecal catheters deliver drugs into the spinal fluid, and intracavitary catheters are placed in the abdomen, pelvis, or chest. Drugs administered in this way tend to stay in the area in which they are introduced and do not affect cells in other parts of the body.

Sometimes the catheter is attached to a port—a small round plastic or metal disk placed under the skin, which is used throughout treatment.

A pump (either external or internal) is used to control the rate at which the drug enters a catheter or port. Catheters, ports, and pumps cause no pain if they are properly placed, although the patient is aware of them.

Frequency

The duration and frequency of chemotherapy depend on the type of cancer, the treatment goals, the specific drugs, and the patient's body's response to treatment. Patients may have chemotherapy every day, every week, or every month. In any case, chemotherapy is often administered in cycles of treatment periods with rest periods in between, to give the body a chance to repair healthy new cells and regain strength.

Chemotherapy on the Job

Most people can continue working while receiving chemotherapy, although they may need to change their work schedule if the drugs make them feel tired or sick. Federal and state laws require employers to let patients work a flexible schedule to meet treatment needs. Social workers and congressional or state representatives can provide information on state and federal laws guaranteeing patient protections.

Side Effects

Chemotherapy drugs cause a variety of side effects that may vary from person to person and treatment to treatment. Almost all side effects are short term and gradually disappear once treatment has stopped. The main areas of the body that may be affected by chemotherapy are those where normal cells rapidly divide and grow, such as the lining of the mouth, digestive system, skin, hair, and BONE MARROW.

However, sometimes chemotherapy can cause permanent changes or damage to the heart, lungs, nerves, kidneys, or reproductive or other organs. Certain types of chemotherapy may have delayed effects (such as a second type of cancer) that do not appear for many years. Patients need to balance their concerns about permanent effects with the immediate threat of cancer.

Great progress has been made in preventing and treating some of chemotherapy's common as well as rare severe side effects. Many new drugs and treatment methods destroy cancer more effectively while doing less harm to the body's healthy cells.

FATIGUE, infection, and unusual bleeding are all very common side effects because chemotherapy lowers the number of blood cells produced by the bone marrow—white blood cells essential for fighting infections, red blood cells that carry oxygen, and platelets that help clot the blood and prevent bleeding.

Fatigue Fatigue is a very common side effect of chemotherapy; patients report that it is quite different from normal tiredness. Fatigue caused by chemotherapy can begin suddenly and may be experienced as lack of energy, weakness, and complete inability to work or think. Moreover, it seems unrelated to activity and does not improve with rest. It has been described as a total lack of energy that makes patients feel worn out and drained.

Fatigue associated with chemotherapy is related to low blood cell counts, stress, depression, poor appetite, lack of exercise, and many other factors. Chemotherapy can interfere with the bone marrow's ability to make red blood cells, which carry oxygen to all parts of the body. When there are too few red blood cells, body tissues do not receive enough oxygen to do their work. If the level of red blood cells in the blood is too low, patients may become tired and lethargic. Because the amount of oxygen being carried around the body is lower, patients also may become breathless. These are all symptoms of anemia (a lack of hemoglobin in the blood). People who have anemia may also feel dizzy and light-headed and have aching muscles and joints. The tiredness fades gradually once the chemotherapy ends, but some people find that they still feel tired a year or more afterward.

Oncologists order regular blood tests to measure hemoglobin during chemotherapy, and a blood transfusion can be given if the hemoglobin falls too low. The extra red cells in the blood transfusion very quickly pick up the oxygen from the lungs and take it around the body so that patients feel more energetic and breathlessness improves. Some studies have also suggested that maintaining a moderate level of physical exercise (such as walking) can help prevent fatigue.

Nausea and vomiting   Although many patients fear the NAUSEA and vomiting that have historically been reported as side effects of chemotherapy, in fact modern drugs have made these side effects far less common.

Because of very effective antinausea medications, many men do not become sick at all during their treatment, and if they do, sickness is quite mild. It is particularly important that patients closely follow their physicians' guidelines regarding antinausea medication, which is usually given together with IV chemotherapy; patients can then take additional antinausea medication at home, before nausea begins. Once nausea starts, it is far more difficult to control. Low dosages of steroids can be helpful in reducing nausea and vomiting.

Antinausea medications that are highly effective include lorazepam (Ativan), prochlorperazine (Compazine), promethazine (Anergan), metoclopramide (Reglan), dexamethasone (DECADRON), ondansetron (Zofran), and granisetron (Kytril).

Chemotherapy drugs cause nausea and vomiting because they tend to irritate the stomach lining, and the irritation stimulates nerves in the vomiting center in the brain. Certain chemotherapy medications are more likely to cause nausea and vomiting:

- Carboplatin
- Carmustine
- Cisplatin
- Cyclophosphamide
- Cytarabine
- Dacarbazine
- Dactinomycin
- Doxorubicin
- Etoposide
- Lomustine
- Mechlorethamine
- Melphalan
- Methotrexate
- Plicamycin
- Procarbazine
- Streptozocin

If patients sickness occurs, it usually begins a few minutes to several hours after chemotherapy, depending on the drugs given. The sickness may last for a few hours or for several days. This reaction to chemotherapy varies from person to person and from drug to drug. For example, some people never vomit or feel nauseous; others feel mildly nauseated most of the time; some become severely nauseated for a limited time during or after a treatment. Their symptoms may start soon after a treatment or hours later. They may feel sick for just a few hours or for about a day. Certain risk factors that influence the intensity of nausea and vomiting include the patient's previous experience with motion sickness, youth, alcohol use, and bad experiences with nausea and vomiting.

The following methods may help. To prevent problems, men should do the following:

- Avoid big meals so the stomach does not feel overfull. Eating small meals throughout the day is better than eating a few large meals.

- Drink liquids at least an hour before or after mealtime, instead of with meals.

- Eat and drink slowly.

- Avoid sweet, fried, or fatty foods.

- Eat foods cold or at room temperature to prevent strong odors (many patients swear by "cold white" foods, such as cold chicken or ice cream).

- Chew food well for easier digestion.

- Drink cool, clear, unsweetened fruit juices, such as apple or grape juice. Avoid carbonated beverages, which can burn a sensitive throat.

- Suck on ice cubes.

- Avoid bothersome odors such as cooking smells, smoke, or perfume.

- Prepare and freeze meals in advance.
- Rest in a chair after eating but avoid lying flat for at least two hours after a meal.
- Breathe deeply and slowly during bouts of nausea.
- Use relaxation techniques.
- Avoid eating for at least a few hours before treatment if nausea usually occurs during chemotherapy.

Appetite loss and weight loss Chemotherapy patients may lose their appetite and lose weight because of nausea and vomiting. Drugs used also can directly influence appetite by affecting the body's metabolism. In severe cases, loss of appetite can lead to CACHEXIA, a form of malnutrition. In general, appetite returns a few weeks after chemotherapy is completed. If loss of appetite is severe, doctors can prescribe medications that may improve the loss of interest in eating.

Bone marrow suppression Chemotherapy damages the blood cell–producing tissues of the BONE MARROW, triggering a condition called bone marrow suppression. Chemotherapy targets rapidly dividing cancerous cells and also affects normal rapidly dividing cells in the body, such as those produced in bone marrow tissue. Until the bone marrow recovers from the damage, the patient has abnormally low numbers of white blood cells, red blood cells, and platelets. For this reason, the patient's blood is monitored weekly during chemotherapy.

Blood cell counts do not drop as soon as chemotherapy is given, because the drugs do not target cells circulating in the blood. Instead, formation of new blood cells in the marrow is temporarily prevented.

Normally, blood cells are constantly replaced as they wear out: white blood cells last about six hours, platelets last about 10 days, and red blood cells last about four months. When chemotherapy is given, however, as these cells wear out they are not replaced, so blood counts begin to drop. The type of chemotherapy drug and the strength of the dosage influence the effect on blood cells.

In general, white blood cells and platelets drop to their lowest level within one or two weeks after chemotherapy. Because red blood cells last longer, their levels drop later. The side effects that result from low levels of various types of blood cells peak when the blood counts are lowest.

Low white blood cell count Because white blood cells fight infection, when a man's white cell count drops during chemotherapy, he becomes more vulnerable to infection. Neutrophils, the most common subtype of white blood cells, provide important defense against infection. The normal range of neutrophils is between 2,500 and 6,000 cells per cubic millimeter; a patient who has a neutrophil count of 1,000 or less is considered to be at risk for infection, and a count of less than 500 is considered to be severely low. Because the risk of infection is great, chemotherapy treatments are delayed if a person has a very low white blood count.

When counts are low during chemotherapy, an infection can begin in almost any part of the body, including the mouth, skin, lungs, urinary tract, rectum, and reproductive tract. Fever is an important first sign of infection; for this reason, patients are usually told to call their doctor or nurse when they have a fever of 100.5°F or above. Other signs of infection include sore throat, cough, shortness of breath, nasal congestion, shaking chills, burning during urination, and redness or swelling of the skin.

If patients contract an infection when their white blood cell level is very low, they may need antibiotics administered directly into the bloodstream. Sometimes, drugs called hematopoietic growth factors can help bone marrow make more white blood cells. Growth factors are sometimes administered after chemotherapy to stimulate the bone marrow to produce new white cells quickly, thereby reducing the risk of infection. There are several naturally occurring growth factors, which are also called colony-stimulating factors. Because scientists have recently discovered how to produce these in the lab, they are now available as drugs.

The two growth factors that boost production of white blood cells are granulocyte-macrophage colony-stimulating factor (Leukine) and granulocyte colony-stimulating factor (filgrastim, Neupogen).

Most infections a cancer patient may contract are due to the bacteria normally found on the skin and in the intestines and genital tract. In some cases, the cause of an infection may not be known. When the white blood cell count is lower than normal, patients can try to prevent infections by taking the following steps:

- Washing hands often during the day, especially before meals or use of the bathroom

- Cleaning the rectal area gently but thoroughly after each bowel movement

- Avoiding people who have communicable diseases (colds, flu, measles, or chickenpox)

- Avoiding crowds

- Avoiding people who have received recent immunizations, such as vaccines for polio, measles, mumps, and rubella (German measles)

- Preventing nicks when using scissors, needles, or knives, for example, by an electric shaver instead of a razor

- Using a soft toothbrush that does not cut the gums

- Taking a warm (not hot) bath, shower, or sponge bath every day

- Cleaning cuts and scrapes immediately with warm water, soap, and an antiseptic

Low red blood cell count   Lack of sufficient red blood cells is ANEMIA. Normally, blood has four to five million red blood cells per cubic millimeter. Another measurement of red blood cells is the hematocrit—the percentage of total blood volume occupied by red blood cells. A normal hematocrit range is between 36 percent and 42 percent.

Patients who have anemia feel tired, dizzy, and irritable and experience headaches, shortness of breath, and rapid breathing. Anemia that results from chemotherapy is a temporary condition, but sometimes blood transfusions are needed until the bone marrow can begin producing red blood cells again. Alternatively, doctors may prescribe ERYTHROPOEITIN (Procrit), a naturally occurring growth factor that boosts production of red blood cells in the bone marrow. Erythropoeitin is usually given three times a week until the hematocrit rises to normal level.

Low platelet count   Anticancer drugs also can affect the bone marrow's ability to make platelets, the blood cells that help stop bleeding by making blood clot. Low platelet count (called thrombocytopenia) may cause a patient to bruise easily, bleed longer than usual after a minor cut, have bleeding gums or nose bleeds, and experience severe internal bleeding. Low platelet counts are temporary, but they can cause serious blood loss if an injury occurs. If counts are very low, a platelet transfusion can be given. Transfused platelets do not last long, but a platelet growth factor can be given as a drug for patients who have severe thrombocytopenia.

Patients should report to their doctor any symptoms of unexpected bruising, small red spots under the skin, reddish or pinkish urine, black or bloody bowel movements, or bleeding from gums or nose. If the platelet count becomes very low, patients may need a platelet transfusion. Regular blood tests are also used to count the number of platelets in the blood.

Diarrhea or constipation   Up to 75 percent of people who receive chemotherapy may experience DIARRHEA as a result of damage to rapidly dividing cells in the lining of the digestive system. The amount and duration of diarrhea depend in part on the type, dosage and duration of drugs. Some of the chemotherapy drugs that cause diarrhea are 5-fluorouracil, methotrexate, docetaxel, and actinomycin D.

Although many patients consider diarrhea merely an annoyance, in fact in severe cases it can be life-threatening if accompanied by dehydration, malnutrition, or electrolyte imbalance. In severe cases, the doctor may prescribe an antidiarrheal medicine. Patients with diarrhea should do the following:

- Eat smaller amounts of food, but eat more often.

- Avoid high-fiber foods, such as whole grain breads and cereals, raw vegetables, beans, nuts, seeds, popcorn, and fresh and dried fruit.

- Eat low-fiber foods, such as white bread, white rice or noodles, creamed cereals, ripe bananas, canned or cooked fruit without skins, cottage cheese, yogurt, eggs, mashed or baked potatoes without skin, pureed vegetables, chicken or turkey without skin, and fish.

- Avoid coffee, tea, alcohol, sweets, and fried, greasy, highly spiced foods.
- Avoid milk and milk products.
- Eat more potassium-rich foods (bananas, oranges, potatoes, and peach and apricot nectars).
- Drink plenty of fluids to replace those lost through diarrhea. Mild clear liquids such as apple juice, water, weak tea, or clear broth are best.

Some chemotherapy drugs can cause constipation. Some patients become constipated because of the drugs they are taking (especially narcotic pain medications); others become constipated because they are less active or less well nourished than usual. Dehydration, decreased fluid intake, depression, and specific chemotherapy drugs (such as vinblastine and vincristine) all can cause constipation. Patients can drink warm or hot fluids to help loosen the bowels, eat high-fiber foods (such as whole wheat bread or fresh fruit), and exercise. Exercise—even just walking around the block—can help, as can a more structured exercise program.

Sore mouth Good oral care is important during cancer treatment, because chemotherapy drugs can cause STOMATITIS and ESOPHAGITIS—sores in the mouth and throat. In addition to being painful and affecting the appetite, these sores can become infected by the germs in the mouth. Because infections can be hard to fight during chemotherapy and can lead to serious problems, it is important to take every possible step to prevent them.

Sores in the throat and mouth usually occur about five to 10 days after treatment and clear up within three to four weeks. Patients who have not been eating well since beginning chemotherapy are more likely to have mouth sores. Mouth sores usually begin with a pale, dry lining of the mouth, followed by inflamed gums, mouth, and throat. The tongue may begin to swell, and swallowing and eating may become painful and difficult.

If possible, patients should see a dentist before starting chemotherapy to have teeth cleaned and to take care of any existing dental problems, such as cavities, abscesses, gum disease, or poorly fitting dentures. Because chemotherapy can make a patient more likely to have cavities, a dentist may suggest using a fluoride rinse or gel each day to help prevent decay. Cleaning the teeth regularly and gently with a soft toothbrush helps to keep the mouth clean. If the mouth is very sore, gels, creams, or pastes can be painted over the ulcers to reduce soreness.

Chemotherapy also can alter a person's sense of taste; food may seem more salty, bitter, or metallic. This change can affect appetite and nutrition. Some common taste changes are a metallic or medicinal taste and sudden dislike of tomato products, beef and pork, sweet foods, or bitter tastes. Typically, normal taste returns after chemotherapy treatment ends.

Hair loss Hair loss is one of the most common and worrisome side effects of chemotherapy. Although a few drugs used to treat cancer do not cause hair loss (or cause an amount of hair loss that is slight), most do cause partial or complete hair loss for a time. Chemotherapy affects the rapidly dividing cells of the hair follicles, making hair brittle so that it may break off near the scalp or spontaneously release. This usually occurs two to three weeks after the first chemotherapy treatment.

The amount of hair lost depends on the type of drug or combination of drugs used, the dosage given, and the person's individual reaction to the drug. If hair loss happens it usually starts within a few weeks of beginning treatment, although rarely it can start within a few days. Body hair may be lost as well, and some drugs even trigger loss of the eyelashes and eyebrows. If patients do lose hair as a result of chemotherapy, it almost always regrows once treatment is over.

Patients who lose their hair during chemotherapy need to take special care of their scalp and any remaining hair. Patients should use mild shampoos, soft hair brushes, and low heat when drying hair.

Once hair loss occurs, patients should use a sunscreen, sunblock, or hat to protect the scalp from the sun. Although hair loss is not life threatening, as are some other side effects of chemotherapy, it can have an emotional and psychological impact on a person's life. Hair loss can cause depression, loss of self-esteem, and even grief reactions.

Skin and nail changes Some drugs can affect the skin, making it drier or slightly discolored. These changes may be worsened by swimming, especially in chlorinated water. The drugs may also make skin more sensitive to sunlight during and after treatment. Nails may grow more slowly, and white lines may appear on them. Nails also may become more brittle and flaky.

Nerves Some chemotherapy drugs can affect the nerves in the hands and feet, causing tingling, numbness, or a sensation of pins and needles known as peripheral neuropathy. This sensation gradually fades after chemotherapy ends, but when severe can damage nerves permanently.

Nervous system Some drugs can directly affect the central nervous system (the brain and spinal cord), causing feelings of anxiety and restlessness, dizziness, sleeplessness, headaches, or concentration and memory problems. Other drugs can lead to a loss of the ability to hear high-pitched sound or cause a continuous noise in the ears known as tinnitus.

Chemotherapy also can affect the cranial nerves, which influence movement and sensation of the head, face, and neck and vision, or the peripheral nerves (those important in touch and movement).

Vaccinations Travelers should keep in mind that patients undergoing chemotherapy should not have any live virus vaccines, including polio; measles; rubella (German measles); measles, mumps, and rubella (MMR); bacille Calmette-Guérin (BCG); (tuberculosis); yellow fever; and typhoid vaccines. Other vaccines, such as diphtheria, tetanus, flu, hepatitis B, hepatitis A, rabies, cholera, and typhoid, should not cause problems.

Radiation recall Some people who have had radiation therapy have a skin problem during chemotherapy known as radiation recall during or shortly after certain anticancer drugs are given. The skin over an area that has received radiation turns red and may blister and peel. This reaction may last hours or even days.

Kidney and bladder problems Some anticancer drugs can irritate the bladder or cause temporary or permanent damage to the bladder or kidneys, because breakdown products from these drugs are excreted through the kidneys. Some anticancer drugs turn the urine orange, red, green, or yellow or give it a strong or medicinelike odor for 24 to 72 hours, although these color changes are harmless. Symptoms of kidney damage include

headache, lower back pain, weakness, nausea and vomiting, fatigue, high blood pressure, change in urination pattern, urgent need to urinate, or swelling. Patients who have had kidney problems in the past are at higher risk for development of problems during chemotherapy, especially if the drugs include high-dose methotrexate, ifosfamide, or streptozocin. Patients should always drink plenty of fluids to ensure good urine flow and help prevent problems.

Flu symptoms Symptoms of flu may bother some patients a few hours to a few days after chemotherapy, especially if they are receiving chemotherapy together with biological therapy. Aching muscles and joints, headache, fatigue, nausea, slight fever (less than 100°F), chills, and poor appetite may last one to three days. An infection or the cancer itself can also cause these symptoms.

Liver damage Chemotherapy drugs are broken down by the liver, which occasionally can become damaged during treatment. However, this problem is temporary and usually improves once treatment is stopped. Symptoms of liver damage include jaundice (yellowed skin and eyes), fatigue, and pain in the lower right ribs or right upper abdomen.

Older patients and those who have had hepatitis are more likely to experience liver problems after chemotherapy, especially if they are taking drugs such as methotrexate, cytarabine (Ara-C), high-dose cisplatin or cyclophosphamide (Cytoxan), vincristine, vinblastine, or doxorubicin (Adriamycin).

Heart problems About 10 percent of patients experience heart damage caused by certain chemotherapy drugs, especially daunorubicin and doxorubicin (Adriamycin). Symptoms of heart damage may include dry cough, ankle swelling, shortness of breath, puffiness, or erratic heartbeat. Patients at higher risk for heart damage include those who have had previous heart problems, high blood pressure, or prior radiation to the chest and those who smoke.

Because of the small risk of heart damage, assessments are done before and during chemotherapy to check for problems.

Fluid retention During chemotherapy the body may retain fluid as a result of hormonal changes caused by therapy, the drugs themselves, or the cancer. Patients may need to avoid table salt and foods that contain a high level of salt. If the problem is severe, a doctor may prescribe a diuretic to help the body get rid of excess fluids.

Infertility   Chemotherapy treatments may cause temporary or permanent infertility because the drugs can destroy both healthy and unhealthy cells, damaging the reproductive system. Risks vary with individual treatment regimens; alkylating and platinum-based agents carry the greatest risk to the reproductive system. Data on the prevalence and duration of infertility are not yet available for most types of chemotherapy.

Long-term problems   Although most side effects of chemotherapy end when treatment does, some patients experience long-term problems related to treatment for cancer. These long-term effects depend on the type of drugs used and whether other treatments (such as radiation) are given.

Some drugs can permanently damage internal organs, such as the heart or reproductive system. Changes in the nervous system can appear months or years after chemotherapy, and may involve fatigue, sleepiness, memory problems, personality changes, shortened attention span, reduced intellect, or seizures. Long-term effects of nerve damage may include numbness, tingling, or prickling sensations.

Finally, it is also possible that some types of chemotherapy can lead to the development of a second type of cancer, including Hodgkin's disease and non-Hodgkin's lymphoma, leukemia, and a few types of solid tumors.

Cost

The cost of chemotherapy varies with the types and dosages of drugs used, the duration and frequency of treatment, and the location of treatment, at home, in an office, or in a hospital. Most health insurance policies cover at least part of the cost of many kinds of chemotherapy. There are also organizations that help with the cost of chemotherapy and with transportation costs. Nurses and social workers have information about these organizations. In some states, Medicaid (which makes health care services available to

people who have financial need) may help pay for certain treatments.

Chemotherapy Foundation   A public foundation established in 1968, dedicated to the control, cure, and prevention of cancer through innovative medical therapies including CHEMOTHERAPY, chemoimmunotherapy, chemohormonal therapy, chemoprevention, and biotechnologies. The foundation is also dedicated to the education of physicians, patients, and the public through publications. The foundation currently sponsors selected basic and clinical research initiatives at six major New York City metropolitan medical centers. For contact information, see Appendix I.

childhood cancers   Cancers of the reproductive system may occasionally occur in young boys, who rarely may be diagnosed with GERM CELL TUMORS or TESTICULAR CANCER. Over the last half of the 20th century, progress in childhood cancer diagnosis and treatment transformed a once uniformly fatal disease into a group of malignancies that are now curable in most children.

childhood malignant testicular germ cell tumor   A type of TESTICULAR CANCER that occurs in childhood, usually in boys younger than four years of age. Surgery is the most common treatment for testicular GERM CELL *TUMORS*; the tumor and one or both testicles are removed through an incision in the groin. This is called a radical inguinal orchiectomy. Treatment for boys younger than five years of age is radical inguinal orchiectomy with or without chemotherapy.

choriocarcinoma   A rare, highly malignant GERM CELL cancer that is a type of NONSEMINOMA that arises within the testicles. Unlike in other testicular tumors, the most common symptoms, are related to metastasis rather than a testicular mass, and may include abdominal or back pain, or lung symptoms such as coughing up of blood.

When seen as a small component of mixed GERM CELL TUMORS, it has little effect on prognosis. In its pure form, however (seen in less than 1 percent of all germ cell tumors) it requires intensive chemotherapy. "Pure" choriocarcinoma does not usually occur in the testicles.

This very rare and aggressive type of TESTICULAR CANCER contains two types of cells—cytotrophoblasts and syncytiotrophoblasts. Such cancers are likely to spread rapidly to distant organs of the body such as the lungs or central nervous system.

chylous ascites An accumulation of lymphatic fluid in the spaces between tissues and organs in the cavity of the abdomen. This is an uncommon side effect of RETROPERITONEAL LYMPH NODE DISSECTION surgery. The development of these ascites cannot be predicted, and the usual treatment is to drain the fluid, restrict intake of fats in the diet, and wait for the fluid to recede.

Cialis See TADALAFIL.

cigarettes and penile cancer Smoking exposes the body to many cancer-causing chemicals that affect many organs in addition to the lungs. These harmful substances are absorbed into blood and carried in the bloodstream throughout the body. Researchers believe that these substances can damage the DNA of cells in the penis and contribute to the development of PENILE CANCER, especially in men who also have HUMAN PAPILLOMAVIRUS (HPV) infections.

circumcision The surgical removal of part or all of the foreskin of the penis, usually shortly after birth. Circumcision is often performed on newborn boys because of purported health benefits and protection against the development of cancer. However, according to the AMERICAN CANCER SOCIETY, circumcision does not help prevent cancer of the penis. Studies note that the PENILE CANCER risk is low in some uncircumcised populations, and the practice of circumcision is strongly associated with socioethnic factors that in turn are associated with lessened risk.

Many experts believe that it is important that the issue of circumcision not distract the public's attention from avoiding known penile cancer risk factors, such as smoking cigarettes and having unprotected sex with multiple partners (increasing the likelihood of HUMAN PAPILLOMAVIRUS infection).

Circumcision is required by the religions of about one-sixth of the people of the world.

In any case, boys who are not circumcised should be taught at an early age the importance of cleaning beneath the foreskin as part of their personal hygiene. Good personal hygiene and safer sexual practices, such as abstinence, limiting of the number of sexual partners, and use of condoms to prevent genital herpes infection, may decrease the risk of development of penile cancer.

See also HERPES, GENITAL.

cisplatin (Platinol) A type of CHEMOTHERAPY used in the treatment of TESTICULAR CANCER in several different regimen combinations. Cisplatin is used together with:

- VP-16 and BLEOMYCIN every three weeks
- Bleomycin and VINBLASTINE every three weeks for four courses
- Bleomycin, VP-16, IFOSFAMIDE, every three weeks

clear margins An area of tissue surrounding a tumor that is free of cancer cells. During cancer surgery, the surgeon tries to remove the tumor and a wide margin of healthy tissue. If no cancer cells are found near the edges of the sample, it is said to have clear margins. After surgery, if the excised tissue is found by the lab to have cancer cells near the margin of healthy tissue, the surgeon may operate again to remove a wider margin of healthy tissue around the original tumor. If additional surgery is not feasible, other treatment (such as radiation or chemotherapy) may be suggested.

clinical cancer centers Cancer centers sponsored by the NATIONAL CANCER INSTITUTE that conduct programs in clinical research and may also have programs in other research areas such as basic research or prevention, control, and population-based research. The centers focus on both laboratory research and clinical research within the same institutional framework, a distinguishing characteristic of many clinical cancer centers. For contact information for individual clinical cancer centers, see Appendix II.

clinical trial   A kind of research study that compares a specific treatment currently recognized as the best available (called the standard of care) with a new treatment that the study's researchers believe is safer or more effective. If clinical trials prove a new treatment to be more effective than current therapies, it may become the new standard of care.

Some patients agree to participate in clinical trials as a way to obtain high-quality cancer care with constant monitoring. If patients are in a study and do not receive the new treatment being tested, they still receive the best standard treatment, which may be as good as or better than the new approach. If a new treatment approach is proved effective, patients who are having this treatment in the clinical trial may be among the first to benefit. Some patients also like the idea that they are helping to further research that may benefit future patients.

On the other hand, there is no way to be sure whether the new treatment will work. New treatments being studied are not always better than (or even as good as) standard care, and they may have side effects that doctors do not expect or that are worse than those of standard treatment. Moreover, not everyone benefits from a new treatment. Even standard treatments, proven effective for many people, do not help everyone. In addition, patients in the control group receive only standard therapy. If patients receive standard treatment instead of the new treatment being tested, it may not be as effective as the new approach.

However, placebos (sugar pills) are not always used in cancer treatment studies. No one is ever given a placebo when an effective treatment is available to treat the cancer. In very rare cases, a placebo may be used when testing a new drug if there is no known effective treatment, but if a study does use a placebo, patients are always informed before taking part.

Phase I

Clinical trials move through phases, from Phase I to Phase III, before the final outcome leads to a potential new treatment.

Phase I trials are small studies that are the first step in testing new treatments in patients and are designed to determine the method and dosages of treatment. Because less is known about the possible risks and benefits in Phase I trials, these studies usually include only a small number of patients who would not be helped by other known treatments.

Phase II

In Phase II, researchers examine possible side effects and the effectiveness of the treatment (for example, how much a tumor shrinks). Although they are larger than Phase I trials, still only a small number of patients enter Phase II trials because the usefulness and the side effects of the new treatments are still unknown.

Phase III

Phase III trials compare the results of people taking the new treatment with results of people taking standard treatment to see which group has a better survival rate and fewer side effects. Patients are randomly divided into two treatment groups, one receiving the new treatment and the other receiving the current standard of care treatment. Sometimes patients do not know which group they are in.

Usually studies move into Phase III testing only after a treatment has shown promise in Phases I and II. Phase III trials may include many hundreds of people around the country.

Safety

Cancer clinical trials are tightly regulated and closely monitored by the U.S. federal government to make sure each phase of the study is as safe as possible. All clinical trials must follow a detailed plan (the protocol) written by the researchers and approved by the institutional review board at each institution. This board, which includes consumers, clergy, and health professionals, reviews the protocol to try to be sure that the research will not expose patients to extreme or unethical risks.

In addition, each patient must be informed of all the facts about a study before deciding whether to take part, including details about treatments, tests, possible benefits, and risks. Each patient must sign an informed consent form that highlights key facts.

The informed consent process continues throughout the study. (For instance, if new risks of the treatment are discovered during a trial, the patients are told of any new findings and must sign a new consent form to continue in the study.) Signing a consent form does not require patients to continue to participate in the study; patients can withdraw at any time.

Costs

Clinical studies at many hospitals and cancer centers require patients to pay for at least some of their medical care, and coverage varies, depending on private insurance policies and state legislation. However, at the NATIONAL CANCER INSTITUTE (NCI) Bethesda campus, all study-related medical services are provided at no charge to study participants. Patients are responsible only for travel costs related to the initial screening visit. Once they are enrolled, NCI arranges and pays for travel to the center, if necessary. However, patients may incur lodging costs if the study does not require hospital admission. A social worker with the study team reviews existing lodging options and provides a small stipend if the study is conducted on an outpatient basis.

Finding a Clinical Trial

Anyone who meets the medical eligibility requirements can participate in a clinical trial, but U.S. citizens and permanent residents are given first priority. Comprehensive information on clinical studies taking place on the National Cancer Institute campus in Bethesda is provided by the Clinical Studies Support Center (CSSC). The CSSC aims to provide the latest information on cancer-related clinical studies at NCI through a toll-free telephone service at (888) NCI-1937 and through its community outreach program.

CSSC staff can tell callers about studies for a particular type of cancer, who can join, methods of treatment being studied, and how to take the next step if the caller is interested in participating in a study.

CSSC serves hundreds of callers each month, including those who have just been diagnosed with cancer, those who have already received treatment, and those whose cancer has recurred. People who have a family member or friend who has cancer and want to help or become familiar with clinical studies as a treatment option also may contact CSSC.

On the basis of the medical history the caller provides, the CSSC staff sends summaries of clinical studies that appear to be a possible option for the caller. Each study summary includes study objectives, eligibility, and the name and phone number of the physician leading the study.

After receiving this information, the caller should consult his or her personal physician to review the information from CSSC. The physician should contact the study's principal investigator to discuss the patient's medical history and current health status. If the patient meets eligibility requirements, a National Cancer Institute screening visit is scheduled.

There is no charge for medical services provided at the National Institutes of Health (NIH) Clinical Center. Before the screening visit, the patient receives a packet of information containing maps, travel and hotel information, instructions on paperwork to supply (usually including medical and treatment summaries, pathology reports and slides, and radiology reports). The screening visit is very similar to a consultation with a medical specialist. During the visit, a patient may be asked to take several diagnostic tests such as routine blood tests, chest X-ray, and an electrocardiogram (ECG). The patient also has the opportunity to meet and speak with the physicians and the nurses and social workers who make up the research team, learn about the risks and benefits of the study, and ask questions. The screening visit is designed to determine whether a patient is a candidate for a particular study; no one expects the patient to make a decision to participate at that time.

When deciding to enroll in a clinical trial, a patient should consider possible risks and benefits, potential effect of the study to his everyday life, and the potential of the study to contribute to the overall improvement of cancer treatment for future generations. Inpatient studies require patients to stay at the NIH Clinical Center for a few days or longer; outpatient studies allow patients to receive treatment and go home the same day.

Patients who decide to participate are asked to sign an informed consent form, a document that describes the treatment schedule and possible benefits and side effects. Signing an informed consent document does not constitute signing away any personal rights or protections. It simply indicates that the person has read and understood the basic purpose and elements of a study and is voluntarily participating. The patient may withdraw from the study at any time. Someone who chooses to leave the study has the opportunity to discuss other treatment options or concerns with the study team.

A complete list of clinical trials relating to men's reproductive cancer is available in Appendix IV and on the Web site of the NATIONAL CANCER INSTITUTE: http://www.cancer.gov/clinical_trials/finding/

Coalition of National Cancer Cooperative Groups The nation's premier network of cancer clinical trials specialists. Members include CANCER CENTERS, academic medical centers, community hospitals, physician practices, and patient advocate groups who represent the interests of more than 17,000 cancer investigators, hundreds of patient advocates, and thousands of patients around the world.

The coalition was created to address serious issues facing the cooperative groups, such as improvement of the clinical trial experience for patients and doctors, regulatory requirements, competition for federal funding, and work under the managed care system. The coalition offers a variety of programs and information for doctors, payers, patient advocate groups, and patients, designed to improve the entire clinical trial process. For contact information, see Appendix I.

coenzyme Q10 (ubiquinone, ubidecarenone) A compound produced naturally in the body that helps cells produce energy needed for cell growth and maintenance. Coenzyme Q10 is found in most body tissues, especially in the heart, liver, kidneys, and pancreas. Low blood levels of coenzyme Q10 have been found in patients who have PROSTATE CANCER (and in those who have other types of cancer as well). Coenzyme Q10 is also an antioxidant (a substance that protects cells from harmful chemicals called FREE RADICALS).

Studies of cancer patients have shown that coenzyme Q10 decreases the harmful effects of the CHEMOTHERAPY drug doxorubicin on the heart. However, no report of a randomized clinical trial of coenzyme Q10 as a treatment for cancer itself has been published in a peer-reviewed scientific journal.

Coenzyme Q10 was first identified in 1957, but scientists did not consider its use as a potential cancer drug until 1961, when a deficiency of the enzyme was noted in the blood of cancer patients. Some studies have suggested that coenzyme Q10 stimulates the immune system and increases resistance to disease. In part because of this, researchers have theorized that coenzyme Q10 may be useful as an ADJUVANT TREATMENT for cancer. Animal studies have found that coenzyme Q10 stimulated the immune system and increased resistance to disease; it also helped protect the heart of animals given doxorubicin, which can damage heart muscle.

No serious side effects of the use of coenzyme Q10 have been reported. Some patients using coenzyme Q10 have experienced mild insomnia, higher levels of liver enzymes, rashes, nausea, and upper abdominal pain. Other reported side effects have included dizziness, sensitivity to light, irritability, headache, heartburn, and fatigue.

Patients should discuss with their health-care provider possible interactions between coenzyme Q10 and prescription drugs they may be taking. Certain drugs, such as those that are used to lower cholesterol or blood sugar levels, may also reduce the effects of coenzyme Q10. Coenzyme Q10 may also alter the body's response to warfarin (a drug that prevents blood clotting) and insulin.

Coenzyme Q10 is used by the body as an antioxidant, to protect cells from free radicals, the highly reactive chemicals that can damage cells. Some conventional cancer therapies, such as chemotherapy and RADIATION THERAPY, are designed to kill cancer cells in part by triggering formation of free radicals. Researchers are studying whether combining coenzyme Q10 with conventional therapies is effective or harmful in fighting cancer.

Several companies distribute coenzyme Q10 as a dietary supplement, which is regulated as a food, not a drug. This means that evaluation and approval by the U.S. Food and Drug Administration (FDA) are not required before marketing, unless specific health claims are made about the supplement. Because dietary supplements are not formally reviewed for manufacturing consistency, there may be variations in the composition of the supplement from one batch to another.

colony-stimulating factor (hematopoietic growth factor)

Substance that usually does not directly kill tumor cells but encourages BONE MARROW STEM CELLS to divide and develop into white blood cells, platelets, and red blood cells. Doctors use colony-stimulating factors (CSFs) to help patients undergoing cancer treatment boost their blood count.

Because CHEMOTHERAPY drugs can damage the body's ability to make white blood cells, red blood cells, and platelets, patients who receive these drugs have a higher risk of development of infections, become anemic, and bleed more readily than normally. By using CSFs to stimulate blood cell production, doctors can increase the dosage of anticancer drugs without increasing the risk of infection or the need for transfusion with blood products. As a result, researchers have found CSFs particularly useful when combined with high-dose chemotherapy.

The following are examples of CSFs and their use in cancer therapy:

- Granulocyte colony-stimulating factor (G-CSF) (filgrastim) and granulocyte-macrophage colony-stimulating factor (GM-CSF) (sargramostim) increase the number of white blood cells, reducing the risk of infection in patients who receive chemotherapy. They can also stimulate the production of stem cells in preparation for stem cell or BONE MARROW TRANSPLANTS.

- ERYTHROPOIETIN increases the number of red blood cells and reduces the need for red blood cell transfusions in patients who receive chemotherapy.

- Oprelvekin reduces the need for platelet transfusions in patients who have chemotherapy.

combined modality therapy

Use of two or more types of treatments as supplements. For instance, surgery, radiation therapy, CHEMOTHER-APY, hormonal therapy, or immunotherapy may be used alternatively or together for maximal effectiveness.

Compazine (prochlorperazine)

A relatively inexpensive drug that is administered either intravenously or orally to help control the delayed episodes of NAUSEA and vomiting that occur more than 48 hours after CHEMOTHERAPY. This drug belongs to a general class of drugs called phenothiazines, which work by blocking messages to the part of the brain that controls nausea and vomiting.

Prochlorperazine can cause sleepiness, dry mouth, constipation, blurred vision, restlessness, weight gain, or increased heart rate. Rarely, it may cause jaundice, sensitivity to light, rash, or hives.

See also ANTINAUSEA MEDICATION.

complementary and alternative medicine (CAM)

A broad group of healing philosophies, approaches, and products (also referred to as integrative medicine) that are not presently considered to be part of conventional medicine.

Complementary treatment is generally considered to be therapy used in addition to conventional treatments; *alternative* treatment usually is used instead of conventional treatment. *Conventional* treatments are those that are widely accepted and practiced by the mainstream medical community.

Although there is scientific evidence for the effectiveness and safety of some CAM therapies, in general many of these therapies have not been scientifically tested. As CAM therapies are proved safe and effective through rigorous studies, they are adopted into conventional health care. Though grouped together, complementary and alternative medicines are different. Complementary medicine is used together with conventional medicine; an example of complementary therapy is the use of aromatherapy to help lessen a patient's discomfort after surgery. Alternative medicine is used in place of conventional medicine, for example, use of a special diet to treat cancer instead of surgery, radiation therapy or chemotherapy recommended by a conventional health care practitioner.

The National Center for Complementary and Alternative Medicine (NCCAM) has classified CAM therapies into five groups:

- Alternative medical systems (for example, homeopathic medicine and traditional Chinese medicine)
- Mind–body interventions, such as visualization or relaxation
- Manipulative and body-based methods such as chiropractic and massage
- Biologically based therapies such as vitamins and herbal products
- Energy therapies such as *qi gong* and therapeutic touch

Research indicates that the use of CAM therapies is increasing. A large-scale study published November 11, 1998, in the *Journal of the American Medical Association* found that CAM use by the general public increased from 34 percent in 1990 to 42 percent in 1997. Several surveys of CAM use by cancer patients have been conducted with small numbers of patients. One study published in the February 2000 in the journal *Cancer* reported that 37 percent of 46 prostate cancer patients used one or more CAM therapies as part of their cancer treatment. These therapies included herbal remedies, old-time remedies, vitamins, and special diets. A larger study of CAM use by patients who had different types of cancer published in July 2000 in the *Journal of Clinical Oncology* found that 83 percent of 453 cancer patients had used at least one CAM therapy as part of their cancer treatment. The study included CAM therapies such as special diets, psychotherapy, spiritual practices, and vitamin supplements. When psychotherapy and spiritual practices were excluded, 69 percent of patients had used at least one CAM therapy in their cancer treatment.

Cancer patients who are considering complementary or alternative therapy should discuss this decision with their doctor, because some complementary and alternative therapies may interfere with standard treatment or may be harmful when used with conventional treatment. It is also a good idea to become informed about the therapy, including whether results of scientific studies support the claims that are made for it. Unlike conventional treatments for cancer, complementary and alternative therapies are often not covered by insurance companies.

comprehensive cancer centers   Cancer institutions sponsored by the NATIONAL CANCER INSTITUTE (NCI) that conducts programs in all three areas of research—basic research, clinical research, and prevention and control research—as well as programs in community outreach and education.

In 1990 there were 19 comprehensive cancer centers across the country; today more than 40 cancer centers meet the NCI criteria for comprehensive status.

Each type of CANCER CENTER has specific characteristics and capabilities for organizing new programs of research. To be recognized by the NCI as a comprehensive cancer center, an institution must pass rigorous peer review and must perform research in three major areas: basic research; clinical research; and cancer prevention, control, and population-based research. It must also have a strong body of interactive research that bridges these research areas.

In addition, a comprehensive cancer center must provide outreach, education, and information directed to and accessible to both health-care professionals and the lay community.

All NCI-designated cancer centers are reevaluated each time their grant is to be renewed (generally every three to five years). For contact information on individual comprehensive cancer centers, see Appendix II.

conformal external beam radiation therapy   A new way of delivering RADIATION THERAPY to the prostate gland to treat PROSTATE CANCER, using computed tomography (CT) scanning to achieve an improved focus of maximal radiation on the glans and less on surrounding tissue. This method may decrease side effects and produce better results than traditional radiation therapy.

coping behavior   The ability to handle life circumstances may affect the progression of cancer, and although the stress of the diagnosis may worsen disease, some studies suggest that good coping style may aid treatment and outcome.

Interventions focused on improving the ability to cope with a cancer diagnosis, treatment, and recovery may have beneficial effects on emotional adjustment, and perhaps on physiological processes, since mental state and coping style work together to affect biological factors such as immune function and hormone levels, both of which play roles in cancer progression.

Whereas stress, distress, depression, anxiety, and posttraumatic stress disorder have all been linked to reduced immune function and altered hormone balance, healthy coping has been shown to improve these factors and potentially to affect cancer outcomes.

Researchers define *coping* as the conscious, volitional effort to regulate cognitive, behavioral, emotional, and physiological responses to stress and stressful aspects of the environment. A person who *actively copes* takes a direct and rational approach to dealing with a problem. *Passive coping* involves indirect approaches such as avoidance, withdrawal, and wishful thinking. Studies have shown that people who adopt active coping strategies have better immune function and lower cortisol levels; people who use passive coping strategies have the opposite results.

Some researchers believe there is clear evidence that interventions can have positive effects on emotional adjustment, functional adjustment, and treatment of disease-related symptoms (such as pain or nausea). A more limited body of research suggests that such interventions have a measurable effect on immune function and cortisol levels. Likewise, there is some preliminary evidence that psychotherapeutic approaches can reduce recurrence rate and improve survival time. Survival benefits of psychological treatment have not been clearly demonstrated, however, suggesting the need for further research.

Some researchers believe that both active coping and effective psychological treatment can also aid cancer treatment by ensuring that patients more closely follow their cancer treatment regimens.

core biopsy Removal (by a large needle) of a piece of tissue to be sent to a lab for microscopic analysis.

See also BIOPSY.

Corporate Angel Network The only charitable organization in the United States whose sole mission is to ease the emotional stress, physical discomfort, and financial burden of travel for cancer patients by arranging free flights to treatment centers, using the empty seats on corporate aircraft flying on routine business.

Based in White Plains, New York, in an office donated by the Westchester County Airport, 50 part-time volunteers and five paid staff work with patients, physicians, corporations, flight departments, and leading treatment facilities to arrange 1,200 flights a year. Participation in the program is open to all cancer patients, bone marrow donors, and bone marrow recipients who can walk and who do not need medical support while traveling.

Eligibility is not based on financial need, and patients may travel as often as necessary. Because of the cooperation of 500 of America's top corporations, including more than half of the top 100 in the Fortune 500, Corporate Angel Network has coordinated more than 14,000 flights since its founding in 1981. For contact information, see Appendix I.

cryotherapy A minimally invasive and relatively new procedure used to treat localized PROSTATE CANCER that uses very low temperatures to "freeze" cancer cells. The procedure is also known as cryosurgery or cryoablation.

In this technique, the surgeon (with the help of a transrectal ultrasound) places five to eight probes through the patient's skin into the prostate gland. Once the probes are positioned correctly, the physician administers liquid nitrogen through the probes to freeze the prostate. The liquid nitrogen forms a ball of ice in the prostate; once it melts, it ruptures the cancer cells, killing them. Typically, physicians administer two freezing-and-melting cycles during one procedure to be sure all the cancer is eliminated.

The doctor normally inserts a warming catheter into the urethra (which travels through the prostate gland) to prevent the urethra from freezing.

Usually after this procedure, the cancer is eliminated and the PROSTATE-SPECIFIC ANTIGEN (PSA) level returns to normal. The procedure does not involve incisions; therefore, recovery is quick.

On the other hand, if the procedure is not performed carefully by a very experienced physician, healthy tissue surrounding the prostate may be damaged, producing unwanted side effects. Moreover, if the nerve bundles that control erection are frozen during this procedure, impotence may result. Although some doctors can freeze the prostate and spare the nerve bundles in a process known as nerve-sparing cryosurgery, that more difficult procedure is not always successful.

Although the method has been used by some physicians since the 1970s, it was not widely used until 20 years later, as new types of probes and more advanced ultrasound technology were developed. However, many doctors remain unconvinced of the benefits of this type of treatment, and very few physicians perform this technique.

Cryosurgery may be a good choice for someone who does not want radiation or surgery but wants some form of therapy for cancer. This method is also sometimes used as a follow-up treatment for a patient who has not responded to the initial treatment. It is more accepted as a form of salvage therapy used after men have failed initial radiation therapy. When used after radiation, the technique can produce uncomfortable side effects such as burning, incontinence, and rectal injury, but these risks are lower than those with surgery after previous prostate radiation.

Cryosurgery is covered by most insurance companies and by Medicare.

cryptorchidism The medical term for undescended testicles, from the Greek words *kryptos*, meaning "hidden," and *orchis*, meaning "testicle." In a fetus, the testicles normally develop inside the abdomen and move through the groin and into the scrotum before birth. However, in about 3 percent of boys the testicles do not make this descent. Sometimes the testicle remains in the abdomen, and sometimes the testicle starts to move into place but instead becomes trapped in the groin area.

Men who have had a testicle that did not move down into the scrotum are at greater risk for development of TESTICULAR CANCER, even if surgery was performed to move the testicle in the scrotum. In fact, cryptorchidism is the only clearly established risk factor for testicular cancer.

About 14 percent of cases of testicle cancer occur in men who have a history of cryptorchidism. The risk of testicle cancer is somewhat higher for a testicle that was positioned in the abdomen, as opposed to one that descended at least partway. Of men who have a history of cryptorchidism, most cancers develop in the testicle that did not descend, but up to 25 percent of cases occur in the normally descended testicle. On the basis of these facts, some doctors conclude that cryptorchidism is not the direct cause of testicular cancer, and that some other disorder is responsible for increasing the testicular cancer risk and preventing normal positioning of one or both testicles. Most undescended testicles eventually move into the proper position during the child's first year of life.

If they do not, a surgical procedure known as ORCHIDOPEXY may be necessary to move the testicle down into the scrotum. Some experts believe that performing orchidopexy before puberty may reduce the risk of development of certain types of GERM CELL TUMORS, although this is not widely accepted. The greatest benefit from orchidopexy is that the testicle is put into the scrotum where it can be readily examined for development of a testicular tumor.

cyclophosphamide See CYTOXAN.

cystoscopy The examination of the bladder and urethra by using a thin lighted instrument (cystoscope) inserted into the urethra. Tissue samples can be removed and examined under a microscope to diagnose cancer, such as urethral, bladder, or PROSTATE CANCER.

cytokines A class of substances that are produced by cells of the immune system and can affect the immune response. Cytokines can also be produced in the laboratory by recombinant DNA technology and given to people to affect immune responses.

cytotoxic Characteristic of causing the death of cells, including cancer cells. The term usually refers to drugs used in CHEMOTHERAPY treatments.

cytotoxic T cells White blood cells that can directly destroy specific cells. T cells can be separated from other blood cells, grown in the laboratory, and then administered to a patient to destroy tumor cells. Certain CYTOKINES can also be used to help form cytotoxic T cells in a patient's body.

Cytoxan (cyclophosphamide) An alkylating agent used to treat several types of cancer (including PROSTATE CANCER) that works by disrupting the growth of cancer cells.

Side effects include NAUSEA and vomiting, HAIR LOSS, APPETITE LOSS, mouth or lip sores, DIARRHEA, decreased sperm production, and decreased white blood cell count. Less common side effects include presence of blood in urine, acne, fatigue, and decreased platelet count. Rarely, heart changes may occur at high dosages.

Decadron (dexamethasone) An ANTINAUSEA MEDICATION that is also a steroid and a strong anti-inflammatory agent, used in combination with other medications to prevent nausea and vomiting after CHEMOTHERAPY treatments.

Side effects include depression, weight gain, increased appetite, sleep problems, skin bruising, mood changes, delayed wound healing, increased risk of infection, increased blood sugar level, and sodium or fluid retention. Less common side effects include bone fractures, sweating, diarrhea, nausea, headache, increased heart rate, fungal infections, and decrease in potassium level. Rarely, the drug may cause cataracts, personality changes, blurry vision, or stomach ulcer.

dexamethasone See DECADRON.

diarrhea Passage of loose or watery stools at least three times a day that may or may not be painful. Often, it is accompanied by gas, bloating, and cramps. Diarrhea occurs in about 75 percent of CHEMOTHERAPY patients because the drugs used damage the rapidly dividing cells in the gastrointestinal tract. The severity of diarrhea depends on the type and dosage of chemotherapy. Some drugs that cause diarrhea are 5-FLUOROURACIL, methotrexate, DOCETAXEL, and actinomycin D. It can be life threatening if it triggers dehydration, malnutrition, and electrolyte imbalances.

diet Some evidence suggests a link between diet and some types of cancer, such as PROSTATE CANCER. For example, some studies suggest that a diet high in animal fat (saturated fat) may increase the risk of prostate cancer, and that a diet high in fruits and vegetables may decrease the risk. Men who eat a lot of red meat and a lot of fat in their diet appear to have a greater risk of development of prostate cancer. These men also tend to eat fewer fruits and vegetables and more dairy products. Doctors are not sure which of these factors is responsible for increasing risk.

Fiber

Fiber, found in whole grain foods, seeds, nuts, and vegetables, is associated with the production of lower levels of ANDROGENS (male HORMONES). In comparison, foods that contain fat increase the production of hormones such as TESTOSTERONE, which then stimulates the growth of prostate cells. This growth may be a risk for development of cancer. Fiber also binds to androgens and both are excreted from the body.

Studies are in progress to learn whether men can reduce their risk of prostate cancer by taking certain dietary supplements. Although experts do not know whether a diet low in fat prevents prostate cancer, a low-fat diet may have many other health benefits. For example, soy foods are high in ISOFLAVONES, which block some hormonal activity in cells. Diets high in soy products have been associated with lower rates of cancers of the prostate.

Several substances, including LYCOPENES (found in high levels in some fruits and vegetables, such as tomatoes, grapefruit, and watermelon), vitamin E, and the mineral selenium, may lower prostate cancer risk. Some studies suggest that a diet high in tomatoes has been associated with a decreased risk of prostate cancer.

Current studies are assessing whether or not these substances actually reduce risk. Until such studies are completed, the best advice to lower prostate cancer risk is to eat fewer red meats and high-fat dairy products and to eat five or more servings of vegetables and fruits each day.

Dietary Fat

In addition, a high-fat diet has been associated with an increased risk of development of cancer of the prostate, among others. Low-fat foods are usually lower in calories than high-fat foods and are low in fat as well. There are three types of dietary fats—saturated, monounsaturated, and polyunsaturated fats:

- *Saturated fats* are almost exclusively from animal products such as meat, milk, and cheese and have been linked to an increased risk of cancer.
- *Monounsaturated fats* are found in olive oil and canola oil.
- *Polyunsaturated fats* are found in vegetable oils.

The latter two types of fat are less closely linked to disease; however, since overall fat intake is associated with cancer, it is a good idea to limit all three kinds. Dietitians generally recommend tub margarine as a better choice than butter, since butter is rich in both saturated fat and cholesterol, and the hazards of saturated fats are better documented and appear to be more severe than the hazards of the hydrogenated fats in margarine. Most margarine is made from vegetable fat and has no cholesterol.

The usual recommendation is that people consume no more than 10 percent of daily calories as saturated fats and that total fat intake not exceed 30 percent of the day's calories.

Dietary fat intake can be reduced by limiting the consumption of red meat, choosing low-fat or no-fat varieties of milk and cheese, removing skin from chicken and turkey, choosing pretzels instead of potato chips, and decreasing or eliminating fried foods, butter, and margarine. Cooking with small amounts of olive oil instead of butter significantly cuts saturated fat intake.

Antioxidants

Antioxidants seek out and destroy the naturally occurring toxic molecules called FREE RADICALS that can cause extensive damage to the body's cells that is thought to be involved in cancer development. Antioxidants reduce the number of free radicals, prevent tissue damage, and, quite possibly, prevent cancer. The antioxidants that have generated most interest and research to date are vitamin C, vitamin E, BETA-CAROTENE and SELENIUM.

Good sources of vitamin C include citrus fruits, kiwi, cantaloupe, strawberries, peppers, tomatoes, potatoes, mangos, and cruciferous vegetables. Vitamin E can be found in green leafy vegetables, wheat germ, whole grain products, nuts, seeds, and vegetable oil. Beta-carotene often (but not always) is identified by its yellow, orange, or deep green color; it occurs in carrots, cantaloupe, sweet potatoes, apricots, broccoli, spinach, and other green leafy vegetables. Selenium is found in seafood, meat, and grains.

Phytochemicals

These plant chemicals contribute to the color and flavor of vegetables and when eaten may suppress cancer development. Phytochemicals that may help prevent cancer include the following:

- The antioxidant beta-carotene
- Lutein in spinach, kale, and other green leafy vegetables
- Limonen and phenols in citrus fruits
- Allyl sulfides in garlic and onions
- Sulforaphane
- Indoles
- Isothiocyanates in broccoli, cauliflower, and other cruciferous vegetables

Pesticides

Health experts recommend eating a variety of fruits and vegetables for a healthy diet; doing so can also reduce the likelihood of ingesting excessive amounts of pesticides used to grow produce. Most experts believe that eating the small amount of synthetic pesticides in produce is not harmful; eating a wide variety of foods guarantees that a person does not consume an excessive amount of any one additive.

Preparation

Whenever possible, consumers should choose foods that are eaten in a form as close to their natural state as possible—eating whole wheat bread rather than refined flour breads, fresh fruits and vegetables instead of canned, whole grain cereals rather than cereals that are heavily sugared.

Refined products, such as white rice and white bread, often have had most of the nutritious part of the grain removed during processing. These products may then be enriched by having certain vitamins and minerals reintroduced. Although "enriched" foods sound good, many valuable nutrients (such as fiber) removed during the refining process are never readded. In addition, many refined products add other undesirable ingredients, such as salt or fats.

diethylstilbestrol (DES)   A synthetic estrogen tablet used to treat advanced PROSTATE CANCER that works by preventing the release of LHRH (luteinizing hormone-releasing hormone), which stimulates the production of TESTOSTERONE.

In order to grow, many prostate cancers need the male hormone testosterone, which is produced by the testes and the adrenal glands. Diethylstilbestrol works by reducing the level of testosterone by boosting the female hormone estrogen. When this occurs, production of testosterone is turned off, because the brain senses that too many sex hormones are circulating in the body. This drop in testosterone can help to slow down the growth of the cancer cells and may cause the cancer to shrink in size.

Although diethylstilbestrol (DES) was the first medicine that was used as an alternative to an ORCHIECTOMY (testicle removal), it is less popular today because of the complications it may cause.

Side Effects

Some men may experience side effects, including fatigue, lethargy, blood clots, nausea and vomiting, fluid retention, weight gain, breast tenderness or fullness, and decreased sex drive. If impotence occurs, sexual function may return to normal after stopping the drug.

Uncommon side effects include headaches, thinning hair, skin rashes, or discolored skin.

diethylstilbestrol and testicular cancer   Although men whose mother took the synthetic estrogen DIETHYLSTILBESTROL (DES) during pregnancy have an increased risk of certain congenital reproductive system malformations, there is no convincing evidence that DES exposure significantly increases a man's risk for development of TESTICULAR CANCER.

differentiation   The maturity of the cancer cells in a tumor. Differentiated tumor cells resemble normal cells and tend to grow and spread at a slower rate than undifferentiated or poorly differentiated tumor cells, which lack the structure and function of normal cells and grow uncontrollably.

digital rectal exam (DRE)   An annual test for men older than age 50 that can detect abnormalities of the prostate and rectum. In a digital rectal examination, the physician feels the prostate through the wall of the rectum. Hard or lumpy areas may indicate that cancer is present.

dihydrotestosterone (DHT)   A breakdown product of TESTOSTERONE that stimulates the growth of the PROSTATE GLAND.

3,3′-diindolylmethane (DIM)   A chemical in broccoli and cauliflower that may help doctors treat PROSTATE CANCER. Men who eat plenty of vegetables seem less likely to develop prostate cancer, but no one has tested the chemical on humans yet. It may not be manufactured as usable drug for many years.

Researchers in the past have found that prostate cancer rates are lower in countries where people eat plenty of fruits and vegetables, although the exact link between diet and the disease is not clear. Researchers at the University of California at Berkeley decided to investigate the cancer-fighting effects of chemicals in cruciferous vegetables such as broccoli, cauliflower, kale, brussels sprouts, and cabbage. The researchers found that DIM, a chemical by-product of consumption of cruciferous vegetables, appeared to prevent the growth of breast cancer cells and that prostate cancer cells treated with DIM grew 70 percent more slowly than untreated cells.

The chemical appears to prevent cancer cells from receiving signals from the hormone testosterone, thereby preventing the cells from growing. By contrast, traditional hormone therapy for prostate cancer patients is designed to prevent testosterone from entering the cells.

It is possible that DIM could be used in combination with hormone therapy, helping to dampen the side effects of lowering testosterone levels. Producing drugs from the vegetables may be easy and inexpensive: Broccoli and cabbage are commonly used vegetables, and it should be possible to obtain a large amount of this chemical at a very cheap price.

Some researchers believe that chemicals derived from vegetables may be more important in preventing prostate cancer than treating it once it appears. These compounds may be of greater importance for prostate cancer prevention at the early stages of cancer development than at later stages when the cancer is advanced. However, it is still not clear how much of the vegetables men would have to consume to protect themselves from prostate cancer.

docetaxel (Taxotere) A type of taxane that when used alone or together with estramustine can aid treatment of PROSTATE CANCER. Docetaxel works by disrupting the growth of cancer cells.

Side effects include NAUSEA and vomiting, rash, APPETITE LOSS, DIARRHEA, hair thinning or loss, and decreased platelet and white cell counts. Steroids are usually at the time of use to minimize side effects.

do not resuscitate order (DNR order) A legal directive by a physician that instructs hospital staff not to try to help a patient whose heart has stopped or who has stopped breathing. A patient can request a DNR order either by filling out an ADVANCE DIRECTIVE form or by telling the doctor that cardiopulmonary resuscitation (CPR) should not be performed. DNR orders are accepted by doctors and hospitals in all states.

doubling time The time required for a cell to double in number.

doxorubicin See ADRIAMYCIN.

edrecolomab A type of MONOCLONAL ANTIBODY used in cancer detection and therapy. Monoclonal antibodies are laboratory-produced substances that can locate and bind to cancer cells.

ejaculation The release of semen through the penis during orgasm. Painful ejaculation is one symptom of PROSTATE CANCER. After radical PROSTATECTOMY, no fluid is released during orgasm. After TRANSURETHRAL PROSTATECTOMY (TURP), the fluid released into the prostate through the ejaculatory ducts may go back into the bladder rather than towards the tip of the penis. This is called RETROGRADE EJACULATION.

embryonal cell carcinoma A fast-spreading type of GERM CELL TUMOR called a NONSEMINOMA that usually grows in gonads (especially testicles). It usually is found as a component of a mixed germ cell tumor.

Embryonal carcinoma causes a firm lumpy mass with many bleeding areas. When viewed under a microscope, these tumors can resemble tissues of very early embryos. This type of nonseminoma tends to be aggressive and is likely to spread and grow rapidly.

About 20 percent of TESTICULAR CANCERS are embryonal carcinomas. They often occur in 20- to 30-year-olds and are highly malignant. In about 30 percent of cases, this type of cancer spreads beyond the testes (often to the lung and liver).

endodermal sinus tumor See YOLK SAC TUMOR.

end-of-life care The medical and psychological care given during the terminal stages of cancer. ADVANCE DIRECTIVES, including a LIVING WILL, durable POWER OF ATTORNEY, and HEALTH CARE PROXY, allow people to express their decisions about end-of-life care before the need arises. Advance directives provide a way for patients to let family, friends, and health-care professionals know their wishes, thus preventing misunderstanding later should they become unable to communicate.

endorectal magnetic resonance imaging A type of MAGNETIC RESONANCE IMAGING (MRI) study of the PROSTATE GLAND in which a probe is placed into the rectum to allow better visualization of the prostate.

endostatin A drug known as an ANGIOGENESIS INHIBITOR that was heralded in 1998 for its ability, demonstrated in animal research, to starve a malignant tumor by drying up its source of blood. Angiogenesis inhibitors are drugs that kill prostate cancer cells by interfering with their blood supply. Human tests of endostatin were launched in 1999 at M. D. Anderson Cancer Center, the University of Wisconsin, and Dana-Farber Cancer Center. Endostatin can decrease blood flow to some tumors and promote the death of cancer and blood vessel cells.

endothelin-1 receptor antagonists A family of drugs that block the hormone endothelin and may prevent PROSTATE CANCER from spreading to the bones.

environmental estrogen Some studies suggest that fetal overexposure to environmental chemicals that have estrogenlike effects can lead to later reproductive cancers in men. Such chemicals include pesticides such as DDT (dichlorodiphenyltrichloroethane), aldrin, dieldrin, parachlorophenyls (PCPs), dioxins, and furans. Although tests of single chemicals containing estrogen have reported little danger, other studies indicate that combinations of estrogen-containing chemicals may be very harmful.

For example, overexposure to estrogen reduces the number of Sertoli's cells (the cells necessary for the initial development of sperm) and thereby may contribute to TESTICULAR CANCER.

Environmental estrogens are chemicals in the environment that mimic natural estrogens and other hormones, which are the chemical messengers of the body's endocrine system. These estrogenlike chemicals may occur naturally in plants and in the human diet; others are synthetic and may be found in plastics or insecticides. Another synthetic chemical that mimics estrogen is DIETHYLSTILBESTROL (DES), which was used in the past to prevent miscarriage and to promote growth in livestock and poultry.

It is important to understand the effects of these compounds because they may remain in the body for a long time and mimic the action of natural hormones. Environmental chemicals may alter the function of the endocrine system by mimicking hormone actions and either triggering or blocking a response to the body's natural hormones.

The body's natural hormonal balance maintains normal body activities by binding to receptor molecules in cell tissues such as the prostate, brain, and skin. Then, the receptor acts as the translator of the hormone in the cell. When synthetic compounds mimic these hormones, they also bind to the receptor. Some foreign chemicals interact with the estrogen receptor and produce estrogenlike effects on the development of the brain and male reproductive organs, causing a variety of disorders.

epididymis   A soft, tubelike structure behind the testicle that collects and carries sperm for several weeks, as they complete their maturation and develop their powerful swimming capabilities. The matured sperm leave the epididymis through the vas deferens.

Cancer of the epididymis is extremely uncommon, although lumps and bumps associated with it are quite common. Spermatoceles are collections of sperm that arise from the epididymis and become walled-off bumps. They are completely benign. Hydroceles are collections of fluid around the testicles that are also completely benign. They can occur for a variety of reasons, including surgery, trauma, and infection. They are not part of the epididymis although they are adjacent to them.

erectile dysfunction   The inability to achieve or maintain an erection in order to complete sexual intercourse.

Causes

All of the treatments for PROSTATE CANCER carry the risk of causing erectile dysfunction.

Prostatectomy   The likelihood of development of erectile problems after a radical PROSTATECTOMY varies with age, erectile function before surgery, sparing or nonsparing of nerves during surgery, and the surgeon's ability. In general, the incidence of erectile dysfunction after a nerve-sparing radical prostatectomy ranges from 16 percent to 82 percent. Erectile dysfunction after a prostatectomy occurs immediately after surgery and is caused by damage to the pelvic nerves along the outside of the prostate. Patients who have had a nerve-sparing prostatectomy may experience a return of erectile function at some point up to a year after surgery.

External beam radiation therapy (EBRT) Between 32 percent and 67 percent of men who have had EBRT experience erectile dysfunction as a result of radiation damage to the arteries. This dysfunction may not occur until a year or more after radiation therapy. The incidence of dysfunction is between 15 percent and 31 percent in the first year after treatment and rises to between 40 percent and 62 percent five years later.

Erectile dysfunction may occur in 6 percent to 50 percent of patients after interstitial seed therapy with or without medium-dose EBRT. This dysfunction also tends to occur months after treatment ends.

Hormone therapy   Hormone therapy also may cause erectile dysfunction as well as loss of interest in sex, which is related to the drop in TESTOSTERONE level.

Treatment

There are several ways to treat erectile dysfunction, including PENILE PROSTHESIS, vacuum devices, medication, injections, or intraurethral treatments. Researchers are also studying the efficacy of nerve grafting, in which a nerve is removed from another part of the body and placed into the area where the pelvic nerve was removed during surgery for prostate cancer.

Medication Much progress has been made with the availability of new drugs to treat erectile dysfunction, such as Viagra, Levitra, and Cialis. The drugs are taken by mouth 15 minutes to 36 hours before intercourse to accentuate the natural process of erection. Success rates vary widely— from 15 percent to 71 percent. Viagra may cause headaches, flushing, or heartburn. Painful erection (priapism) is uncommon. They should never be given to men taking nitroglycerin, because the combination can cause low blood pressure, heart attack, and death.

Apomorphine is a type of medication placed under the tongue that is reported to work very quickly (within 20 minutes), improving erectile function in up to 54 percent of men. It is not currently available in the United States.

Intraurethral alprostadil (Muse) A small suppository preloaded into a syringe, which is inserted into the urethra. When the suppository is released, it enters the urethra, where it quickly dissolves so that the medication can be absorbed. This method is successful in between 20 percent and 40 percent of men who have postradical prostatectomy or post-EBRT erectile dysfunction. It can cause urethral or penile pain in 33 percent of users (especially those who have had a radical prostatectomy). It also may lower blood pressure in a few patients and may cause priapism or vaginal irritation in the partners of 10 percent of patients.

A new form of intraurethral therapy that is being studied combines prazosin with alprostadil, improving erections in up to 60 percent of patients (compared to 52 percent in men who are using alprostadil alone).

Prostaglandin injections Injection of prostaglandins into the side of the penis sounds uncomfortable, but the needle is very small and the amount of fluid is tiny. Injections should be given in alternate sides of the penis and should not be given more often than every 48 to 72 hours to prevent formation of scar tissue.

Those men who experience discomfort may try a combination of medications such as triple P/trimix (prostaglandin, papaverine and phentolamine) which contains less prostaglandin. This combination of chemicals helps the blood vessels expand so that more blood flows into the penis. Ideally, an erection occurs about 10 or 20 minutes after the injection and lasts about an hour.

Injection treatments work in up to 85 percent of men who have erectile dysfunction as a result of a radical prostatectomy. It also may be temporarily helpful for men who have had nerve-sparing radical prostatectomy, until nerve function returns. Injection treatments also work well for men who have erectile dysfunction after EBRT and seed placement treatments.

However, it may cause prolonged erections (longer than four to six hours) in up to 1.3 percent of patients, and a painful erection in 15 percent to 30 percent.

Other types of injectable drugs currently under investigation include vasoactive intestinal peptide, which works together with phentolamine. Linsidomine is another drug, which, when injected, may increase the level of nitric oxide in the penis, opening the blood vessels. Use of this drug does not seem to be more effective than prostaglandin therapy.

Forskolin is another type of injection treatment that increases blood flow when added to trimix, improving the duration and rigidity of erections in up to 61 percent of patients.

Vacuum constriction A vacuum erection device, which costs between $150 and $450, is basically a plastic cylinder with a hand- or battery-operated pump and constricting bands. The tube—with the preloaded constricting band—is placed over the penis. When the pump is activated, it creates suction that pulls blood into the penis; once the penis becomes rigid, the constricting band is pulled off the tube and placed around the base of the penis so that the blood cannot escape. This band keeps the penis erect so that intercourse can occur.

Once intercourse is completed, the band is removed and the blood is allowed to drain from the penis back into the body. (The band should not remain on the penis longer than 30 minutes, to prevent damage of the penis.) Although the band may interfere with ejaculation, it does not prevent orgasm. Men who have had a radical prostatectomy do not ejaculate any fluid; men who have had EBRT or interstitial seed therapy do ejaculate, although the volume may be lower than before surgery.

The vacuum method results in a satisfaction rate of between 68 percent and 83 percent. It may cause painful ejaculations in between 3 percent and 16 percent of users and an inability to ejaculate in between 12 percent and 30 percent. A few patients notice numbness during erection.

Topical gel   Scientists are studying a new treatment for erectile dysfunction involving a topical prostaglandin gel that is applied to the penis, increasing blood flow to the area.

Nerve grafts   Researchers are studying the possibility of grafting nerves to treat erectile dysfunction after non–nerve sparing radical prostatectomy. In this method, during prostatectomy surgery, a segment of a nerve located in the leg is removed and sewn into the place where the neurovascular bundle has been removed. Initial results suggest that this nerve grafting technique may improve erectile function after surgery in men whose usual nerves have been removed during surgery.

Penile prosthesis   The penile prosthesis is a permanent device that is surgically inserted into the penis. There are several different types, of implants ranging from semirigid to inflatable.

The semirigid device maintains the same width, but it is bent up for intercourse and down at other times. This type of prosthesis is the easiest to insert and entails the fewest mechanical problems, but it is also the least natural-looking of all the prostheses.

Inflatable prostheses look quite natural, since when deflated the penis is flaccid, and when inflated the penis is erect. The two-piece inflatable unit includes two cylinders, one in each side of the penis, with a small pump in the scrotum. Squeezing the pump pushes fluid into the cylinders, making the penis erect. The three-piece unit includes a reservoir inside the abdominal wall near the bladder that contains additional fluid; this fluid allows for a more rigid penis.

The more complex the device, the more likely that mechanical problems can occur. Today the failure rate is about 10 percent at 10 years. The major risk of use of the penile implant is infection; if this occurs, often the entire device must be removed. Moreover, once a prosthesis has been implanted and then removed, other forms of treatment usually do not work. This is why it is important to try other treatment methods before choosing surgical prostheses.

Still, although this option is expensive and requires surgery, up to 90 percent of patients are satisfied with the inflatable prosthesis.

erythroplasia of Queyrat   A clearly defined reddish area that develops on the penis, usually on or at the base of the head, usually in uncircumcised men. It is a CARCINOMA IN SITU, and if untreated, the area can become cancerous.

The diagnosis is made by a biopsy of a small sample of skin. The condition is treated with FLUOROURACIL cream followed by reexamination every few months, because of the risk of cancer in the area. Alternatively, the abnormal tissue may be removed.

erythropoietin (Epogen, Procrit)   Produced in the adult kidney, this substance triggers the production of red blood cells. When given as a drug to supplement the body's natural supply, it can reverse ANEMIA in cancer patients who are receiving CHEMOTHERAPY.

esophagitis   Inflammation of the esophagus that is a direct result of taking CHEMOTHERAPY drugs for cancer and that usually develops between five to 14 days after receiving chemotherapy. Esophagitis can lead to bleeding, painful ulcers, and infection. However, sores in the esophagus are usually temporary and heal completely once chemotherapy is finished.

Symptoms
Symptoms include intermittent or constant chest pain or a burning feeling in the throat that can be heavy or sharp and that may worsen when swallowing. Less often, there may be bleeding in the vomit or stools.

Prognosis
In most cases symptoms begin to improve within a week or two after the chemotherapy treatment ends.

estramustine phosphate (Emyct, Estracyt, Estracyte) A type of CHEMOTHERAPY drug sometimes used to treat PROSTATE CANCER. Estramustine is an ALKYLATING AGENT, which may cause nausea and vomiting.

European Organisation for Research and Treatment of Cancer An international nonprofit group that conducts, coordinates, and stimulates laboratory and clinical research in Europe to improve the management of cancer. Because comprehensive research in this field is often beyond the means of individual European laboratories and hospitals, the organization coordinates multidisciplinary, multinational efforts of basic research scientists and clinicians on the European continent.

The ultimate goals of the European Organisation for Research and Treatment of Cancer (EORTC) are to improve the standard of cancer treatment in Europe through the development of new drugs and innovative approaches, and to test more effective treatments with drugs, surgery, and RADIATION THERAPY.

The organization was founded as an international organization under Belgian law in 1962 by eminent oncologists working in the main cancer research institutes of the European Union countries and Switzerland. It was named Groupe Européen de Chimiothérapie Anticancéreuse (GECA); it was renamed the EORTC in 1968. For contact information, see Appendix I.

Exceptional Cancer Patient (EcaP) A nonprofit organization dedicated to promoting a comprehensive integrative philosophy of the importance of the mind–body connection in health care for cancer patients and others who have chronic illnesses.

Exceptional Cancer Patients was founded in 1978 by Bernie Siegel, M.D., and successfully operated for many years; it was acquired in 1999 by the Mind–Body Wellness Center in order to build upon and advance the organization and its principles. Today it is owned and operated by Meadville Medical Center and MMC Health Systems, Inc., to offer comprehensive, integrative whole-person programs in a traditional medical setting. Through a combination of outcome-based clinical studies and basic science research, the cen-

ter promotes the concept of integrative healing in mind, body, and spirit.

The center provides resources, comprehensive professional training programs, and interdisciplinary retreats to help people facing the challenges of cancer discover their inner healing resources. These programs are based on mind–body–spirit medicine. For contact information, see Appendix I.

exercise Exercise in general is extremely beneficial to overall health; however, little research suggests that it is particularly helpful in preventing male reproductive cancers such as PROSTATE CANCER.

Exercise helps the body function properly so that the food is used optimally to build lean muscle and burn calories. A sedentary lifestyle contributes to obesity, which is a risk factor for many cancers. The amount of exercise that is enough is controversial, however: Some studies recommend that even only 30 minutes of exercise a day—not even at one time—is enough; others indicate that benefit may result only from vigorous exercise. A brisk walk of 30 to 40 minutes on most days of the week is probably the level that people should be trying to achieve, scientists suggest.

The AMERICAN CANCER SOCIETY is also putting a new emphasis on exercise as a way to reduce the risk of developing and dying of cancer. The society's minimal recommendation for cancer prevention in adults is at least 30 minutes of moderate activity, such as a brisk walk, five days a week. In addition, 45 minutes or more of moderate to vigorous activity five or more days a week may enhance reductions in cancer risk. Vigorous activity may include activities such as jogging, martial arts, or basketball.

expectant therapy Close monitoring of PROSTATE CANCER by a doctor instead of immediate treatment, also called watchful waiting. Expectant therapy may be recommended if prostate cancer is in a very early stage, especially in the cases of older men who have small tumors that are expected to grow very slowly, that are confined to one area of the prostate, and that are not causing any symptoms or other medical problems. Because prostate cancer cells often spread very slowly, many older men who have the disease may not need more extensive treatment. Expectant therapy usually includes routine physician examinations, including the DIGITAL RECTAL EXAM and the PROSTATE-SPECIFIC ANTIGEN (PSA) BLOOD TEST.

external beam radiation therapy (EBRT) The use of radiation therapy from outside the body to kill cancer cells.

In PROSTATE CANCER and PENILE CANCER, external beam radiation therapy (EBRT) is sometimes recommended when the tumor has spread to immediate surrounding tissues. In the case of TESTICULAR CANCER, external beam radiation is aimed at lymph nodes in the abdomen. SEMINOMAS (a type of testicular cancer) are highly sensitive to radiation; NONSEMINOMAS are less sensitive to radiation, so men who have this type of cancer usually do not undergo radiation.

Most EBRT is given by the three-dimensional (3-D) conformal radiation technique, using a computer to focus the radiation close on the prostate. A new modification is intensity modulated radiation therapy (IMRT), which is a more intensive 3-D mode that confines the radiation more closely to the prostate, decreasing side effects.

EBRT usually is given on an outpatient basis for seven to eight weeks to destroy cancer cells and shrink tumors. The results are similar to those of surgery after the first 10 years, but after that time surgical treatment shows a slight advantage.

Impotence eventually occurs in about 50 percent of those receiving radiation treatment, but incontinence is rare unless there has been prior prostate surgery. Other complications include urination discomfort, urinary urgency, and DIARRHEA (especially during the late stages of treatment). Frequently a patient feels very tired during the later stages of radiation, and temporary or long-term bladder or bowel irritability or bleeding may occur.

extragonadal germ cell tumor A primary GERM CELL TUMOR located outside the testicles that may not respond as well to therapy as a primary testicular tumor. Germ cell tumors develop from testicular cells.

Extragonadal germ cell tumors can be malignant or benign. Noncancerous extragonadal germ cell tumors are often very large and are removed surgically. The cancerous tumors are divided into two types—SEMINOMA and NONSEMINOMA. Nonseminoma cancers include EMBRYONAL CARCINOMA, malignant TERATOMA, ENDODERMAL SINUS TUMOR, CHORIOCARCINOMA, and mixed germ cell tumors. These tumors are aggressive and usually occur in young men. Nonseminomas can develop anywhere but usually appear in the chest, abdomen, or brain.

Seminomas
Seminomas are very sensitive to RADIATION THERAPY; about 60 percent to 80 percent of patients who undergo radiation therapy remain disease-free. CHEMOTHERAPY is also very effective for seminomas. Patients whose cancer has not spread are usually treated first with radiation therapy. Patients who have large tumors or tumors that are spreading may be treated with etoposide- and CISPLATIN-based anticancer drugs.

For many patients, treatment does not totally remove the tumor. Small masses should be closely monitored but are not treated until symptoms appear or change. Larger masses may be monitored or surgically removed.

Nonseminomas
Patients who have nonseminomas receive chemotherapy when the cancer is diagnosed. Nonseminomas are typically very large, but early surgery is seldom useful; however, those whose tumor does not respond to chemotherapy may have surgery.

Nonseminomas that occur in the chest occur more frequently in those who have KLINEFELTER SYNDROME. These patients are also at risk for cancer of the blood.

Treatment is more successful for patients who have small tumors that respond to chemotherapy and who are not likely to have other cancers. Patients who have nonseminoma that occurs near the kidneys generally respond well to treatment, depending on the size of the tumor.

extratesticular Outside the testicle, involving the EPIDIDYMIS, SPERMATIC CORD, VAS DEFERENS, TUNICA VAGINALIS, and RETE TESTIS. TESTICULAR CANCER does not originate in the extratesticular region.

Family and Medical Leave Act (FMLA) A 1993 law that requires most employers to allow their workers up to 12 weeks off without pay for illnesses. (For example, men recovering from prostatectomy need to take between four and six weeks off from work.)

The employer of a man taking medical leave as a result of cancer must either hold the job open or provide a similar job when the man returns to work. FMLA leave may be either intermittent or continuous.

The Equal Employment Opportunity Commission in Washington, D.C., can provide information on the FMLA.

family history of cancer A man's risk for developing PROSTATE CANCER is higher if his father or brother has had the disease. Men who have a family history of TESTICULAR CANCER also may have an increased risk of development of testicular cancer as well.

See also GENES.

fat Some evidence suggests there may be a link between consumption of saturated fat (animal fat) and PROSTATE CANCER or TESTICULAR CANCER—and that a DIET high in fruits and vegetables may decrease the risk.

Studies are in progress to learn whether men can reduce their risk of prostate cancer by taking certain dietary supplements. Although experts do not know whether a diet low in fat prevents prostate cancer, such a diet may have many other health benefits.

In addition, a few studies have found that increasing total fat, saturated fat, and cholesterol consumption was associated with increasing risk of nonseminoma testicular cancer. Studies also found that the risk for seminoma testicular cancer marginally increased with increasing intake of total fat and saturated fat.

fatigue The most common side effect experienced by cancer patients, usually as a result of surgery, RADIATION THERAPY, CHEMOTHERAPY, or BIOLOGICAL THERAPY. Although it occurs most frequently in those undergoing treatment, overwhelming fatigue may continue after treatment ends.

Scientists are not sure of its exact cause; some researchers believe fatigue may be caused by the waste products produced as a tumor shrinks or may be related to the energy the body needs to fight cancer. Others believe fatigue may be related to interruptions in the signals sent through the nervous system. A low blood count (ANEMIA) caused by chemotherapy, sleep disturbances, stress, depression, poor DIET, infection, and other medication side effects can all contribute to this exhaustion.

Symptoms

The symptoms of cancer-related fatigue are different from normal sensations of tiredness. Fatigue can begin suddenly and can be all-consuming; naps may not help. Fatigue can be physically and emotionally draining on the patient as well as the family. General weakness may be accompanied by limb heaviness, decreased ability to concentrate, sleeplessness, and/or irritability.

Diagnosis

Patients who experience this type of extreme tiredness should consult a health-care provider, who will conduct a few simple tests, including a blood count to check for anemia or infection, and a physical examination.

Treatment

If symptoms are fatigue related, there are several ways patients can manage those symptoms. It is important to eat healthy, appetite-stimulating foods. The complex carbohydrates found in pasta, fresh fruits, and whole grain breads provide long-term energy. Studies have shown that a moderate amount of exercise may improve energy level as well.

Sleep also is important. Patients should go to bed at a regular time each day and follow a regular routine.

Fertile Hope   A national nonprofit organization that addresses the reproductive needs of cancer patients and survivors. The group provides education, financial help, research, and support.

Fertile Hope also gives financial assistance to patients whose medical treatments threaten reproductive function and offers support to help patients cope with the physical and emotional issues associated with infertility, fertility preservation, assisted reproduction, family planning, genetic counseling, pregnancy, adoption, and related issues. For contact information, see Appendix I.

financial issues   The cost of treating cancer can be very expensive, but health insurance plans usually cover much of the cost. Patients who belong to a health maintenance organization (HMO) or preferred provider organization (PPO) should become familiar with their provider choices and their financial responsibility if they receive care out of network from a doctor not covered by the health plan.

Cancer patients who do not have insurance should contact their local Social Security office to determine whether they qualify for supplemental security income (SSI) or social security disability insurance (SSDI). The medical requirements and disability determination process of both programs are the same. However, whereas eligibility for SSDI is based on employment history, SSI is based on financial need.

Free Hospital Care

Cancer patients who do not have insurance also can receive care from hospitals who receive federal grants from Hill-Burton funds that allow hospitals and nursing homes to provide low-cost or no-cost medical care. To receive a listing of hospitals or nursing homes participating in the Hill-Burton program, patients can call (800) 638-0742 or visit the Hill Burton Web site (www.hrsa.gov/osp/dfcr/).

See also HILL-BURTON FREE HOSPITAL CARE.

Prescription Drugs

Most major pharmaceutical companies have patient assistance programs that offer a free three-month supply of medication to those who cannot afford their prescriptions. To obtain guidelines and a listing of participating companies, patients can call the Pharmaceutical Manufacturers' Association at (800) 762-4636. The medication request must be completed by a physician.

Free Air Transportation

For patients who travel to treatment centers, many nonprofit agencies offer free air transportation provided by private pilots who donate their time and use of their own planes. Patients can obtain a list of these services at http://www.aircareall.org. In addition, major airlines sometimes offer reduced or no-cost travel through an assistance program.

Local Transportation

For local travel assistance to and from treatments, the hospital social worker may be able to provide van service or cab or bus vouchers. Some local AMERICAN CANCER SOCIETY offices run volunteer transportation programs or provide funds to reimburse travel expenses. Others offer vans for those who qualify because of illness or disability. Local nursing homes, park districts, or YMCAs also may offer van transportation to local hospitals. In addition, many communities offer seniors reduced-fare taxi service within the community.

Temporary Housing

Temporary housing is sometimes required by cancer patients who must travel for consultation or treatment or by families who visit hospitalized patients. The American Cancer Society may be able to arrange a low-cost hotel room for those receiving treatment. Many hospitals negotiate discount rates at local hotels or provide dormitory-style housing. In addition, the NATIONAL ASSOCIATION OF HOSPITALITY

HOUSES (800) 542-9730 provides referral information to anyone in need of lodging while undergoing treatment away from home.

Utilities

Assistance programs are offered by many gas, electric, water, and phone companies for cancer patients who may have trouble paying monthly bills. Many states have regulations that prohibit companies from turning off utilities; a doctor or social worker may need to write letters describing why the services are medically necessary. The regulations do not lessen a patient's responsibility for paying bills but may allow families more time or lower monthly payments. In an emergency, local help lines and social service agencies may be able to provide onc-time emergency help with utility bills.

Home Care and Respite

Some insurance plans offer coverage for home care ranging from skilled nurses to companions. If companion care is not a covered benefit, patients can contact various agencies for assistance. Respite care allows the caregiver a few hours each week to take a break while someone watches over the patient. Many caregivers use this time to run errands, take care of personal health needs, or unwind.

Local respite caregivers can be located by calling the National Respite Locator at (800) 773-5433. The locator service can also provide a listing of qualifying conditions.

In addition, the National Federation of Interfaith Volunteer Caregivers, a not-for-profit group that oversees 400 regional offices, sends volunteers into the homes of people who need care, company, and supervision. They can be reached at (800) 350-7438.

Medical Supplies

The CANCER FUND OF AMERICA (800-578-5284) can provide needed nonprescription medical supplies such as nutritional supplements. Items available vary as the group receives products donated by companies. Patients or family members can call to be placed in their database for specific needs.

Food Programs

Meals on Wheels coordinates thousands of programs throughout the United States dedicated to delivering meals to those who are homebound.

Some programs require a small donation; eligibility is determined by each program. For a local referral to the Meals on Wheels patients can contact the national office at (616) 530-0929.

Income Tax Deductions

Medical costs that are not covered by insurance policies sometimes can be deducted from annual income before taxes. Examples of tax-deductible expenses may include mileage for trips to and from medical appointments, out-of-pocket costs for treatment, prescription drugs or equipment, and cost of meals during lengthy medical visits. The local Internal Revenue Service office, tax consultants, or certified public accountants can determine medical costs that are tax deductible. These telephone numbers are available in the local telephone directory.

Medicaid

Medicaid is a jointly funded federal–state health insurance program for people who need financial assistance for medical expenses, coordinated by the Centers for Medicare & Medicaid Services (CMS) (formerly the Health Care Financing Administration). At a minimum, states must provide home care services to people who receive federal income assistance such as Social Security Income and Aid to Families with Dependent Children. Medicaid coverage includes part-time nursing, home care aide services, and medical supplies and equipment. Information about coverage is available from local state welfare offices, state health departments, state social services agencies, and state Medicaid offices.

Medicare

Medicare is a federal health insurance program administered by the CMS. Eligible individuals include those who are 65 or older, people of any age who have permanent kidney failure, and disabled people younger than age 65. Medicare may offer reimbursement for some home care services. Cancer patients who qualify for Medicare may also be eligible for coverage of HOSPICE services if they are accepted into a Medicare-certified hospice program. To receive information on eligibility, explanations of coverage, and related publications, call Medicare at the number listed or visit their Web site. Some publications are available in Spanish. Toll-free: (800) 633-4227 (800-MEDICARE).

Patient Assistance Programs

The PATIENT ADVOCATE FOUNDATION (PAF) is a national nonprofit organization that provides referrals related to managed care, insurance, financial issues, job discrimination, and debt crisis matters to cancer patients and survivors. For contact information see Appendix I.

Veterans' Benefits

Eligible veterans and their dependents may receive cancer treatment at a Veterans Administration Medical Center. Treatment for service-connected conditions is provided, and treatment for other conditions may be available, depending on the veteran's financial need.

Viatical Settlement Companies

Viatical companies purchase a patient's life insurance policy at a discounted rate and provide money for patients to use as they decide. The seller, in turn, signs over the policy to the viatical company.

In general, any life insurance policy (group or individual) can be sold, but the rate of return and eligibility criteria vary from company to company. However, patients should consider tax implications and the effect of a viatical settlement on assistance programs.

A free brochure, "Viatical Settlements: A Guide for People with Terminal Illnesses," is available at the Federal Trade Commission at (202) 326-2222. The National Viatical Association at (202) 347-7361 offers a listing of viatical companies.

Life Insurance Loans

LifeWise Family Financial Security, Inc., allows patients to take out a loan against their existing life insurance policy if their life expectancy is five years or less. There is no obligation to repay the loan, but the option is available, distinguishing the process from selling an insurance policy to a viatical company. If a patient chooses not to repay the loan, the life insurance policy proceeds are the sole source of repayment. All surplus funds are remitted to the patient's family. LifeWise has counselors available to answer any questions and publishes *The Financial Resource Guide—A Comprehensive, Step-by-Step Refer-*

ence for Individuals Facing Life-Threatening or Terminal Illnesses. Counselors can be contacted and a copy of the guide provided by calling (800) 219-7385.

finasteride A drug that prevents the conversion of testosterone to its active form DHT and therefore prevents action of testosterone on prostate cells. It was studied as a possible preventive medication for PROSTATE CANCER in the seven-year PROSTATE CANCER PREVENTION TRIAL, which involved thousands of men across the United States who participated through 2004.

fine needle aspiration The use of a thin, hollow needle to withdraw tissue from the body. A fine needle aspiration (also called a needle aspiration BIOPSY) is less expensive and less painful and entails less risk of infection than a surgical biopsy. Because of its safety, cost-effectiveness, and accuracy, it is often the biopsy procedure of choice for evaluating a variety of different masses.

A core needle biopsy is similar to needle aspiration but uses a wider needle in order to obtain a larger tissue sample. Fine needle aspiration is less painful than core biopsy, but both can be performed as an outpatient procedure and at periodic intervals for serial follow-up. Many urologists use a bioptic gun with ultrasound guidance to diagnose prostate cancer. This procedure is not painful and has a low risk of complications. A transperineal, ultrasound-guided approach can be used for patients who may be at increased risk of complications through a transrectal approach.

five-year survival rate The percentage of people who have cancer who are expected to survive five years or longer with the disease. Although the rates are based on the most recent information available, they may include data from patients treated several years earlier. Although statistically valid, five-year survival rates may not reflect advances in cancer treatment, which often occur very quickly. They should not be seen as predictive in an individual case.

flaxseed and prostate cancer Flaxseed is the richest plant source of omega-3 fatty acids and is high in dietary fiber. A diet rich in flaxseed seems to block the growth and development of PROSTATE CANCER in mice, according to Duke University researchers. The flaxseed diet reduced the size, aggressiveness, and severity of tumors in mice genetically engineered to have PROSTATE CANCER and prevented prostate cancer in 3 percent of the animals.

A current Duke clinical trial is studying 160 men who have prostate cancer to determine whether prostate cancer cells can be prevented from dividing when exposed to a low-fat diet, flaxseed supplementation, or a combination of both.

flow cytometry   A procedure that assesses cellular DNA, which can be used to assess the aggressiveness of a malignant cell. Flow cytometry is used to assess the likelihood of a recurrence of PROSTATE CANCER, among other types of cancer.

Flow cytometry is an important test that can determine the number of sets of chromosomes in a cell and the percentage of cells in active DNA synthesis. In this test, suspected cancer cells are removed and then stained with a special dye. They are then analyzed in a flow cytometer by using a laser beam to measure their fluorescence; the results are charted to show the distribution of DNA in the cells.

Tumors with an abnormal number of chromosomes are more likely to be aggressive than tumors that have the normal two sets of chromosomes. Likewise, tumors with a low number of cells in active DNA synthesis (S-phase) have a better prognosis.

Results of flow cytometry are helpful to determine prognosis, monitor treatment response, and document tumor recurrence.

See also ANEUPLOID CELLS.

fluorouracil (5-FU, Adrucil, Efudex)   An antimetabolite that is applied as a cream to treat very small surface cancers of the penis. 5-FU interferes with nucleic acid synthesis, preventing cells from making DNA and RNA. Side effects include DIARRHEA, NAUSEA and vomiting, and mouth sores.

flutamide (Eulexin)   An anticancer drug that belongs to the family of drugs called ANTIANDROGENS, used to treat PROSTATE CANCER. These drugs block the action of ANDROGENS that help fuel the growth of malignant cells. Taking it three times a day in combination with a luteinizing hormone–releasing agonist provides total androgen blockade.

free radicals   Highly charged destructive forms of oxygen generated by each cell in the body that destroy cellular membranes through the oxidation process. Free radicals can damage important cellular molecules such as DNA or lipids in other parts of the cell.

Because free radicals are essential to many reactions in the body (they are generated by the immune system to fend off microbes and help the digestive system break down food), they should not be entirely destroyed. It is only when their levels become too high that damage can occur.

Free radical damage can be offset by molecules called ANTIOXIDANTS, which neutralize free radicals, preventing them from damaging cells. Antioxidants include BETA-CAROTENE, SELENIUM, and vitamins E and C. Although there are no guarantees of the effectiveness of the dietary supplements of antioxidants in preventing cell damage, many doctors recommend the antioxidants beta-carotene and vitamins C and E to their patients.

frozen section   A technique in which part of BIOPSY tissue is frozen immediately and a thin slice is then mounted on a microscope slide, enabling a pathologist to analyze it in just a few minutes for a diagnosis.

garlic The edible bulb of a plant in the lily family (*Allium* genus) that research suggests may effectively inhibit the cancer process. Studies reveal that the benefits of garlic are not limited to a specific species, to a particular tissue, or to a specific carcinogen. Of 37 observational studies in humans using garlic and related allyl sulfur components, 28 studies showed some cancer preventive effect. The evidence is particularly strong for a link between garlic and prevention of PROSTATE CANCER. However, all of the available information is from observational studies comparing cancer incidence in populations who eat or do not eat garlic or using animal models or observations with cells in culture. These findings have not yet been verified by clinical trials in humans.

Although the health benefits of garlic are frequently reported, eating excessive quantities can have unpleasant effects, such as garlic odor on breath and skin, occasional allergic reactions, stomach disorders, diarrhea, decrease in protein and calcium levels, association with bronchial asthma, and contact dermatitis.

Because garlic preparations vary in concentration and in the number of active compounds they contain, quality control is important when considering the use of garlic as a cancer-fighting agent.

Several compounds are involved in garlic's possible anticancer effects. Garlic contains allyl sulfur and other compounds that slow or prevent the growth of tumor cells. Allyl sulfur compounds, which occur naturally in garlic and onions, make cells vulnerable to the stress created by products of cell division. Because cancer cells divide very quickly, they generate more stressors than most normal cells do. Thus, cancer cells are damaged by the presence of allyl sulfur compounds to a much greater extent than normal cells. However, the chemical properties of garlic are complicated, and the ultimate quality of garlic products depends on the manufacturing process.

Peeling garlic and processing garlic into oil or powder can increase the number and variety of active compounds. Peeling garlic releases an enzyme called allinase and starts a series of chemical reactions that produce diallyl disulfide (DADS). DADS is also formed when raw garlic is cut or crushed. However, if garlic is cooked immediately after peeling, the allinase is inactivated and the cancer-fighting benefit of DADS is lost. This is why scientists recommend waiting 15 minutes between peeling and cooking garlic to allow the allinase reaction to occur.

Processing garlic into powder or garlic oil releases other cancer-fighting agents; the inconsistent results of garlic research may be due, at least in part, to problems standardizing all of the active compounds within garlic preparations. Some of the garlic compounds currently under investigation are allin (responsible for the typical garlic odor), alline (odorless compound), ajoene (naturally occurring disulfide), diallyl sulfide (DAS), diallyl disulfide (DADS), diallyl trisulfide (DAT), *S*-allylcysteine (SAC), organosulfur compounds, and allyl sulfur compounds.

granulocyte colony-stimulating factor (G-CSF, filgrastim, Neupogen) A natural chemical in the body that helps to control the production of white blood cells in the BONE MARROW.

G-CSF is sometimes given as medication with or after CHEMOTHERAPY, as a way of stimulating the production of white blood cells to decrease the risk of infection.

G-CSF was one of the first HEMATOPOIETIC GROWTH FACTORS approved and is an important part of BIOLOGICAL THERAPY. G-CSF also may allow patients to tolerate stronger chemotherapy regimens and enhance the effectiveness of chemotherapy drugs.

genes   Some genes appear to increase a man's risk of developing many different types of cancer, including PROSTATE CANCER and TESTICULAR CANCER.

Prostate Cancer

Genes have been linked to prostate cancer, especially in those men who were diagnosed with prostate cancer at a relatively young age (younger than 55 years old). The younger the person is when he is diagnosed, the higher the risk is for male relatives to have prostate cancer at a young age. Prostate cancer seems to run in some families, suggesting an inherited or genetic factor. Having a father or brother who has prostate cancer almost doubles a man's risk of developing this disease. The risk is even higher for men who have several affected relatives, particularly if their relatives were young at the time of diagnosis.

The causes of prostate cancer are still poorly understood, and reflect complex interactions between genetic and environmental factors. Still, genes are clearly important, because a man whose father and grandfather had prostate cancer is two to three times more likely to have the disease than a man with no such family history. The ethnic and family contributions to the probability of developing prostate cancer reveal that there is a strong genetic basis for this disease, as there is for most cancers.

Scientists have identified several inherited genes that seem to increase prostate cancer risk, although the genes probably account for only a small fraction of cases.

Some inherited genes increase the risk for more than one type of cancer. For example, inherited mutations of the *BRCA1* or *BRCA2* gene cause a higher risk of breast and ovarian cancers in women who inherit them. A man who inherits one of these gene mutations also has a higher prostate cancer risk; however, the mutations are responsible for a very small percentage of prostate cancer cases.

The genetics of inherited prostate cancer are complex, and family linkage studies suggest that mutations in at least six different genes may be involved. So far, scientists have identified a few genes that appear to be responsible for a man's inherited tendency to have prostate cancer:

- *HPC1* (hereditary prostate cancer gene 1)
- *HPC2* (also known as *ELAC2*)
- *HPCX* (found on the X chromosome)
- *CAPB* (named because of its connection to cancers of the prostate and brain)

Research on these genes is still preliminary, and genetic tests are not yet available.

Most gene mutations related to prostate cancer develop during a man's life rather than before birth. Every time a cell prepares to divide into two new cells, it must make a copy of its DNA. This process is not perfect, and sometimes errors occur. Fortunately, cells have repair enzymes that correct mistakes in the DNA. But some errors may slip past (especially if the cells are growing rapidly), leaving the DNA in the new cell with a mutation. Exposure to radiation or cancer-causing chemicals may cause DNA mutations in many organs of the body, but these factors have not been proved to be important causes of mutations in prostate cells.

Further studies of these genes could help shed light on the biological features of prostate cancer, which may provide suggestions for developing new treatments. Men who have a family history of prostate cancer who are concerned about an inherited risk for this disease should talk with their doctor, who may suggest consulting a health professional trained in genetics. Much more work is needed, however, before scientists can say exactly how changes in these genes are related to prostate cancer.

Testicular Cancer

HIWI, discovered at Duke University Medical Center in 2002, is the first gene known to be linked to testicular cancer. The Duke research shows that 63 percent of men who inherit the overactive form of the *hiwi* gene could develop SEMINOMA.

Testicular cancers are grouped into two main classes: seminoma and NONSEMINOMA. Nonseminomas tend to be more aggressive than seminomas and in most cases quickly spread to the lymph nodes.

Although *hiwi* is the first gene known to be highly correlated to seminoma, scientists are close to identifying other genes suspected of playing a role in other testicular cancers. Cancer researchers in the United Kingdom announced in February 2000 they had located (but not yet identified) a gene on a region of chromosome X associated with testicular cancer. The gene, *TGCT1*, can increase a men's risk of testicular cancer by up to 50 times. Other researchers have located testicular cancer susceptibility on chromosome 19 in mice.

gene therapy   A procedure in which healthy genes are inserted into a patient's blood to treat cancer, including PROSTATE CANCER. Prostate cells become malignant as a result of genetic changes within the cells; the goal of gene therapy is to place into the cancerous cells genes that cause the cancer cells to stop growing, be more susceptible to other therapy, or die.

There are several ways to insert the genes into cancer cells. The most popular method is to insert the gene into a modified harmless virus, which is then inserted into the prostate gland. Once inside the prostate, the virus transfers the gene to the prostate cells, including the malignant cells. This gene destroys the cancer cells.

Alternatively, the gene-containing viruses may be inserted into cancer cells that have been removed from the patient's body. After the gene has been transferred into the cancer cells by the virus, the cells are then returned to the patient. When the patient's own immune cells approach the cancer cells, they recognize the cancer cells as "foreign" and destroy them.

Clinical cancer centers across the United States are currently participating in gene therapy studies in the treatment of prostate cancer, including Johns Hopkins University School of Medicine, M. D. Anderson Cancer Center, and Duke University Medical Center.

germ cell   The cells within the testicle that in a male divides to produce the immature sperm cells. *Germ* means "seed"; the term refers to the role of male germ cells in producing sperm cells. The male germ cell remains intact throughout a man's reproductive life. Many types of male reproductive cancers, including 95 percent of all TESTICULAR CANCERS, are GERM CELL TUMORS.

germ cell tumors   Tumor that arise from GERM CELLS (the testicular cells that divide to produce

immature sperm). Up to 95 percent of all TESTICULAR CANCERS are germ cell tumors.

There are two main types of germ cell tumors in men: SEMINOMAS and NONSEMINOMAS. (The suffix *-oma* means "tumor.") Many testicle tumors contain features of both types. Because of the way these "mixed" tumors grow, spread, and respond to treatment, they are classified as being nonseminomas. Most invasive testicular germ cell cancers begin as a noninvasive form of the disease called CARCINOMA IN SITU (CIS) or INTRATUBULAR GERM CELL NEOPLASIA. Researchers have estimated that CIS takes about five years to progress to the invasive form of germ cell cancer. When a cancer becomes invasive, its cells have penetrated the surrounding tissues and may have spread through either the blood circulation or the lymph nodes to other parts of the body.

Blood tests including measures of ALPHA-FETO-PROTEIN and HUMAN CHORIONIC GONADOTROPIN can be used to help diagnose germ cell tumors.

germinoma   A type of tumor that develops from cells that normally make sperm (GERM CELLS) and may form in the testicles, among other locations. They occur most commonly in young people.

Gilda's Clubs   Nonprofit places where all patients who have any type of cancer (including male reproductive cancers) and their families and friends build social and emotional support as a supplement to medical care. Gilda's Clubs offer free support and networking groups, lectures, workshops and social events in a nonresidential, homelike setting. Funding is solicited from private individuals, corporations, and foundations. The Gilda's Club philosophy is to provide an emotional and social support community as an essential complement to medical treatment for people with cancer.

The Gilda's Club program is composed of the following elements that take place in every clubhouse:

• Support and networking groups, including weekly Wellness Groups for those living with cancer, Family Groups for family members and friends, and monthly Networking Groups focusing on a particular kind of cancer or topic of common interest (such as PROSTATE CANCER, cancer in young adults, and living solo with cancer).

- Lectures and workshops: Typical lecture topics, which are selected on the basis of members' interests, include stress reduction, nutrition, talking to children about cancer, and management of pain. Major workshop areas include art and other forms of self-expression, meditation, exercise and yoga, and cooking.

- Social activities: A range of gatherings from potluck suppers with music to karaoke nights to joke fests or comedy nights to major celebrations around special holidays.

- Team convene: Two-hour sessions requested by a person who has cancer or a family member to create an active support network at the time of diagnosis and for any challenging situations that may follow. Sessions include all significant friends and family in a member's life, who join together to provide support for transportation, food preparation, and child care.

- Family focus: A family meeting facilitated by a staff member designed to enlist the entire family as a resource and help them learn together how to live with cancer. It seeks to identify and discuss family beliefs about cancer, critical family issues, and immediate practical problems as well as solutions.

Gilda's Clubs are named in memory of comedian Gilda Radner, who died of ovarian cancer in 1989. Radner is best known for her work on NBC's *Saturday Night Live;* her book, *It's Always Something,* describes her life with cancer. Gilda's Clubs was founded by Joanna Bull, Radner's cancer psychotherapist, with the help of Radner's husband, Gene Wilder; Joel Siegel; and other friends.

All Gilda's Clubs have a warm and welcoming homelike atmosphere with a living room for reading and relaxing; support group rooms for weekly sessions led by licensed professionals; a workshop area for meditation, nutrition, stress reduction, and art projects; an It's Always Something room, a quiet place for personal time; and a large Community Meeting Room for potluck suppers, joke fests, and lectures. For contact information, see Appendix I.

Gleason grading system   A widely used method for classifying aggressive or malignant PROSTATE CANCER tumors by using a score from 1 to 10. A doctor uses this system to grade a tumor by describing how closely it resembles normal tissue. The less the cancerous cells resemble normal cells, the more malignant the cancer is. On the basis of the microscopic appearance of a tumor, pathologists may describe it as low-, medium-, or high-grade cancer. The higher the score, the higher the grade of tumor.

Because the cancer cells may be composed of many different grades, the pathologist assigns a value to the most common grades found in biopsy specimens. Two numbers (each from 1 to 5) are assigned successively to the two predominant patterns of differentiation present in the tissue sample examined; added together, these produce the Gleason score. The pathologist checks prostate tissue under a microscope to determine where the tumor is most prominent (the primary grade) and second-most prominent (secondary grade). The pathologist scores each of these two areas and adds the two together to derive the Gleason score (the primary grade is usually the first number). The range can thus be anywhere from a low of 2 (grade 1 and grade 1) to a high of 10 (grade 5 and grade 5). However, not all Gleason scores are equal. If two men both have a combined Gleason score of 7, the breakdown of those scores may be different. If the first man's score breaks down to a primary grade 3 and a secondary grade 4 and the second man has a primary grade 4 and a secondary grade 3, the first man may have better outlook because his cancer is more likely to be cured.

In general, however, the lower the combined Gleason score, the better. Numbers of 2, 3, and 4 indicate a well-differentiated cancer; 5 and 6 indicate a mildly aggressive cancer; grade 7 is considered moderately aggressive. High numbers (8, 9 and 10), indicate a highly aggressive tumor.

The system was devised by a pathologist, Dr. Donald Gleason, in 1966; Gleason invented the scale by studying the biopsy findings of more than 3,000 patients with prostate cancer. The Gleason score is used by pathologists throughout the world to grade prostate cancer tumors and is considered to be quite reliable.

Prostate cancer can be graded both before and after surgery, but the grading done after a prostate gland is removed may be more accurate because the pathologist has the entire gland to assess.

Grading done before surgery is performed on just a sliver of tissue from a biopsy. This means that after surgery, a man's grade may change (for better or worse).

glutathione *S*-transferase gene   A gene that directs the formation of glutathione *S*-transferase (GSTP1), an enzyme that detoxifies environmental carcinogens and protects against cancer. GSTP1 plays a key role in preventing precancerous prostate lesions (called PIA [proliferative inflammatory atrophy lesions] LESIONS) from becoming malignant. Investigators are studying the use of novel compounds and drugs to restore and/or compensate for missing or low levels of the enzyme. In fact, many of these compounds are found naturally in diets associated with lower prostate cancer risk.

Scientists have found that measuring the level of *GSTP1* could greatly strengthen standard detection of early-stage curable disease.

In PROSTATE CANCER patients, the *GSTP1* gene has probably been deactivated through a cellular process known as HYPERMETHYLATION. Methylation functions much as a cellular punctuation mark would: When levels of this substance are too low or too high, affected genes no longer function properly. In hypermethylation, high levels of methylation inactivate the *GSTP1* gene, shutting off its cancer-preventing properties. The altered *GTSP1* gene may cause the prostate to stop producing critical protective enzymes and as a result become defenseless against an ongoing onslaught of carcinogens that eventually results in prostate cancer. It is most often seen in early-stage prostate cancers and rarely in normal or benign prostate disease. Hypermethylation is known to be the most common genetic error in prostate cancer.

Finding a mutant *GSTP1* gene could be a genetic marker that would be found in early-stage prostate cancers.

GnRH antagonist (gonadotropin-releasing hormone antagonist)   A type of HORMONE THERAPY that directly suppresses the production of TESTOSTERONE without first raising the testosterone level, unlike LHRH (LUTEINIZING HORMONE–RELEASING HORMONE) ANALOGS. An example of a GnRH antagonist is ABARELIX.

gonadal aplasia   Failure of the testes to grow during fetal development. Scientists believe there may be a link between this condition and the later development of TESTICULAR CANCER.

gonads   The parts of the reproductive system that produce and release sperm (also called the TESTICLES or TESTES).

goserelin acetate (Zoladex)   A drug that belongs to the family of drugs called gonadotropin-releasing hormone analogs. Goserelin is used to block hormone production in the testicles.

grading   A laboratory diagnostic process that determines the aggressiveness of cells taken from a malignant tumor. The cancer cells' aggression is assessed by how similar to normal cells they appear to be, which provides their degree of DIFFERENTIATION or histologic tumor grade. The more normal the cell (that is, the more differentiated), the lower the grade and the better the prognosis. Tumor grade often plays a role in treatment decisions.

granulocyte   A type of white blood cell that is produced in bone marrow; granulocytes include neutrophils, basophils, and eosinophils. These white blood cells fight infectious organisms by engulfing them; these actions may contribute to inflammation and are responsible for allergic reactions.

gynecomastia   Excessive development of the breast in men. In rare cases, men who have GERM CELL cancer notice breast growth or tenderness. This symptom occurs when certain types of germ cell tumors secrete high levels of a hormone called HUMAN CHORIONIC GONADOTROPIN (hCG). BLOOD TESTS can measure hCG levels; these tests are important in diagnosis, staging, and follow-up of some of these cancers. This condition also may be a side effect of hormonal therapy for prostate cancers.

hair loss One of the most common (and upsetting) side effects of CHEMOTHERAPY. Although a few drugs used to treat cancer do not affect the hair, most cause partial or complete hair loss during treatment. Chemotherapy affects the rapidly dividing cells of the hair follicle, making hair brittle so that it may break off near the scalp or spontaneously release. This usually begins two to three weeks after the first chemotherapy treatment.

The amount of hair lost depends on the type of drug or combination of drugs used, the dosage given, and the person's individual reaction to the drug. Body hair may be lost as well, and a few drugs even trigger loss of the eyelashes and eyebrows. If patients do lose hair as a result of chemotherapy, it almost always regrows once treatment is over.

Patients who have lost their hair during chemotherapy need to take special care of their scalp and any remaining hair. They should use mild shampoos and soft hair brushes. Hair should be cut short, because a shorter style makes remaining hair appear thicker and fuller; it also makes any hair loss easier to manage.

Once hair loss occurs, patients should use a sunscreen, sunblock, hat, or scarf to protect the scalp from the sun. Although hair loss is not life threatening, it can have an emotional and psychological impact, causing depression, loss of self-esteem, and even grief reactions.

hCG See HUMAN CHORIONIC GONADOTROPIN.

health care proxy A legal type of ADVANCE DIRECTIVE (also called a health care POWER OF ATTORNEY) that gives another person the authority to make decisions related to health care for a patient who has become unable to do so. Patients usually choose as proxy someone whom they trust to represent their preferences when they can no longer communicate their wishes.

A patient should be sure to ask whether this person is willing to serve as proxy, since an agent may have to exercise judgment in the event of a medical decision for which the patient's wishes are not known.

The health care proxy is a legal document that should be signed, dated, witnessed, notarized, copied, distributed, and incorporated into the patient's medical record.

Patients also may want to appoint someone to manage their financial affairs if they cannot. The durable power of attorney for finances is a different legal document from the healthy care proxy. Patients may choose the same person or another to act as their agent in financial matters.

health insurance The cost of treating cancer can be high, but health insurance plans will usually cover much of the cost. Patients who belong to a health maintenance organization (HMO) or preferred provider organization (PPO) should become familiar with their provider choices and their financial responsibility if they receive care "out of network" from a doctor not covered by the health plan.

Cancer patients who do not have insurance should contact their local Social Security Office to determine if they qualify for SUPPLEMENTAL SECURITY INCOME (SSI) or SOCIAL SECURITY DISABILITY INSURANCE (SSDI). The medical requirements and disability determination process are the same under both programs. However, while eligibility for SSDI is based on employment history, SSI is based on financial need.

Cancer patients without insurance also can receive care from hospitals who receive federal grants from Hill-Burton funds that allow hospitals and nursing homes to provide low-cost or no-cost medical care. To receive a listing of hospitals or nursing homes participating in the Hill-Burton program, patients can call (800) 638-0742.

See also FINANCIAL ISSUES.

hematospermia Presence of blood in the semen. This condition is only rarely associated with malignant cancers of the testicles or prostate. The cause of hematospermia is often poorly understood, but may be caused by inflammation of the urethra, prostate, or seminal vesicles.

Semen is produced by many organs, including the testicles, EPIDIDYMIS, vas deferens, seminal vesicles, and prostate. Most semen originates in the seminal vesicles and prostate, and it is probably from these two organs that most blood finds its way into semen. Infection or inflammation of the organs listed accounts for most of the other cases of hematospermia. In addition, up to a third of patients who have an ultrasound-guided prostate biopsy experience hematospermia afterward. Cancer accounts for only a very small percentage of hemospermic diagnoses.

In primary hematospermia, the patient's only symptom is blood in the ejaculate (there is no blood in the urine); the patient has no symptoms of urinary irritation or infection, and physical exam findings are completely normal. In patients who have this type of hematospermia with no other symptoms, the blood recedes in time without treatment. About 17 percent of patients have one episode and no recurrence.

Secondary hematospermia is diagnosed when the cause of bleeding is known or suspected, such as blood that appears immediately after a prostate biopsy or in the presence of a urinary or prostate infection or cancer. Rarely, the blood may be linked to tuberculosis, parasitic infections, or diseases that affect blood clotting, such as hemophilia and chronic liver disease.

Patients who have hematospermia associated with symptoms of urinary infection or blood in the urine, or who have persistent hematospermia for longer than three weeks, should have further urologic evaluation to identify the specific cause. The physical exam should include a genital and rectal exam, as well as a blood pressure test, because high blood pressure can be associated with hematospermia.

Some urologists recommend TRANSRECTAL ULTRASOUND to look for stones and cysts in the prostate, seminal vesicles, and ejaculatory ducts and to rule out PROSTATE CANCER. Other urologists recommend CYSTOSCOPY because hematospermia can be related to urethral and prostate problems.

In general, however, hematospermia almost always fades away spontaneously and rarely is associated with significant problems.

hemibody radiation A type of RADIATION THERAPY utilizing larger areas of the body in an attempt to halt the spread of painful PROSTATE CANCER in the bones. Hemibody radiation is administered in several different treatment sessions that may help control bone pain up to a year for most patients.

Because this type of radiation affects a larger portion of the body, it usually causes more side effects, such as lowered blood pressure, NAUSEA and vomiting, DIARRHEA, lung irritation, HAIR LOSS, and low blood cell counts.

heredity and cancer See GENES.

herpes, genital A sexually transmitted viral infection characterized by repeated attacks of small, painful blisters on the genitals, around the rectum, or on adjacent areas of skin. Men who have genital herpes are at higher risk for PENILE CANCER.

high-intensity focused ultrasound (HIFU) An experimental technique used to treat localized PROSTATE CANCER in which a device administers heat-producing ultrasound to destroy local cancer cells within the prostate. This experimental technique is less invasive than other types of heat-producing probes.

See also CRYOTHERAPY; MICROWAVE THERAPY.

Hill-Burton Free Hospital Care A program sponsored by the U.S. government in which certain medical facilities or hospitals must provide free or low-cost care to patients who meet certain low-income guidelines. Hill-Burton facilities also are responsible for providing emergency treatment and for treating all patients who live in the service area, regardless of race, color, national origin, creed or Medicare or Medicaid status.

Each facility chooses which services it will provide at no or reduced cost. Services fully covered by third-party insurance or a government program such as Medicare or Medicaid are not eligible for Hill-Burton coverage. However, Hill-Burton may pay for services not included in government programs.

Private pharmacy and private physician fees are not covered by this program, but services provided by doctors may be covered under the Hill-Burton program.

Hill-Burton facilities include hospitals, nursing homes, and clinics. To find local Hill-Burton facilities, patients can check the state-by-state directory listing at the Hill-Burton Web site (www.hrsa.gov/osp/dfcr). Although a facility may be listed in the directory, patients still must call the facility to be certain that it has funds available and that the service desired is still covered. A patient interested in free care should apply at the admissions, business, or patient accounts office. Eligibility is based on a person's family size and income, calculated on actual income for the past 12 months (or last three months' income multiplied by four, whichever is less). Patients may qualify if their income falls within the federal poverty guidelines or their income is up to double (or triple, for nursing home services) the poverty guidelines. Gross income includes interest and dividends earned and child support payments, but not assets, food stamps, gifts, loans, or one-time insurance payments. (For self-employed people, income is determined after deductions for business expenses.)

Patients may apply for Hill-Burton assistance at any time before or after receiving care—even after a bill has been sent to a collection agency. If a hospital obtains a court judgment before the patient applies for Hill-Burton assistance, the solution must be worked out within the judicial system, but if patients applied for Hill-Burton before a judgment was rendered and they are found eligible, they receive Hill-Burton aid even if a judgment is given while waiting for a response to their application. The program is open to both citizens and noncitizens who have lived in the United States for at least three months.

Patients who believe they were unfairly denied services or discriminated against should contact the Office for Civil Rights (OCR) at (800) 368-1019.

Hispanics/Latinos Cancer affects different racial and ethnic groups differently. As of 2003, compared to non-Hispanic Caucasians, Hispanic/Latino-American men have lower incidence and mortality from PROSTATE CANCER, but are less likely to use screening tests for this condition, according to the journal of the American Cancer Society. (People from Cuba, Mexico, Puerto Rico, South or Central America, and other Spanish cultures—regardless of race—are considered Hispanic.)

Many of the differences in prostate cancer incidence and mortality rates among racial and ethnic groups may be due to factors associated with social class rather than ethnicity. Socioeconomic status in particular appears to play a major role in the differences in cancer incidence and mortality rates, risk factors, and screening prevalence among racial and ethnic minorities. Moreover, studies have found that socioeconomic status more than race predicts the likelihood of a group's access to education, certain jobs, and health insurance, as well as income level and living conditions. All of these factors are associated with a person's probability of cancer development and survival.

HLA See HUMAN LEUKOCYTE ANTIGEN.

hormonal ablation therapy See HORMONAL THERAPY.

hormonal therapy A type of treatment that interrupts the supply of male hormones (such as TESTOSTERONE) that encourage cancer growth, either by medication or by surgery to remove the testicles (the main source of testosterone). This treatment is used in some types of male reproductive cancer (such as PROSTATE CANCER). Hormonal therapy may be used in combination with RADIATION TREATMENT or PROSTATECTOMY (removal of the prostate) in both early and advanced prostate cancers.

Hormonal therapy also may be used to relieve the pain and other symptoms of advanced disease. Although hormonal therapy cannot cure cancer, it usually shrinks the tumor and slows the advance of disease.

In SURGICAL CASTRATION, surgeons remove the testicles (ORCHIECTOMY) through a small incision in the scrotum. The surgery is permanent and the effects cannot be reversed. In MEDICAL CASTRATION (or chemical castration), doctors administer a luteinizing hormone–releasing hormone analog (LHRHa) such as leuprolide, goserelin, or buserelin. These drugs work by switching off the production of male hormones in the testicles by reducing the level of luteinizing hormone. This hormone is produced by the pituitary gland at the base of the brain. This type of castration is reversible; if treatment is stopped, testosterone is produced once again. Most men who undergo castration (surgical or medical) experience a loss of sexual desire and hot flushes.

After surgery to remove the testicles, or treatment with an LHRH analog, the testicles no longer produce testosterone. However, the adrenal glands still produce small amounts of male hormones. For this reason, the patient also may be given antiandrogens such as KETOCONAZOLE or aminoglutethimide, FLUTAMIDE or BICALUTAMIDE to block the effects of any remaining male hormones. Combination hormone therapy involving a complete blockage of androgen production including orchiectomy or LHRH analogs, plus the use of antiandrogens drugs is also called total hormonal ablation, total androgen blockade, or total androgen ablation.

Doctors are not sure whether total androgen blockade is more effective than orchiectomy or LHRH analogs alone. Prostate cancer that has spread to other parts of the body usually can be controlled with a hormonal therapy for some time (often years). Although hormone therapy may delay the progression of prostate cancer, however, its influence on survival is not well known. Eventually, most prostate cancers are able to grow with very little or no male hormones. When this happens, hormonal therapy is no longer effective, and the doctor may suggest other forms of treatment that are under study.

Men who have high-grade prostate cancer (Gleason score above 7) or cancer in the seminal vesicles or lymph nodes at surgery and who experience a rise in prostate-specific antigen (PSA) level within two years of prostatectomy probably have metastatic disease and are candidates for hormone therapy.

Side Effects

The side effects of hormonal therapy depend largely on the type of treatment. Orchiectomy and LHRH analogs often cause side effects such as impotence, HOT FLASHES, and loss of sexual desire. When first used, an LHRH analog may make a patient's symptoms worse for a short time; this temporary problem is called flare. Gradually, however, the treatment causes the testosterone level to fall. Without testosterone, tumor growth slows and the patient's condition improves. (To prevent flare, the doctor may give the man an antiandrogen for a while along with the LHRH analog.)

Antiandrogens can cause NAUSEA, vomiting, DIARRHEA, or breast growth or tenderness. If used over a long period, ketoconazole may cause liver problems, and aminoglutethimide can cause skin rashes. Men who receive total androgen blockade may experience more side effects than men who receive a single method of hormonal therapy. Any method of hormonal therapy that lowers androgen levels can contribute to weakening of the bones in older men.

Hormone-Refractory Prostate Cancer

When a man's PSA level continues to increase despite all forms of hormone therapy, the cancer is called hormone refractory, meaning it is resistant to hormone therapy. In this case, a doctor may prescribe chemotherapy.

Hormonal therapy may be given *before* prostatectomy or radiation therapy to reduce the size of the prostate; this is called neoadjuvant hormone therapy. The treatment also may be used *after* prostatectomy or radiation (adjuvant hormone therapy) to affect any cancer cells that remain after prostatectomy or radiation therapy.

hormones Chemical substances produced in one organ that influences activity of cells or another organ in another part of the body. Many hormones are believed to stimulate the growth of a variety of cancers. For example, PROSTATE CANCER is stimulated by the hormones TESTOSTERONE and DIHYDROTESTOSTERONE (a chemical made from testosterone by the body). This is why HORMONE THERAPY is sometimes used to try to block the hormones that the prostate cancer cells need to grow.

hospice A concept, rather than a place of care, that focuses on a holistic model of services designed neither to hasten nor to postpone death, but rather to make a patient's final days as positive and symptom-free as possible. It is based on a philosophy of caring that respects and values the dignity and worth of each person. Although hospices care for people who are approaching death, they cherish and emphasize life by helping patients and families live each day to the fullest. There are almost 3,000 hospice and palliative care organizations in the United States. Hospice services can be provided to a terminally ill person even in a nursing home, so that the patient receives visits from hospice nurses, home health aides, chaplains, social workers, and volunteers, in addition to other care and services provided by the nursing home.

A few hospice programs have their own facilities or have arrangements with freestanding hospice houses, hospitals, or inpatient residential centers to care for patients who cannot live in a private residence. These patients may require an alternative place to live during this final phase of their life when they need extra care.

The modern American hospice movement began in 1974 when the Connecticut Hospice was established in New Haven. It was founded on a care model outlined by Dame Cicely Saunders, M.D., who opened the Saint Christopher's Hospice in 1967 in Sydenham, England. This center became the model for hospice care around the world.

How It Works

Hospice care usually starts as soon as a formal referral is made by the patient's doctor. Often a hospice program representative tries to visit the patient on the day the referral is made; in any case, care begins within a day or two of a referral.

Typically, a family member serves as the primary caregiver and, when appropriate, helps make decisions for the terminally ill individual. Hospice is a medical benefit covered by most insurance plans, enabling patients to stay at home at the end of their life and receive care from an integrated hospice team of nurses, medical social workers, physical and occupational therapists, nutritionists, home aide workers, pastoral counselors, and trained volunteers.

Patients can continue to be treated by their own physician or by the hospice physician. If the hospice patient chooses to have the family doctor involved in the medical care, the patient's physician and the hospice medical director may work together to coordinate the patient's medical care, especially when symptoms are difficult to manage.

Members of the hospice staff make regular visits to assess the patient and provide additional care or other services and are on call 24 hours a day, seven days a week. Every hospice patient can take advantage of services offered by a registered nurse, social worker, home health aide, and chaplain. Typically, full-time registered nurses provide care to about 12 different families, and social workers usually handle about twice that number. If needed, home health aides who can provide personal care to the patient visit most often; all visits are subject to the needs described in the care plan and the condition of the patient during the course of the illness. The availability and frequency of spiritual care often depend on the family request.

In addition, hospice volunteers enhance quality of life and ease the burden of caregiving. Volunteers usually can provide different types of support to patients and their family, including running errands, preparing light meals, staying with a patient to give family members a break, lending emotional support and companionship, and helping out with light housekeeping.

Care Plan

The hospice team develops a care plan that meets each patient's individual needs for pain management and symptom control and outlines the medical and support services required, such as nursing care, personal care (dressing, bathing), social services, physician visits, counseling, and homemaker services. It also identifies the medical equipment, tests, procedures, medication, and treatments necessary to provide high-quality comfort care.

While patients are at home, all necessary symptom-relieving medications are provided by hospice workers, along with any necessary special medical equipment. In emergencies, hospice workers take patients to a hospital or hospice inpatient unit designed to be as homelike as possible. Inpatient respite care is also available to provide a break for families.

Other Services

Besides medical aid, hospice workers help patients with practical support (such as shopping) and emotional support, including life closure, grief, and spiritual counseling. Depending on the hospice's resources, it may also provide other services such as art, touch, and music therapy.

Paying for Hospice

Medicare, private health insurance, and Medicaid (in 43 states) cover hospice care for patients who meet eligibility criteria. As in any health-care program, there may be copayments and deductibles that families pay to receive care, but many hospices also rely on community support for donations. Each hospice has its own policies about payment, but traditionally hospice offers services based on need, rather than ability to pay.

Hospice care is available as a benefit under Medicare Part A, which is designed to give patients who have terminal illness and their family special support and services not otherwise covered by Medicare. Under the Medicare Hospice Benefit, beneficiaries choose to receive noncurative treatment and services for their terminal illness by waiving the standard Medicare benefits for treatment of a terminal illness. However, the beneficiary may continue to access standard Medicare benefits for treatment of conditions unrelated to the terminal illness. Medicare law states that to qualify for hospice care, a patient must have "a medical prognosis that life expectancy is six months or less if the illness runs its normal course." However, it is difficult to predict how much time is left to a patient with cancer, and ben-

eficiaries are not restricted to six months of coverage by hospice rules.

Finding a Program

Patients and families can get information about local hospices from health-care professionals, social workers, clergy, counselors, friends or neighbors, their local or state Office on Aging or senior centers, health-related Web sites, or the phone book. Alternatively, patients may contact the NATIONAL HOSPICE AND PALLIATIVE CARE ORGANIZATION (NHPCO), which represents most hospice programs in the United States, at (800) 658-8898 or http://www.nhpco.org/database.htm.

See also HOSPICE FOUNDATION OF AMERICA.

Hospice Education Institute An independent nonprofit organization founded in 1985 that serves a wide range of individuals and organizations interested in improving and expanding HOSPICE and palliative care throughout the United States and around the world. The institute works to educate and support people seeking or providing care for the dying and the bereaved or those coping with loss or advanced illness.

The institute offers a range of programs, including HOSPICELINK, which maintains a directory of hospice programs; a gift program offering small gifts to patients and their families; and seminars, books, and pamphlets. For contact information, see Appendix I.

Hospice Foundation of America A nonprofit organization that promotes HOSPICE care and educates professionals and those they serve about caregiving, terminal illness, loss, and bereavement. The foundation provides leadership in the development and application of hospice and its philosophy of care. Hospice Foundation, Inc., was chartered in 1982 as a way to help raise money for hospices operating in South Florida, before passage of the Medicare hospice benefit. In 1990 the foundation expanded its scope to a national level in order to provide leadership in the entire spectrum of end-of-life issues.

To reflect its national scope more accurately, in 1992 the foundation opened a Washington, D.C., office and in 1994 changed its name to Hospice

Foundation of America. For contact information, see Appendix I.

HospiceLink   A service offered by the HOSPICE EDUCATION INSTITUTE that maintains a computerized directory of all hospice and palliative care programs in the United States. The toll-free telephone number, (800) 331-1620, provides referrals to hospice and palliative care programs and general information about the principles and practices of good hospice and palliative care. For contact information, see Appendix I.

hot flashes   A sensation of heat and flushing that occurs suddenly during HORMONE THERAPY. Although hot flashes are usually associated with menopause in women, they also may occur in men during treatment with many types of hormone therapy. The reason hot flashes are associated with hormone therapy is not well understood, but they appear to be linked to the sudden drop in TESTOSTERONE level and the effect of testosterone on blood vessels.

For example, in one study of men receiving hormone therapy before radical PROSTATECTOMY, 80 percent experienced hot flashes, which continued for more than three months in 10 percent of cases. Men taking hormone therapy for more than four months were more likely to experience hot flashes. About 75 percent of all men being treated with hormone therapy for prostate cancer report hot flashes that began between a month and a year after the beginning of hormone therapy.

There are different treatments for the hot flashes associated with hormone therapy. Medications include the blood pressure medicine clonidine (Catapres) and the hormones megestrol acetate (Megace), medroxyprogesterone acetate (Provera or Depo-Provera), the antidepressant venlafaxine, and diethylstilbestrol (DES).

Limiting caffeine intake and avoiding very warm temperatures and excessive exercise also may help.

HPC-1   A specific location on chromosome 1 of a gene that scientists believe may be the place where the familial PROSTATE CANCER gene is found. The existence of a prostate cancer gene has been sus-

pected because of a clear link between a family history of prostate cancer and a man's risk of developing the disease. Prostate cancer that is believed to have a genetic basis is called hereditary prostate cancer (HPC).

Investigators at the Brady Urological Institute at Johns Hopkins Hospital, the National Human Genome Research Institute, and Umea University in Sweden first linked the disease to a gene located at *HPC-1*. The specific gene has not been isolated, but scientists believe it probably is responsible for about one-third to half of all cases of hereditary prostate cancer.

Only about 10 percent of all cases of prostate cancer are thought to be predominantly hereditary, but many scientists believe that the defective gene or mechanisms involved in hereditary cancer are the same ones that somehow go awry in the more common sporadic cancer that develops over the course of a lifetime.

Most scientists believe that cancer is triggered by a combination of mutations of a variety of genes that may be inherited or acquired as a result of environmental factors such as diet or smoking or of random mistakes in the replication or repair of DNA.

Researchers hope that identifying the chromosomal location associated with some cases of hereditary prostate cancer will lead to the identification of a specific gene involved in the development of prostate cancer. This should enable doctors to identify families who carry this mutated form of the gene and men who are at high risk for prostate cancer. Ultimately, the goal is either to develop treatments to prevent prostate cancer or to develop tests that help doctors detect prostate cancer in time to cure it.

Men who have hereditary prostate cancer tend to develop the disease far sooner than other men— even as young as the late 30s or early 40s. By the time these men start routine screening for prostate cancer, it may already be too late to cure.

An estimated 250,000 American men may have a genetic defect at the *HPC-1* location on chromosome 1.

The gene may be active over a wide variety of geographic regions and ethnic backgrounds. In the study, susceptibility was found in Caucasian and black men scattered throughout the United States, as well as Caucasians in Canada and Sweden.

Until more is learned about hereditary prostate cancer, men who have a family history of the disease should have a DIGITAL RECTAL EXAM (DRE) and a prostate-specific antigen (PSA) BLOOD TEST every year beginning at age 40.

human chorionic gonadotropin (hCG) A hormone whose level rises significantly in men with TROPHOBLASTIC TUMOR or nonseminomatous GERM CELL TUMORS. For this reason, it is used as a TUMOR MARKER for a number of different cancers, including TESTICULAR CANCER. High levels of beta-human chorionic gonadotropin (beta-hCG) are found in 100 percent of patients with trophoblastic tumors and 40 to 60 percent of patients with nonseminomatous germ cell tumors, all patients with CHORIOCARCINOMA, 80 percent of patients with EMBRYONAL CARCINOMA, and 10 to 25 percent of patients with pure SEMINOMA.

Because half of the beta-hCG in the blood disappears after 24 to 36 hours, the inference is that high levels should return to normal within five to seven days after surgery if all tumor is removed.

A normal hCG level is usually less than 5 mIU/ml. However, it is also possible that the hCG level can become elevated (a false positive finding) as a result of abnormally low levels of testosterone or of marijuana use.

See also IMMUNE SYSTEM.

human immunodeficiency virus and testicular cancer There is some evidence that men who are infected with the human immunodeficiency virus (HIV)—and especially those men who have developed full-blown AIDS—are at increased risk for development of TESTICULAR CANCER. If they do have testicle cancer, most of these men can be cured by using standard treatment (ORCHIECTOMY, CHEMOTHERAPY, and RADIATION THERAPY) and can experience improved quality of life despite their HIV status.

human papillomavirus (HPV) A virus that causes the common wart on hands and feet, as well as warts in the genital area. Infection by human papillomavirus (HPV) is believed by many researchers to

be the most important preventable risk factor for PENILE CANCER.

HPVs are a group of more than 70 types of viruses called papillomaviruses because they can cause warts (papillomas). Different HPV types cause different types of warts in different parts of the body. Some types cause common warts on the hands and feet, on lips or tongue; certain other types of HPV types can infect the genitals and the anal area. These HPV types are passed from one person to another during sexual contact. Having sex at an early age, having multiple sexual partners, having sex with a partner who has had multiple other partners, and having unprotected sex at any age increase a person's risk of HPV infection.

When HPV infects the skin of the external genital organs and anal area, the virus often causes raised bumpy warts that range from barely visible to several inches across. The medical term for genital warts is *condyloma acuminatum.* Most genital warts are caused by two HPV types, HPV-6 and HPV-11. These rarely develop into cancer and are called low-risk viruses. However, other sexually transmitted HPVs have been linked with genital or anal cancers in both men and women. These high-risk HPV types include HPV-16, HPV-18, HPV-33, HPV-35, and HPV-45.

Many studies have shown the presence of HPV types 16 and 18 in penile carcinoma. In an examination of 30 specimens of penile cancer, the HPV-16 genome was found in 15 patients (65 percent), HPV-30 in three patients (13 percent), and HPV-6 or HPV-11 in two patients (9 percent).

The mechanism by which HPV transforms a cell into a malignancy is probably mediated through two viral genes (E6 and E7) that are actively transcribed in HPV-infected cells. The E6 and E7 proteins bind to and inactivate the host cell's tumor suppressor gene products, leading to uncontrolled growth.

In men, HPVs can also cause flat warts on the penis that are not visible and cause no symptoms. Flat warts caused by low-risk HPV types have little or no effect on cancer risk, but flat warts caused by high-risk types can develop into cancers.

Treatment

There is currently no cure for human papillomavirus infection. However, the warts and abnormal cell growth caused by these viruses can be effectively destroyed, preventing them from developing into cancers. New tests that are now available can directly identify the DNA from HPVs and identify the exact HPV type causing the infection. At this time, it is not clear how treatment should be affected by this information. HPV testing and typing are not presently routinely recommended and most health-care providers do not use this testing. However, scientists are searching for ways to determine the potential role of this test in preventing cancers of the male and female genital organs.

hyperechoic   A part of an ultrasound image where the echoes are brighter than normal or brighter than the surrounding structures. Hyperechoic areas are generally denser than surrounding structures and appear brighter on ultrasound image. Calcifications are commonly seen as hyperechoic signals.

hypermethylation   A biochemical process that causes a gene to stop working. Hypermethylation on certain prostate genes can shut off its cancer-preventing properties so that the prostate stops producing critical protective enzymes. This can lead to the development of prostate cancer.

In PROSTATE CANCER patients, hypermethylation can lead to the deactivation of the GLUTATHIONE S-TRANSFERASE gene, shutting off its cancer-preventing properties. Scientists suspect the altered gene may cause the prostate to stop producing critical protective enzymes and, as a result, become defenseless against an ongoing onslaught of carcinogens that eventually results in prostate cancer. It is most often seen in early-stage prostate cancers and rarely in normal or benign prostate disease. Hypermethylation is the most common genetic error in prostate cancer.

hyperplasia   Enlargement of an organ or tissue caused by an increase in the number of constituent cells.

See also BENIGN PROSTATIC HYPERPLASIA.

hypoechoic   A part of an ultrasound image where the echoes are not as bright as normal or are less bright than the surrounding structures. Hypoechoic structures in the testicle usually indicate the presence of a solid mass inside the testicle and indicate that the mass is very likely to be cancerous and should be removed.

ifosfamide (Ifex) An anticancer drug related to the nitrogen mustards that is active in a number of cancers, including GERM CELL TUMORS.

immune system and cancer The body's immune system plays a critical role in controlling cancerous cell development, in addition to attacking and killing a range of foreign substances such as viruses and bacteria. The immune system attacks cancer cells, not because they are foreign—which they are not—but because the cells' biological function has gone awry so that it cannot respond to the body's normal methods of controlling cell growth and reproduction. As a result, the abnormal cells continue to grow, leading to cancer. This is why cancer is 100 times more likely to occur in people who take drugs that suppress the immune system (such as someone who has had an organ transplant) than in people who have a normal immune system.

Most of the time, the body is protected against cancer by the immune system, which can detect the appearance of tumor antigens (a foreign substance that the immune system recognizes and targets for destruction) on cancer cells. These antigens attract the attention of certain kinds of white blood cells responsible for destroying cancer cells.

Antigens are found on the surface of all cells; when a cell becomes cancerous, new antigens that the immune system does not recognize suddenly appear on the cell's surface. With luck, the immune system may regard these new "tumor antigens" as foreign and may be able to contain or destroy the cancer cells. Unfortunately, even a very healthy immune system cannot always destroy every cancer cell.

So far, tumor antigens have been identified in several types of cancer, including malignant melanoma, bone cancer (osteosarcoma), and some gastrointestinal cancers. People who have these cancers may have antibodies against the tumor antigens, but the antigens generally do not trigger a strong enough immune response to control the cancer. For some reason, the immune system's antibodies do not seem to be able to destroy the cancer; sometimes, they even seem to stimulate the tumor's growth.

Certain tumor antigens can be used to help diagnose cancer, however. Antigens released into the bloodstream by some cancers can be detected with blood tests; in this case, they are called tumor markers because their presence in the blood indicates that a tumor is growing. Scientists are trying to determine whether tumor markers can be used to screen healthy people for cancer. Because the tests are expensive and not very specific, their routine use is not recommended. On the other hand, tumor markers are quite valuable in both diagnosis and treatment of cancer. Blood tests can help determine whether a cancer treatment is effective, because after treatment if the tumor marker no longer appears in the blood, experts assume that the cancerous cells are gone. If the marker disappears and later reappears, the doctor assumes the cancer has recurred.

There are several types of tumor antigen markers present in male reproductive cancers.

ALPHA-FETOPROTEIN (AFP), normally produced by fetal liver cells, is also found in the blood of people who have certain types of TESTICULAR CANCER.

HUMAN CHORIONIC GONADOTROPIN (hCG) is a hormone produced during pregnancy that also appears in men who have various types of testicular cancer. Beta-hCG is a very sensitive tumor marker used to monitor the effects of treatment.

PROSTATE-SPECIFIC ANTIGEN (PSA) level is high in men who have benign prostate gland enlargement, and considerably higher in men who have PROSTATE CANCER. Experts still are not sure exactly how high a level must be before it becomes significant, but men who have a raised PSA level should be tested further for prostate cancer. In addition, monitoring the blood level of PSA after treatment for prostate or testicular cancer can indicate whether the cancer has recurred.

High levels of LACTATE DEHYDROGENASE (LDH) occur in testicular cancer, but tests for this antigen are not currently recommended for cancer screening. However, LDH levels are useful in monitoring the response to treatment of a person already diagnosed with cancer.

immune therapy A type of treatment that boosts the patient's ability to fight off cancer. It is currently being tested as a possible treatment for PROSTATE CANCER; the patient's immune cells are removed from the blood and mixed with prostate cancer cells. After the immune cells are mixed with the malignant cells, they are re-injected into the patient's body, where they theoretically should help fight cancer.

In another type of immune therapy, substances from the patient's prostate cells or prostate cancer cells are injected into the patient's body in the hope that the body will become immune to the substances in the cancer cells.

implant radiation See BRACHYTHERAPY.

impotence See ERECTILE DYSFUNCTION.

infection Patients undergoing CHEMOTHERAPY are at greater risk for developing life-threatening infections because the drugs affect the bone marrow, inhibiting production of infection-fighting white blood cells. The blood cells are usually at their lowest level from seven to 14 days after the chemotherapy treatment, although this will vary depending on the type of chemotherapy. As the number of white cells in the blood fall, patients will be more likely to get an infection. For this reason, oncologists order regular blood tests to show the number of white cells in the blood.

Most infections come from bacteria normally found on the skin and in the mouth, intestines, and genital tract. Sometimes, the cause of an infection may not be known. Symptoms include the following:

- fever above 100°F or 38°C.
- shaking chills
- sweating
- diarrhea
- urgency to urinate or burning urination
- severe cough or sore throat
- unusual vaginal discharge or itching
- redness, swelling, or tenderness, especially around a wound, sore, pimple, rectal area or catheter site
- sinus pain or pressure
- earaches, headaches, or stiff neck
- blisters on the lips or skin or mouth sores

Treatment

If patients get an infection when their white blood cell level is very low, they may need antibiotics given directly into the bloodstream. Sometimes, drugs called growth factors can help the bone marrow make more white blood cells. Growth factors are sometimes given after chemotherapy treatment to stimulate the bone marrow to produce new white cells quickly, thereby reducing the risk of infection.

Prevention

Chemotherapy patients can prevent a great many infections by being very careful not to injure themselves or eat potentially tainted food. Patients should wash their hands often during the day, especially before meals, and after using the toilet or touching animals. The rectal area should be cleaned gently but thoroughly after each bowel movement.

Patients should avoid crowds during those periods when their white counts are lowest and should stay away from people with contagious diseases, such as colds, the flu, measles, or chicken pox. Patients should also avoid contact with children who have recently received "live virus" vaccines, such as chicken pox and oral polio, because they may be contagious to people with a low blood cell count.

Patients should be careful to avoid breaking the skin when using scissors or nail scissors, knives or razors, and should not squeeze or scratch pimples or insect bites. Cuts and scrapes that do occur should be cleaned daily until healed with warm water, soap, and an antiseptic. Good oral hygiene and daily baths can help prevent infections, and lotion or oil can soften and heal skin that has become dry and cracked. Protective gloves should be worn when gardening or cleaning up after others.

Patients should avoid contact with animal litter boxes and waste, bird cages, and fish tanks and avoid standing water in bird baths, flower vases, or humidifiers. They should not get any immunizations, such as flu or pneumonia shots, without checking with a doctor first and should avoid raw fish, seafood, meat, and eggs.

infertility and cancer Certain cancers (especially TESTICULAR CANCER) can severely impair sperm production, and cancer treatment (CHEMOTHERAPY, SURGERY, and RADIATION THERAPY) can harm sperm cells. Cancer survivors typically have more problems with fertility than do couples who have never had cancer, and birth rates among cancer survivors are only 40 percent to 85 percent of the expected rates. Today, as millions of men of childbearing age are surviving cancer, the question of reproduction is arising as a paramount consideration in planning treatment.

In some cases, infertility also may be a symptom of some types of cancer, such as testicular cancer. Men who develop testicular cancer father fewer children and are more likely to have been diagnosed with infertility problems before their cancer diagnosis. Scientists suspect that inability to impregnate a woman may be a manifestation of unhealthy testes in which cancer eventually develops.

Danish researchers examining the relationship between increasing rates of testicular cancer and decreasing sperm quality also have concluded that men who have infertility problems have an increased risk of developing the disease. The study found a strong association between infertility problems and the subsequent risk of testicular cancer: Men in couples who had fertility problems were more than one and a half times more likely to have testicular cancer than other men. Men who had poor overall semen quality were two to three times more likely to develop testicular cancer.

Moreover, men who had a low sperm count who had fathered children in the past had a lower risk of developing testicular cancer than men who had been unable to father children.

In the Danish study, researchers analyzed the sperm quality of semen samples taken from more than 32,000 men in Copenhagen between 1963 and 1995. The risk remained constant over time, suggesting that sperm abnormalities had been present many years before the diagnosis of cancer. Researchers conclude that there may be common risk factors for poor sperm quality and testicular cancer and suggest that these factors may be present in the developing male fetus.

Patients who are concerned about the effects of cancer treatment on their ability to have children should discuss this issue with their doctor before treatment. The doctor can recommend a counselor or fertility specialist who can discuss available options and help patients and their partners through the decision-making process.

Radiation Therapy and Chemotherapy

Radiation therapy and chemotherapy treatments may cause temporary or permanent infertility, depending on a number of factors, including age at time of treatment, specific type and dosage of radiation therapy or chemotherapy, use of single therapy or multiple therapies, and length of time since treatment.

Direct radiation to areas such as the prostate or testicles may cause permanent sterility, and the closer the radiation treatments are to a man's reproductive organs, the higher the risk of infertility. For men who receive radiation therapy to the pelvis, the amount of radiation focused directly on the testes is an important factor.

Fertility may be preserved by the use of modern radiation therapy techniques and of lead shields to protect the testes. Although men may not produce sperm for as long as five years after radiation therapy, sperm production may eventually recover.

In addition, radiation may make men too tired to be interested in sex. This loss of libido is a temporary side effect; once treatment ends and the body begins to return to normal, libido also usually returns.

After treatment for testicular cancer, radiation therapy does not usually cause sterility, although a small dosage of radiation reaches the remaining testicle. There is no evidence that this radiation has any effect on children fathered after the treatment, but men are usually advised to use contraceptives for six to 12 months after treatment has ended.

Chemotherapy drugs (especially alkylating and platinum-based agents) and other drugs that can harm reproductive function tend to affect fertility in men. Age is an important factor for men receiving chemotherapy, and fertility recovery improves the longer the patient is off chemotherapy. Chemotherapy drugs that have been shown to affect fertility include busulfan, melphalan, cyclophosphamide, cisplatin, chlorambucil, mustine, carmustine, lomustine, cytarabine, and procarbazine. However, new combinations of cancer drugs are helping to improve fertility rates among these patients.

Testicular Cancer

Men who have been diagnosed with testicular cancer are not necessarily infertile. The removal of one testicle does not affect sexual performance or ability to father children, as long as the other testicle is healthy, because the remaining healthy testicle produces more testosterone and sperm to compensate for the removal of the affected testicle.

Chemotherapy usually causes infertility for a short time after treatment for testicular cancer; although this is usually temporary, for some men it may be permanent. For this reason, it is usually advisable to store sperm before starting chemotherapy. The rate at which the sperm count recovers varies from person to person, but it generally returns to normal within two to three years.

Because the effect of chemotherapy on semen and sperm is uncertain, experts recommend that men use a condom during treatment and for about a month after treatment ends. This practice protects the man's partner and avoids any stinging sensation.

Although there is no evidence that chemotherapy can harm children fathered after the treatment has finished, doctors usually advise that patients avoid having a child for six to 12 months after treatment.

Some men who have testicular cancer have a low sperm count before they start any treatment; sometimes successful treatment with chemotherapy may actually improve sperm production.

Lymphadenectomy

Sometimes doctors must surgically remove lymph glands in the abdomen if they are still enlarged after radiation therapy or chemotherapy. This removal can affect a man's fertility, since the surgery can damage nerves that control the discharge of sperm through the penis. However, new surgical techniques can usually prevent this problem. If there is a possibility that a patient may need lymph surgery, patients may want to consider storing sperm samples before treatment starts. Although this further surgery may make fathering a child more difficult, it has no physical effect on the ability to have an erection or orgasm.

Preservation of Fertility

There are two ways a man facing treatment for cancer can preserve his fertility—either by banking his sperm before treatment or by attempting TESTICULAR TISSUE PRESERVATION.

Sperm banking Sperm banks are available where sperm are frozen and stored in liquid-nitrogen-cooled refrigerators. Specimens can be stored because the capacity of sperm to fertilize eggs does not change over an extended period.

Before undergoing treatment, patients should collect sperm specimens over at least two weeks. Sperm banks charge fees for freezing, storing, and retrieving sperm for the donor. Costs vary among institutions, and some portions are covered by some insurance companies. Since most physicians want patients to start cancer treatment shortly after diagnosis, it is important to locate a sperm bank as soon as possible so the patient can begin storing sperm.

Testicular tissue preservation Testicular tissue preservation is an experimental procedure that has, as not yet resulted in any live births. In this procedure, testicular tissue and the sperm-producing stem cells are surgically removed, analyzed, and then frozen and stored. They are returned to the patient's testicles after treatment is over. However, experts worry that it may not be easy to repopulate the specialized tubules in the testicles with sufficient stem cells to allow production of sufficient sperm for normal conception.

Testicular sperm extraction Testicular sperm extraction is another method to preserve fertility that has resulted in a small number of births. If after cancer treatment a man is no longer producing sperm, his testicular tissue can be examined to see whether any sperm cells remain in the tissue. If so, the sperm can be removed and used in an in vitro fertilization procedure to produce pregnancy.

Pregnancy after Treatment

Cancer treatment may cause genetic damage to sperm cells exposed to chemotherapy or radiation for up to a year after treatment; therefore, experts recommend that men use a condom during this time. After one year, rates of birth defects in children born after one parent's cancer treatment appear to be similar to those of the general population. No unusual cancer risk has been identified in the children of cancer survivors except in family genetic cancer syndromes.

inguinal orchiectomy See ORCHIECTOMY.

injury and testicular cancer There is no convincing evidence that injury to the testicles increases the risk of developing cancer in that location.

Institutional Review Board A group of scientists, doctors, and consumers who oversee the protocols for clinical trials. The review board is designed to protect patients who take part in studies and must review and approve the protocols for all clinical trials funded by the federal government. The board checks to see that the study is well designed, does not entail undue risks, and includes safeguards for patients.

insurance coverage See FINANCIAL ISSUES.

intensity modulated radiation therapy A fairly new type of external beam RADIATION TREATMENT for PROSTATE CANCER in which beams of radiation are shaped to produce a more intense pattern that can destroy cancer cells without harming surrounding healthy tissue. This more intensive type of radiation confines the radiation more closely to the prostate, decreasing side effects.

Intercultural Cancer Council (ICC) A nonprofit group that promotes policies, programs, partnerships, and research to eliminate the unequal burden of cancer among racial and ethnic minorities and medically underserved populations in the United States and its associated territories.

The council believes that all Americans, particularly minorities, the medically underserved, and cancer survivors, must have access to cancer prevention, detection, diagnosis, treatment, rehabilitation, mental health, and long-term care services. In addition, they believe that minorities must have major roles in developing health policies and programs intended for their communities. The council supports the development of culturally appropriate literature and new programs to promote educational efforts to counteract fatalism and overcome fears.

The group also works to establish survivors' programs to replace denial and ignorance with confidence and the knowledge of how to prevail over cancer. They also believe that much higher priority must be given to research and control programs about cancers that disproportionately affect minorities and the medically underserved and that research must focus on cancer disparities between population groups, as well as relevant risk factors. They support more comprehensive research to document the scope of cancer in minority and medically underserved communities accurately in order to design effective interventions.

The council also tries to ensure that diverse populations are fully represented in clinical studies and research supported by public and private sector funds, which requires third-party coverage of patient care costs associated with these trials, including maximal cooperation with managed care systems.

interleukins Any of several proteins made by the body, and also produced synthetically, that boost the effectiveness of the immune system. Interleukins are produced by the body when stimulated by an infection. They have a variety of functions but most are involved in directing other infection-fighting immune cells to multiply and mature. When produced synthetically, the interleukins are used to help fight cancer. Many interleukins have been identified, and researchers continue to study the benefits of interleukins to treat a number of other cancers, including PROSTATE CANCER.

IL-1a

Interleukin-1-alfa (IL-1a) is a type of BIOLOGICAL RESPONSE MODIFIER (a substance that can improve the body's response to infection and disease). IL-1-alfa stimulates the growth and action of immune system cells that fight disease. IL-1-alfa is normally produced by the body and can be manufactured in the laboratory.

IL-2

Interleukin-2 (IL-2) is a type of biological response modifier that enhances the ability of the immune system to kill tumor cells and may interfere with blood flow to a tumor. These substances are normally produced by the body. Aldesleukin is IL-2 that is made in the laboratory for use in treating cancer and other diseases.

IL-3

Interleukin-3 (IL-3) is a type of biological response modifier that enhances the immune system's ability to fight tumor cells. These substances are normally produced by the body; they are made in the laboratory for use in treating cancer and other diseases.

IL-4

Interleukin-4 (IL-4) is a type of biological response modifier that enhances the immune system's ability to fight tumor cells. These substances are normally produced by the body and are made in the laboratory for use in treating cancer and other diseases.

IL-6

Interleukin-6 (IL-6) is a type of biological response modifier. These substances are normally produced by the body, but they can also be made in the laboratory.

IL-11

Also called oprelvekin, interleukin-11 (IL-11) is a type of biological response modifier that stimulates immune response and may reduce toxicity to the gastrointestinal system that results from cancer therapy. These substances are normally produced by the body; they are made in the laboratory for use in treating cancer and other diseases.

IL-12

Interleukin-12 (IL-12) is a type of biological response modifier that enhances the ability of the immune system to kill tumor cells and may interfere with blood flow to the tumor. These substances are normally produced by the body and are made in the laboratory for use in treating cancer and other diseases.

internal radiation   See BRACHYTHERAPY.

International Cancer Alliance (ICARE)   A nonprofit organization that provides cancer information on a person-to-person basis. International Cancer Alliance (ICARE) has developed several unique patient-centered programs through an extensive process of collection, evaluation, and dissemination of information, putting the cancer patient in contact with top physicians and scientists around the world. This organization is operated by a network of people who include scientists, clinicians, staff, and lay volunteers, many of whom are patients themselves. For contact information, see Appendix I.

International Union against Cancer (UICC)   A nonprofit group devoted exclusively to all aspects of the worldwide fight against cancer. Its objectives are to advance scientific and medical knowledge in research, diagnosis, treatment, and prevention of cancer and to promote all other aspects of the campaign against cancer throughout the world. Particular emphasis is placed on professional and public education. The International Union against Cancer (UICC) is an independent association of more than 290 member organizations in about 85 countries. Members are voluntary cancer leagues and societies, cancer research and/or treatment centers, and, in some countries, ministries of health. For contact information, see Appendix I.

interstitial seed placement   See BRACHYTHERAPY.

intratubular germ cell neoplasia   An abnormal microscopic finding within the seminiferous tubules of the testis that is highly associated with GERM CELL tumor. It is considered CARCINOMA IN SITU of testes. This is commonly found in other areas of the testicle in men with germ cell tumors. Men with this finding are at higher risk for the development of germ cell tumors in the future.

investigational new drug   A drug that is allowed by the U.S. Food and Drug Administration (FDA) to be used in clinical trials but not approved for sale to the general public.

2IT-BAD monoclonal antibody 170   A type of MONOCLONAL ANTIBODY, laboratory-produced substance that can locate and bind to cancer cells, used in cancer detection and therapy.

Japanese men Japanese men have some of the lowest rates of PROSTATE CANCER, TESTICULAR CANCER, and PENILE CANCER in the world.

Whereas prostate cancer is uncommon among Japanese in Japan, Japanese in Hawaii have a prostate cancer rate in between that in Japan and the high incidence among Hawaiian Caucasians. Studies show migrant populations tending toward the prostate cancer risk pattern of their host country, strongly suggest that environmental factors contribute to the large differences in risk found between countries.

This incidence of penile cancer among Japanese men (0.3 per 100,000) is similar to the incidence in other countries where neonatal circumcision is not routinely performed, such as Denmark (1.1 per 100,000).

In Japan, the testicular cancer death rate has always been low, with a peak of 0.3 per 100,000.

Kegel exercises Exercises designed to strengthen the muscle that contracts to control the release of urine. To perform the exercise, the man squeezes the muscles required to stop a urinary stream while voiding in a systematic way. The man should hold each contraction for six to 10 seconds and then allow the muscle to relax completely. This exercise should be repeated four to five times in a series, four to five times a day. These exercises can help men who have prostate problems retain urine better and longer.

ketoconazole An antifungal drug that is also used as a treatment for PROSTATE CANCER because it can block the production of male sex hormones (ANDROGENS). It is used together with AMINO-GLUTETHIMIDE and is classified as a second-line hormonal treatment, recommended for patients who do not have a satisfactory response to LUTEINIZING HORMONE–RELEASING HORMONE (LHRH) ANALOGS or ANTIANDROGENS.

It is most commonly used in men with advanced cancers who present with severe symptoms due to widespread disease. It is a rapid method for lowering hormone levels.

As ketoconazole became widely used as an antifungal agent, doctors noticed that a small number of male patients experienced painful breast tenderness; this observation led to the discovery that the drug inhibited gonadal and adrenal hormone production.

Ketoconazole has been shown to be a useful second-line treatment in advanced prostate cancer, but its use has been limited by concerns about its adverse effects (especially on the liver). Ketoconazole is available in Spain, but is not approved for the treatment of advanced prostate cancer.

Side Effects
Antiandrogens can cause nausea, vomiting, diarrhea, or breast growth or tenderness. If used a long time, ketoconazole may cause liver problems. Men who receive total androgen blockade may experience more side effects than men who receive a single method of hormonal therapy. Any method of hormonal therapy that lowers androgen levels can contribute to weakening of the bones in older men.

killer cells White blood cells that attack tumor cells and body cells that have been invaded by foreign substances.

Klinefelter syndrome A sex chromosome disorder characterized by low levels of male hormones, sterility, breast enlargement, and small testes. Men who have Klinefelter syndrome also are at greater risk of developing TESTICULAR CANCER.

Normal boys have an X chromosome and a Y chromosome (XY); in Klinefelter syndrome, the boy has one Y (male) and two X (female) chromosomes. In Klinefelter the affected boy has a genetic signature of XXY with a total of 47 chromosomes within each cell, instead of the normal 48.

Klinefelter syndrome occurs in about one of every 500 live births; often it is not diagnosed until puberty.

History
In 1942 Dr. Harry Klinefelter and his coworkers at the Massachusetts General Hospital in Boston published a report about nine men who had enlarged breasts, sparse facial and body hair, small testes, and inability to produce sperm. It was not until the late 1950s that researchers discovered that these men had Klinefelter's syndrome and an extra sex

chromosome. In the early 1970s, researchers around the world sought to identify boys who had the extra chromosome by screening large numbers of newborn babies. One of the largest of these studies, sponsored by the National Institute of Child Health and Human Development (NICHD), checked the chromosomes of more than 40,000 infants. On the basis of these studies, the XXY chromosome arrangement appears to be one of the most common genetic abnormalities known. Although the syndrome's cause (an extra sex chromosome) is common, the syndrome itself—the set of symptoms and characteristics that may result from having the extra chromosome—is not common. In fact, many men live out their lives without ever even suspecting that they have an additional chromosome.

Cause

No one knows what puts a couple at risk for conceiving an XXY child. Advanced maternal age only slightly increases the risk of the XXY chromosome count. Furthermore, recent studies conducted by Case Western Reserve University researchers show that half the time, the extra chromosome is passed on by the father.

In some cases, the X chromosomes—or the X chromosome and Y chromosome—do not pair and do not exchange genetic material. Occasionally, this causes them to move independently to the same cell, producing either an egg that has two Xs or a sperm that has both an X and a Y chromosome. When a sperm that has both an X and a Y chromosome fertilizes an egg that has a single X chromosome, or a normal Y-bearing sperm fertilizes an egg that has two X chromosomes, an XXY male is conceived.

Because these boys often do not appear to be different from anyone else, many XXY males probably never learn of their extra chromosome. They are usually diagnosed before or shortly after birth, during early childhood or adolescence, or as a result of infertility testing in adulthood. In recent years, many XXY males have been diagnosed before birth, through amniocentesis or chorionic villus sampling (CVS).

Cancer Risk

XXY males who have enlarged breasts have the same risk of breast cancer as women—about 50 times the risk of a normal male. For this reason, XXY adolescents and men need to practice regular breast self-examination. XXY males may also wish to consult their physicians about the need for more thorough breast examinations by medical professionals.

Symptoms

This syndrome causes testicular failure that is due to hardening of the tubules within the testes. In some individuals, more complicated genetic patterns (called mosaicism) such as XXYY, XXXY, or XXXXY have been found. Skeletal abnormalities are more common among men who have multiple X chromosomes.

Patients who have chromosomal mosaics (XXY/XY) have a less severe form of Klinefelter's syndrome and may be fertile, since a normal (XY) group of sperm-producing seminiferous tubules may exist within the testes.

In adolescent boys, Klinefelter syndrome may produce small firm testes, overdevelopment of the male breasts, slowed growth of facial hair, and incomplete masculine body build. Most young men who have Klinefelter syndrome are tall (the average height is about six feet), but they may not be coordinated or athletic. Psychological, social and learning problems are common in this group, as is mental retardation. Other associated conditions include glucose intolerance (inability to metabolize sugar) and varicose veins in the legs.

High levels of gonadotropins are usually found in the blood, and there is an imbalance in blood levels of estradiol (a form of the female sex hormone estrogen) and ANDROGEN (male sex hormone).

Although most adult men who have Klinefelter syndrome have normal sexual function with adequate erection and ejaculation, some may be impotent or have a low sex drive, and they may exhibit incomplete development of the scrotum or penis. Sperm are not produced.

Treatment

Counseling can help overcome any related depression or other psychological problems. Testosterone therapy may help boys who have Klinefelter syndrome, especially if their hormonal levels are low. Specialists generally recommend hormone therapy to ensure sexual development, including growth of pubic and facial hair, increased size of the penis and scrotum, deepening of the voice, and increased muscular size and strength. Therapy includes use of synthetic testosterone. Treatment, however, does not repair the sperm production problems nor protect against the development of testicular cancer.

Klinefelter Syndrome and Associates A nonprofit organization founded in 1989 by Melissa Aylstock, mother of a son who had the condition. The organization distributes a newsletter three times a year to more than 1,400 patients, families, physicians, and support organizations. The association also participates actively in research and educational projects about KLINEFELTER'S SYNDROME and other male sex chromosome variations. For contact information, see Appendix I.

lactate dehydrogenase (LDH) An enzyme normally found in the blood that is produced by many tissues. At higher-than-normal levels, it is considered to be a TUMOR MARKER, indicating possible malignancies such as TESTICULAR CANCER and other cancers. However it is also possible for cancer to occur without an increase in LDH level.

laetrile A purified form of the chemical amygdalin, a substance found in the pits of many fruits and in numerous plants, which some people have used as a cancer treatment. However, laetrile has exhibited little anticancer activity in animal studies and no anticancer activity in human clinical trials, and it is not approved for use in the United States.

Used as a poison in ancient Egypt, laetrile was first used as a cancer treatment in Russia in 1845 and in the United States in the 1920s, because some people thought that the cyanide contained in laetrile might fight cancer. In the 1970s, laetrile gained popularity as an anticancer agent, and by 1978 more than 70,000 individuals in the United States were reported to have been treated with it.

The term *laetrile* is an acronym (from *laevorotatory* and *mandelonitrile*) used to describe amygdalin, the plant compound that contains sugar and produces cyanide. Laetrile has been used for cancer treatment both as a single agent and in combination with a metabolic therapy program that consists of a specialized diet, high-dose vitamin supplements, and pancreatic enzymes. It is not available in the United States.

laparoscopic prostatectomy See PROSTATECTOMY, RADICAL.

laparoscopy A surgical procedure in which a viewing tube with camera is inserted through a small incision to allow a doctor to examine internal organs on a video monitor. Other small incisions can be made nearby so that instruments can be inserted to perform procedures. Doctors can use laparoscopy to asses nearby lymph nodes in cases of suspected PROSTATE CANCER. It can be used to remove lymph nodes associated with TESTICULAR CANCER by surgeons with specialized training and experience.

It is less invasive than regular open abdominal surgery (LAPAROTOMY) and usually entails less pain, less risk, less scarring, and faster recovery. Because laparoscopy is much less invasive than traditional abdominal surgery, patients can leave the hospital sooner.

Since the late 1980s, laparoscopy has been a popular diagnostic and treatment tool. As technological advances are made with improved fiber optics, robotics, and more precise instruments, more cancer surgeries are being performed with these techniques.

Diagnosis

As a diagnostic procedure, laparoscopy is useful in taking biopsies of pelvic growths, as well as lymph nodes. It allows the doctor to examine the abdominal area, including reproductive organs.

Cancer Treatment

Laparoscopy is sometimes used as part of a palliative cancer treatment to lessen uncomfortable symptoms. For example, cancer patients may need a feeding tube if they are unable to eat normally; inserting the tube via laparoscopy eliminates the need for open surgery.

Procedure

Laparoscopy is a surgical procedure that is performed in the hospital under general anesthesia. Gas is pumped into the abdomen by using a hollow needle to allow a surgeon a better view of the internal organs. The laparoscope is then inserted through this incision to look at the internal organs. The image from the camera attached to the end of the laparoscope is seen on a video monitor. Sometimes, additional small incisions are made to insert other instruments that are used to manipulate internal organs for examination or to perform surgical procedures.

There may be some slight pain or throbbing at the incision sites in the first day or so after the procedure, and the gas used to expand the abdomen may cause discomfort below the ribs or in the shoulder for a few days. Many patients can return to work within a week of surgery and most do so within two weeks. Laparoscopy is a relatively safe procedure, especially if the physician is experienced.

lasers   A treatment method that uses high-intensity light to destroy malignant cells. Lasers can treat cancer by shrinking or destroying a tumor with heat or by activating a photosensitizing agent that destroys cancer cells. It is a standard treatment for certain stages of PENILE CANCER and can be used to ease the symptoms of cancer (such as bleeding or obstruction), especially when the cancer cannot be cured by other treatments.

The acronym *laser* stands for "light amplification by stimulated emission of radiation." Whereas ordinary light occurs in many wavelengths and spreads in all directions, laser light is focused in a narrow high-energy beam. So powerful that some can cut through steel, lasers also can be used for very precise surgical work.

These high-powered light beams have several advantages over standard surgical tools. Because it is more precise than a scalpel, the laser can make an incision while avoiding tissue around the wound. And because the heat lasers produce sterilizes the surgery site, lasers can reduce the risk of infection. The laser is so precise that only a small incision is needed, making the surgery faster and

recovery quicker because less bleeding, swelling, and scarring occurs.

The light of some lasers can be transmitted through a flexible endoscope fitted with fiber optics so that doctors can see to work in parts of the body that could not otherwise be reached except by surgery. Lasers also may be used with low-power microscopes, giving the doctor a clear view of the site being treated. Used with other instruments, laser systems can produce a cutting area as small as 200 microns in diameter—less than the width of a very fine thread.

Although there are several kinds of lasers, only three have gained wide use in medicine: carbon dioxide (CO_2) lasers, argon lasers, and neodymium:yttrium-aluminum-garnet (Nd:YAG) lasers. CO_2 and Nd:YAG lasers are used to shrink or destroy tumors. Laser-induced interstitial thermotherapy, one of the newest techniques, uses the same principle applied in the cancer treatment hyperthermia, which uses heat to shrink tumors by damaging cells or depriving them of substances they need to live.

leukopenia   A condition in which there are too few white cells in a patient's blood supply as a side effect of chemotherapy treatment.

Levitra   See VARDENAFIL.

Leydig's cell   The testicular cell that produces the male hormone TESTOSTERONE. Leydig's cells are also called interstitial cells or stromal cells.

Leydig's cell tumors   Rare tumors of the testicle. Although some of these tumors are malignant, pathologists are usually not able to determine whether a tumor is malignant simply by looking at it. As a result, a radical ORCHIECTOMY, which usually cures the cancer and eliminates the need for further treatment, is performed.

See also SERTOLI'S CELL TUMOR; TESTICULAR CANCER.

lifestyle and cancer   Scientists have identified many factors that contribute to the development of cancer, including a number of lifestyle factors. Avoiding these risk factors whenever possible may have a significant effect on a person's cancer risk. The main lifestyle risk factors for men's reproductive cancers are DIET and OBESITY.

Diet

Researchers believe that what humans eat makes a difference in the risk of developing a variety of cancers. The content of each meal, as well as the way it is prepared, also influences cancer risk. For example, meat grilled on a barbecue may be more risky than that prepared by baking or boiling. Cured meats containing compounds such as nitrosamines have been liked to higher risk of cancers. Other evidence suggests that people who have diets high in saturated fats have higher cancer risk than those who have lower-fat diets.

In some cases, a lack of certain foods can increase the risk of cancer. Eating a diet rich in fruits, vegetables, whole grains, and other plant-based foods is associated with a reduced risk of developing cancer.

Obesity

Although study results related to cancer have been conflicting, obesity does appear to be linked to some types of cancer, including PROSTATE CANCER.

LiveHelp A new government Internet program that provides information about cancer, provided by the NATIONAL CANCER INSTITUTE (NCI). For general cancer questions or help in navigating NCI web sites, consumers can access LiveHelp online Monday through Friday 9 A.M. through 10 P.M. Eastern Standard Time (EST) at www.nci.nih.gov/Common/popUps/livehelp.aspx.

At the Web site, consumers type questions to NCI information specialists who can provide NCI information, publications, and Web sites, as well as information about cancer and cancer-related resources. However, the information specialists are not health-care providers, and they cannot provide medical advice.

The same information is also available via telephone at the Cancer Information Service (800-4-CANCER), available Monday through Friday, from 9:00 A.M. to 4:30 P.M.

liver cancer Some reproductive cancers can spread to the liver. The five-year survival rate for reproductive cancer that has spread to the liver is very low in the United States (usually less than 10 percent).

Symptoms

Liver cancer is sometimes called a silent disease because at first there may be no symptoms. Eventually, as the disease progresses, it may trigger symptoms such as the following:

- Pain in the right upper abdomen, extending to the back and shoulder
- Swollen abdomen
- Weight loss
- Loss of appetite and feelings of fullness
- Weakness
- FATIGUE
- NAUSEA and vomiting
- Jaundice
- Fever

lung cancer It's very common for a reproductive cancer to spread to the lungs, since all the blood from the heart flows through the lungs. The most common male reproductive cancers that typically spread to the lungs include TESTICULAR CANCER and GERM CELL TUMORS.

Symptoms

Common signs and symptoms of lung cancer include the following:

- A persistent, worsening cough
- Chest pain (constant)
- Coughing up blood
- Shortness of breath, wheezing, or hoarseness
- Pneumonia or bronchitis (repeated episodes)
- Swelling of the neck and face
- Loss of appetite or weight loss
- Fatigue

luteinizing hormone–releasing hormone analogs
A type of medical treatment for PROSTATE CANCER designed to stop the production of male hormones (androgens) by the testicles. Luteinizing hormone–releasing hormone (LHRH) analogs (also

called luteinizing hormone-releasing hormone [LHRH] agonists) are chemicals produced in the brain that trigger the production of another chemical called luteinizing hormone, which directs the testicles to produce TESTOSTERONE. The LHRH analogs override the body's normal regulatory system and shut down production of testosterone.

When a man first takes an LHRH analog, the body responds with a boost in production of luteinizing hormone and subsequent burst of testosterone. This initial increase may affect patients whose cancer has spread to the bone, worsening bone pain in what is called a flare reaction.

The hyperstimulation causes the brain to stop producing LHRH, and so eventually the testicles stop producing testosterone. The LHRH analogs take about a week to lower testosterone level.

LHRH analogs are of two types: leuprolide (Lupron) and goserelin (Zoladex). They work in about the same way, but they are administered differently. Leuprolide is given as an intravenous injection or an implant, and goserelin is given as an injection under the skin.

The benefits of this treatment include the fact that it eliminates the need for testicle removal, but it is expensive and requires return visits to the doctor.

Side Effects

Side effects of LHRH analogs include hot flashes, ERECTILE DYSFUNCTION, low libido, ANEMIA, and osteoporosis.

lycopene   One of more than 600 phytochemicals called carotenoids, which have very powerful disease-fighting capabilities, particularly against PROSTATE CANCER. Lycopene is associated with the red color in tomatoes; tomato-based products such as sauce, soup, and juice have the most concentrated source of lycopene. A number of studies have suggested that eating of tomatoes and tomato products such as sauce, paste, and soup is associated with a lower prostate-cancer risk. Scientists believe that lycopene gives the fruit its anticancer properties.

Cooked tomato sauces are associated with greater health benefits than uncooked because the heating process makes lycopene more easily absorbed by the body. Also, lycopene is fat soluble: in order for the body to absorb it, it has to be eaten with at least a small amount of fat. Lycopene has been associated with a reduced risk of many cancers.

But whereas a tomato a day may help prevent prostate cancer, lycopene as a dietary supplement may not be enough, according to the first animal study that compared the cancer-preventing potential of tomato products to that of lycopene. Rats with prostate cancer survived longer when fed a diet that included whole tomato products, but not when fed the same diet plus lycopene, according to Ohio State University Cancer Center scientists. The effect was most apparent when the animals' food intake was modestly restricted. The study, which was published in the November 4, 2003, issue of the *Journal of the National Cancer Institute,* strongly suggested that risks of poor dietary habits cannot be reversed simply by taking a pill. Instead, researchers recommend that people eat a variety of healthy foods, exercise, and control weight.

In the study, scientists first separated 194 rats with prostate cancer into three groups. A control group was fed a balanced diet containing no detectable lycopene; the second group received the control diet plus lycopene, the third group received a control diet mixed with tomato powder made from tomato paste that included seeds and skins. Each group was subdivided into an energy-restricted group and an energy-unrestricted group. Animals in the unrestricted group received as much food as they wanted; energy-restricted animals received 20 percent less food than the unrestricted group. The experiment continued for about 14 months.

Rats in the tomato-fed, energy-unrestricted group had longer prostate-cancer-free survival; their risk of dying of prostate cancer dropped by 26 percent. Animals in the tomato-fed, energy-restricted group fared even better, showing a 32 percent drop in risk. No benefit of lycopene alone was seen in either the energy-restricted or energy-unrestricted groups. This does not mean that lycopene is useless, but it suggests that if men want the health benefits of tomatoes, they should eat tomatoes or tomato products and not rely on lycopene supplements alone.

lymphadenectomy   Removal and BIOPSY examination of lymph nodes to check for the extent of the spread of cancer. The surgeon performs a biopsy of the lymph nodes to determine whether malignant cells have spread. The presence of cancer cells in the lymph nodes suggests that the cancer has spread from the primary site and is likely to continue to metastasize to other parts of the body. Lymphadenectomy may be performed when cancer recurrence is suspected.

lymphangiography An X-ray examination of a specific part of the body to check for enlarged lymph nodes. In this procedure, a dye is injected into the lymphatic vessels of the legs before X-rays are taken. Any enlarged lymph nodes are revealed by the X-ray, which also may reveal an abnormal pattern of lymph drainage. This method may have been used to help diagnose TESTICULAR CANCER in the past, but it does not appear to significantly improve patient management, and therefore it is not usually performed.

lymphatic system A network of capillaries, vessels, ducts, nodes, and organs that produce, filter, and carry lymph, a colorless liquid that bathes the body's tissues and contains cells that help the body fight infection. As lymph is slowly moved through larger and larger lymphatic vessels, it passes through lymph nodes that filter out substances harmful to the body; these nodes also contain lymphocytes and other cells that activate the immune system to fight disease. Eventually, lymph flows to larger ducts and to the major lymphatic duct in the chest, where the lymph is then moved into the bloodstream. Ultimately, lymph flows into one of two large ducts in the neck. The right lymphatic duct collects lymph from the right arm and the right side of the head and chest and empties into the large vein beneath the right collarbone. The left lymphatic duct collects lymph from both legs, the left arm, and the left side of the head and chest and empties into the large vein beneath the left collarbone.

The lymphatic system collects excess fluid and proteins from the tissues and carries them back to the bloodstream.

lymphedema A fluid buildup that may collect in a person's legs after nearby lymph vessels or lymph nodes are blocked or removed. Although lym-phedema is most often associated with breast cancer, it also can develop after treatment for other types of cancer. Untreated, this stagnant fluid interferes with wound healing and provides a culture medium for bacteria that can lead to lymph node infection (lymphangitis).

If lymph nodes are removed, there is always a risk of developing lymphedema, either immediately after surgery or weeks, months, and even years later. Lymphedema also can develop if CHEMOTHERAPY is unwisely administered to the side of the body on which surgery was performed or after repeated aspiration of fluid in the groin area, which often causes infection and lymphedema. Air travel also has been linked to the onset of lymphedema in patients who have had cancer surgery, probably as a result of decreased cabin pressure. This is why cancer patients should always wear a compression garment when flying.

Risk Factors

There are a number of risk factors for the development of lymphedema:

- Surgical removal of lymph nodes in the groin or pelvic regions
- Radiation therapy to the groin or pelvic region
- Cancer spread to the lymph nodes in the neck, chest, underarm, pelvis, or abdomen
- Tumors in the pelvis or abdomen that block lymph drainage
- Excessive thinness or heaviness, which may delay recovery and increase risk for lymphedema

Symptoms

Lymphedema can develop in any part of the body, causing symptoms such as a full sensation in the limb, tightened skin, or decreased flexibility. In the early stages of lymphedema, a patient may experience swelling that indents with pressure but remains soft. The swelling may improve readily by supporting the leg in a raised position, gently exercising, and wearing elastic support garments.

However, continued problems with the lymphatic system cause the lymphatic vessels to expand; as lymph flows back into the body tissues, the condition worsens. This causes pain, heat, redness, and swelling as the body tries to get rid of the extra fluid. The skin becomes hard and stiff and no longer improves with raised support, gentle exercise, or wearing of elastic support garments.

Stages

Lymphedema develops in a number of stages, from mild to severe, referred to as stages 1, 2, and 3.

Stage 1 (spontaneously reversible): In the initial stage of lymphedema, tissue appears pitted when pressed by fingertips. Typically, on waking in the morning the affected area looks normal.

Stage 2 (spontaneously irreversible): In this intermediate stage, the tissue now has a spongy consistency and bounces back when pressed by fingertips, with no pitting. The area begins to harden and enlarge.

Stage 3 (lymphostatic elephantiasis): In this advanced stage, the swelling is irreversible and the affected area has usually grown quite large. The tissue is hard and unresponsive. Some patients consider reconstructive surgery (debulking) at this stage.

Acute Lymphedema

There are four types of acute lymphedema, which may be treated with different aspects of decongestive therapy, such as manual lymphatic drainage, bandaging, proper skin care and diet, compression garments, or remedial exercises.

The first type of acute lymphedema is mild and lasts only a short time, appearing immediately after surgery to remove the lymph nodes. The affected limb may be warm and slightly red but is usually not painful and improves within a week if the affected leg is supported in a raised position and the muscles in the affected limb are contracted.

The second type of acute lymphedema occurs six to eight weeks after surgery or during radiation therapy. This type may be caused by inflammation of either lymphatic vessels or veins, producing a limb that is tender, warm, and red. It is treated by keeping the limb supported in a raised position and using anti-inflammatory drugs.

The third type of acute lymphedema occurs after an insect bite, minor injury, or burn that causes an infection of the skin and the lymphatic vessels near the skin surface in a leg that is chronically swollen. The affected area becomes hot, red, and very tender. It is treated by supporting the affected leg in a raised position and using antibiotics. A compression pump should not be used and affected area should not be wrapped with elastic bandages during the early stages of infection. Mild redness may continue after the infection.

The fourth and most common type of acute lymphedema develops very slowly and may become noticeable only two years or more after surgery—or not until many years after cancer treatment. The patient may experience discomfort of the skin or aching in the neck and shoulders or spine and hips caused by stretching of the soft tissues, overuse of muscles, or posture changes caused by increased weight of the arm or leg.

Temporary vs. Chronic Lymphedema

Temporary lymphedema lasts less than six months and does not involve hardening of the skin. A patient may be more likely to develop lymphedema as a result of:

- A surgical drain that leaks protein into the surgical site;
- Inflammation;
- Inability to move the limb;
- Temporary loss of lymphatic function; or
- Blockage of a vein by a blood clot or inflammation of a vein.

Chronic (long-term) lymphedema is the most difficult of all types of swelling to treat; it occurs when the damaged lymphatic system of the affected area is not able to handle the increased need for fluid drainage from the body tissues. This may happen:

- After a tumor recurs or spreads to the lymph nodes;
- After an infection of the lymphatic vessels;
- After periods of inability to move the limbs;
- After radiation therapy or surgery;
- When early signs of lymphedema have not been controlled; or
- When a vein is blocked by a blood clot.

Patients with chronic lymphedema are at increased risk of infection. No effective treatment is yet available for advanced chronic lymphedema. Once the body tissues have been repeatedly stretched, lymphedema may recur more readily.

Prevention

Poor drainage of the lymphatic system caused by surgery to remove lymph nodes or RADIATION THERAPY may make an affected leg more susceptible to serious infection. Even a small infection may lead to severe lymphedema.

It is important that patients take precautions to prevent injury and infection in the affected arm or leg, since lymphedema can occur 30 years or more after surgery. Because lymphatic drainage is improved during exercise, exercise can help prevent lymphedema. Those who have surgery have affects pelvic lymph node drainage should do leg and foot exercises.

lymph node dissection The removal of the lymph nodes from a specific area.

macrobiotic diet A semivegetarian DIET whose adherents advocate disease prevention by adjusting food, lifestyle, relationships, and environment. According to the macrobiotic philosophy, everything in the world (including cancer) has two opposite forces: yin and yang. Macrobiotic diet proponents believe that an imbalance of yin and yang may cause cancer, so the diet is planned to correct any imbalances of yin and yang that lead to ill health.

The modern macrobiotic diet contains 50 percent whole cereal and grains, 20 percent to 30 percent vegetables, 5 percent to 10 percent soups, and 5 percent to 10 percent beans and sea vegetables (such as nori, wakame, dulse, and agar-agar). Foods that may occasionally be eaten include fish, seafood, seasonal fruits, nuts, seeds, and other natural snacks. Sugar and meat are not allowed in a macrobiotic diet.

The American Medical Association, the U.S. Food and Drug Administration, and nutrition experts believe a macrobiotic diet can be harmful. The NATIONAL CANCER INSTITUTE (NCI) and the AMERICAN CANCER SOCIETY consider a strict macrobiotic diet ineffective for treating or preventing cancer and indicate that there are possible risks associated with the macrobiotic diet.

Diet critics warn that the modern macrobiotic diet may not provide enough of certain nutrients, including protein, vitamins D and B$_{12}$, and the minerals zinc, calcium, and iron. An earlier version of the macrobiotic diet that included only grains has been associated with severe malnutrition and even death. According to the NCI, no clinical trials have shown the health benefits of the macrobiotic diet.

magnetic resonance imaging (MRI) A body scan produced by combining a computer and a high-powered magnet to show a detailed X-ray image of a specific body part or region. It can be used in some forms of male reproductive cancers; for example, an MRI can detect whether a tumor has penetrated the prostate gland or invaded the seminal vesicles. MRI images also can be used to evaluate whether lymph nodes are enlarged.

Man to Man A support group for men diagnosed with PROSTATE CANCER founded by the AMERICAN CANCER SOCIETY in 1993. Some chapters welcome women (wives, partners, and friends); others prefer to separate the genders. The group offers information and support. For contact information see Appendix I.

margin The surgical edge of a pathology specimen. *Positive margins* indicate that cancer cells were found at the surgical edge of the specimen; their presence implies that not all the cancer cells were removed.

See also CLEAR MARGINS.

marijuana (*Cannabis sativa*) A member of the cannabis plant family that can relax the mind and body, ease NAUSEA, and heighten perception. One component of marijuana, synthetic tetrahydracannabinol (delta-9-THC) (dronabinol), is now available in synthetic form as the drug MARINOL to treat nausea and vomiting after CHEMOTHERAPY patients. Delta-9-THC is also a naturally occurring component of marijuana. Although marijuana use is illegal in the United States, in 1985 the U.S. Food and Drug Administration approved Marinol for the treatment of nausea and vomiting associated with cancer chemotherapy in patients who did not respond to conventional antinausea treatments.

Although research has shown that THC is more quickly absorbed from marijuana smoke than from an oral preparation, antinausea effects of smoking marijuana may not be consistent because of varying potency, depending on the source of the marijuana contained in the cigarette.

Eight states (Alaska, California, Colorado, Hawaii, Maine, Nevada, Oregon, and Washington) already allow severely ill patients to use medical marijuana, usually through a doctor's recommendation and an independent board's certification. A similar bill that would have allowed medical marijuana use in New Mexico was defeated in March 2003.

The Marinol patient assistance program is designed to help find potential insurance coverage for Marinol; for eligible patients with financial need, Marinol may be supplied free of charge. Information about the program is available at (800) 256-8918.

Marinol (dronabinol) The synthetic version of medicinal MARIJUANA used to treat NAUSEA and vomiting after chemotherapy in those who do not respond to other antinausea medication.

maximal androgen blockade See COMBINED ANDROGEN BLOCKADE.

medical castration The use of drugs to cut off supplies of male hormones that PROSTATE CANCER cells require to grow. Typically, drugs called LUTEINIZING HORMONE-RELEASING ANALOGS (LHRH)—including leuprolide, goserelin, and buserelin—are administered. LHRH drugs work by reducing the level of luteinizing hormone, which is produced by the pituitary gland at the base of the brain.

Medical castration is one type of HORMONAL THERAPY. Permanent hormonal control also can be achieved by surgically removing the testicles (the main source of TESTOSTERONE); this is called SURGICAL CASTRATION and is not reversible.

Hormonal therapy targets cancer that has spread beyond the prostate gland and is thus beyond the reach of local treatments such as RADIATION THERAPY. It also can help alleviate the painful and distressing symptoms of advanced disease. It also is being studied as a way to stop prostate cancer before it has a chance to spread.

Although hormonal therapy cannot cure cancer, it can usually shrink or halt the advance of the disease for some years. Unfortunately, hormonal therapy eventually stops working for prostate cancer that has spread. Remissions typically last two to three years. Eventually, cancer cells that do not require testosterone begin to flourish, and cancer growth resumes. When this happens, a variety of other hormonal-type drugs, such as hydrocortisone or progesterone, may be tried.

Side Effects
Medical castration is reversible; if treatment is stopped, testosterone is produced once again. Most men who undergo medical castration experience a loss of sexual desire and hot flashes; they may also experience breast enlargement and have an increased risk of heart attack and stroke.

medical oncologist See ONCOLOGIST.

Medicare A federally subsidized insurance program for citizens older than age 65 was established by the U.S. Congress in 1965. Medicare has two parts: Part A, which is free, pays for 80 percent of inpatient hospital care and a variety of follow-up services. Part B, for which patients pay a monthly premium, pays for 80 percent of doctors' services, outpatient hospital care, and other medical expenses. Some people also decide to buy "Medigap" insurance to cover the unpaid 20 percent of medical costs.

In addition to being older than age 65, those who have permanent kidney failure or who have been receiving SOCIAL SECURITY DISABILITY INSURANCE (SSDI) for 24 months are also eligible to enroll. Cancer patients whose disease has spread are usually considered permanently disabled and are therefore also eligible for Medicare, at any age. Generally, if cancer has spread to a major organ such as the lung, liver, or brain, patients will be accepted into the program.

microlithiasis An uncommon condition usually found during an ultrasound examination of the testes in which layers of material called microliths form and harden in the seminiferous tubules. Some studies indicate that as many as 40 percent of men who have testicular microlithiasis may have a testicular tumor. Since the condition usually appears in both testicles, if one testis is removed because of a tumor, the other should be regularly monitored by ultrasound.

microwave therapy   A new type of treatment for PROSTATE CANCER, also known as thermal ablation therapy, in which very high temperatures are used to kill malignant cells. Microwave therapy has been used for some time as a treatment for BENIGN PROSTATIC HYPERPLASIA. Just as CRYOSURGERY and RADIATION THERAPY do, microwave therapy destroys the prostate gland so as to destroy the malignant cells within the gland, without actually removing the gland.

The best candidates for this type of treatment are men whose cancer has not spread beyond the prostate gland and who do not want to have either radiation therapy or surgery. Microwave therapy, which can be administered more than once, is also a good choice when radiation therapy has not successfully eradicated cancer.

In this procedure, the physician uses a rectal or urethral probe to administer microwaves into the prostate to increase the gland's temperature and destroy it, along with the cancer cells. The microwave devices are designed to avoid the urethra and lower the risk of side effects.

The benefits of this type of treatment are that it can be used several times and that it prevents the side effects of radiation therapy. Usually, little or no anesthesia is needed.

The major disadvantage of this method is that healthy tissue may be destroyed inadvertently. And because this type of treatment is still considered to be experimental in the United States, it can be given only by physicians currently involved in a clinical trial using the method. At this time, sufficient research has not been done to confirm conclusively that this method is as effective in treating prostate cancer as radiation therapy or surgery.

Physicians are also testing a device that administers heat-producing high-intensity focused ultrasound (HIFU) to destroy local cancer cells within the prostate. This experimental technique is less invasive than other types of heat-producing probes.

mistletoe   A semiparasitic plant that has been used for centuries to treat numerous human ail-

ments; more recently, mistletoe extracts have been shown to kill cancer cells in the laboratory and to stimulate the immune system. Mistletoe is used for humans primarily in Europe, where a variety of different extracts are marketed as injectable prescription drugs. These extracts are not available commercially in the United States. Although mistletoe plants and berries are considered poisonous to humans, few serious side effects have been associated with mistletoe extract use.

The use of mistletoe as a treatment for cancer has been investigated in more than 30 clinical studies. Reports of improved survival rate or better quality of life have been common, but nearly all of the studies had major weaknesses that raise doubts about the reliability of the findings, according to U.S. federal researchers. At present, the U.S. government does not recommend the use of mistletoe for the general public.

Meanwhile, experts are investigating two components of mistletoe (viscotoxins and lectins) that they think may be responsible for certain anticancer effects. Viscotoxins are small proteins that can kill cells and possibly stimulate the immune system. Lectins are complex molecules of protein and carbohydrates that can trigger biochemical changes.

Because of mistletoe's ability to stimulate the immune system, it has been classified as a type of BIOLOGICAL RESPONSE MODIFIER (a diverse group of biological molecules that have been used to treat cancer or to lessen the side effects of anticancer drugs).

Commercially available extracts of mistletoe are marketed in Europe under a variety of brand names, including Iscador, Eurixor, Helixor, Isorel, Iscucin, Plenosol, and ABNOBAviscum. Some extracts are marketed under more than one name. For example, Iscador, Isorel, and Plenosol are also sold as Iscar, Vysorel, and Lektinol, respectively. All of these products are prepared from *Viscum album Loranthacea* (*Viscum album L.* or European mistletoe).

Mistletoe grows on several types of trees, and the chemical composition of extracts derived from it depends on the species of the host tree (such as apple, elm, oak, pine, poplar, and spruce), the time of year harvested, the technique by which the extracts are prepared, and the commercial producer.

At present, at least one U.S. investigator has approval to study mistletoe as a treatment for cancer.

Mistletoe is one of the most widely studied complementary and alternative medicine therapies for cancer. Mistletoe extracts have been evaluated in numerous clinical studies, and improvements in survival rates, improvements in quality of life, and/or stimulation of the immune system have been frequently reported. Still, no evidence exists that stimulating the immune system can improve the ability to fight cancer.

Side Effects

Reported side effects, including soreness and inflammation at injection sites, headache, fever, and chills, have generally been mild. A few cases of severe allergic reactions, including anaphylactic shock, have been reported.

However, mistletoe plants and berries are considered poisonous; they cause seizures, vomiting, and death after ingestion. The severity of the toxic effects associated with mistletoe ingestion may depend on the amount consumed and the type of mistletoe plant.

mixed germ cell tumor   A tumor containing more than one type of the GERM CELL TUMOR (for example, TERATOMA and SEMINOMA).

monoclonal antibodies (MOABs)   Synthetic antibodies produced by a single type of cell that are specific to a particular antigen. Researchers are examining ways to create monoclonal antibodies (MOABs) specific to the antigens found on the surface of PROSTATE CANCER cells (among others).

MOABs are made by injecting human cancer cells into mice so that their immune system produces antibodies against these cancer cells. The mouse cells that produce the antibodies are then removed and fused with lab-grown cells to create hybrid cells (hybridomas) that can produce large quantities of pure antibodies. They may be used in cancer treatment in a number of ways:

- They may react with specific types of cancer to enhance a patient's immune response to cancer.
- Programmed to act against cell growth factors, they may interfere with the growth of cancer cells.
- Linked to anticancer drugs, radioisotopes (radioactive substances), or other toxins, the antibodies latch onto cancer cell and deliver these poisons directly to the tumor, helping to destroy it.
- They may aid in diagnosing prostate cancer.

Researchers also are testing MOABs in clinical trials to treat prostate cancer and other types of cancer.

Muse (alprostadil)   A medication inserted internally to treat impotence that results from treatment for PROSTATE CANCER. The drug is administered by inserting a small applicator into the end of the penis and releasing a tiny medicated pellet into the urethra. Muse works to cause relaxation in the smooth muscle cells in the penis and allow blood to enter, thus causing an erection. The transurethral applicator may be applied five or 10 minutes before sex and may be used twice daily. However, this method should not be used when the partner is pregnant.

Side Effects

Some men experience discomfort caused by the applicator. Occasionally an erection may last longer than wanted (a condition known as priapism).

National Bone Marrow Transplant Link A national clearinghouse that provides information about a variety of BONE MARROW TRANSPLANT issues. Services include patient advocacy, research funding, referrals, and a resource guide. For contact information, see Appendix I.

National Cancer Institute (NCI) A component of the National Institutes of Health (NIH), the National Cancer Institute (NCI) was established under the National Cancer Act of 1937 as the U.S. federal government's principal agency for cancer research and training. The National Cancer Act of 1971 broadened the scope and responsibilities of the NCI and created the National Cancer Program, which conducts and supports research, training, health information dissemination, and other programs related to the cause, diagnosis, prevention, and treatment of cancer; rehabilitation from cancer; and continuing care of cancer patients and families of cancer patients. NCI is responsible for coordinating the National Cancer Program.

Services include the NCI's comprehensive database (PDQ), which contains peer-reviewed summaries and the most current information on cancer treatment, screening, prevention, genetics, and supportive care. The NCI also maintains a registry of cancer clinical trials being conducted worldwide and directories of physicians, professionals who provide genetic counseling services, and organizations that provide care to people with cancer. For contact information, see Appendix I.

National Cancer Institute Cancer Centers Program A program that comprises more than 50 NATIONAL CANCER INSTITUTE (NCI)–designated cancer centers engaged in multidisciplinary research to reduce cancer incidence, morbidity, and mortality rates. Through cancer center support grants, this program supports three types of centers:

- COMPREHENSIVE CANCER CENTER conducts programs in all three areas of research—basic research, clinical research, and prevention and control research—as well as in community outreach and education
- CLINICAL CANCER CENTERS conduct programs in clinical research and may also have programs in other research areas
- CANCER CENTERS (formerly called basic science cancer centers) focus on basic research or cancer control research but do not have clinical oncology programs.

Several cancer centers existed in the late 1960s, but it was the National Cancer Act of 1971 that strengthened the program by authorizing the establishment of 15 new cancer centers and continued support of existing ones. The passage of the act also dramatically transformed the centers' structure and broadened the scope of their mission to include all aspects of basic, clinical, and cancer control research. In 1990 there were 19 comprehensive cancer centers in the nation. Today more than 40 cancer centers meet the NCI criteria for comprehensive status. Each type of cancer center has specific characteristics and capabilities for organizing new programs of research that can exploit important new findings and address timely research questions. All NCI-designated cancer centers are reevaluated each time their Cancer Center Support Grant is renewed (generally every three to five years).

Since the passage of the National Cancer Act of 1971, the Cancer Centers Program has continued to expand. Today NCI-designated cancer centers continue to work toward creating new and innovative approaches to cancer research. Through interdisciplinary efforts, cancer centers can effectively move this research from the laboratory into clinical trials and into clinical practice. Patients seeking clinical oncology services (screening, diagnosis, or treatment) can obtain those services at clinical cancer centers or comprehensive cancer centers. They also can participate in clinical trials at these types of cancer centers. Most cancer centers are engaged almost entirely in basic research and do not provide patient care. The following is a list of the NCI-designated types of cancer centers. Information about referral procedures, treatment costs, and services available to patients can be obtained from the individual cancer centers; for contact information, see Appendix II.

Comprehensive Cancer Center

To attain recognition from NCI as a comprehensive cancer center, an institution must pass rigorous peer review. Under guidelines revised in 1997, a comprehensive cancer center must perform research in three major areas: basic research; clinical research; and cancer-prevention, control, and population-based research. It must also have a strong body of interactive research that bridges these research areas. In addition, a comprehensive cancer center must conduct activities in outreach, education, and information provision, which are directed to and accessible to both health-care professionals and the lay community.

Clinical Cancer Center

The clinical cancer center must have active programs in clinical research and may also have programs in another area (such as basic research or prevention, control, and population-based research). Clinical cancer centers focus on both laboratory research and clinical research within the same institutional framework. This interaction of research and clinical activities is a distinguishing characteristic of many clinical cancer centers.

Cancer Center

The general term *cancer center* refers to an organization of scientific disciplines outside the specific qualifications for a comprehensive or clinical cen-

ter. Such centers may, for example, concentrate on basic research, epidemiological and cancer control research, or other areas.

National Coalition for Cancer Survivorship   The only patient-led advocacy organization working on behalf of 8.9 million U.S. survivors of all types of cancer and those who care for them to ensure high-quality cancer care for all Americans. Founded in 1986 the National Coalition for Cancer Survivorship (NCCS) continues to lead the cancer survivorship movement. By educating all those affected by cancer and speaking out on issues related to quality of cancer care, NCCS hopes to empower every survivor. NCCS serves a key role in policy-making in Washington, D.C., as well as acting as a source of support for thousands of survivors and their families. Services include referrals, education, and advocacy. For contact information, see Appendix I.

National Comprehensive Cancer Network   A nonprofit alliance of the world's leading CANCER CENTERS established in 1995 to support member institutions of the evolving managed-care environment. The National Comprehensive Cancer Network (NCCN) tries to strengthen the mission of member institutions by providing state-of-the-art cancer care, cancer prevention, screening, diagnosis, and treatment through excellence in basic and clinical research and to enhance the effectiveness and efficiency of cancer care delivery.

The NCCN develops programs and products that, in partnerships with managed care companies, employers, and unions, offer people greater access to leading doctors, superior treatment, programs that continuously improve the effectiveness of treatment, and management that enhances the efficiency of cancer care delivery. For contact information, see Appendix I.

National Family Caregivers Association (NFCA)   A nonprofit association that provides educational and emotional support for family caregivers. Services include advocacy; education; and individual, family, group, peer, and bereavement counseling. For contact information, see Appendix I.

National Hospice and Palliative Care Organization The largest nonprofit membership organization representing HOSPICE and PALLIATIVE TREATMENT programs and professionals in the United States. The organization is committed to improving end-of-life care and expanding access to hospice care with the goal of profoundly enhancing quality of life of people dying in America and their loved ones.

Considered to be the model for high-quality, compassionate care at the end of life, hospice care offers a team-oriented approach of expert medical care, pain management, and emotional and spiritual support expressly tailored to the patient's wishes. Emotional and spiritual support also is extended to the family and loved ones. Generally, this care is provided in the patient's home or in a homelike setting operated by a hospice program. Medicare, private health insurance, and Medicaid in most states cover hospice care of patients who meet certain criteria. In recent years, many hospice care programs added *palliative care* to their titles to reflect the range of care and services they provide, as hospice care and palliative care share the same core values and philosophies.

Those offering *palliative care* seek to address not only physical pain, but also emotional, social, and spiritual pain to achieve the best possible quality of life for patients and their families. Palliative care extends the principles of hospice care to a broader population who could benefit from receiving this type of care earlier in their illness or disease process.

To better serve individuals who have advanced illness or are terminally ill and their families, many hospice programs encourage early access to care. Health-care professionals who specialize in hospice and palliative care work closely with staff and volunteers to address all of the symptoms of illness, with the aim of promoting comfort and dignity.

The National Hospice and Palliative Care Organization, founded in 1978 as the National Hospice Organization, changed its name in February 2000. With headquarters in Alexandria, Virginia, the organization acts as an advocate for the terminally ill and their families. It also develops public and professional educational programs and materials to enhance understanding and availability of hospice and palliative care; convenes frequent meetings and symposia on emerging issues; provides technical informational resources to its membership; conducts research; monitors congressional and regulatory activities; and works closely with other organizations that share an interest in end-of-life care. For contact information, see Appendix I.

National Kidney and Urologic Diseases Information Clearinghouse A service of the U.S. federal government's National Institute of Diabetes and Digestive and Kidney Diseases that can supply free information about benign PROSTATE ENLARGEMENT and other noncancerous urinary tract problems. For contact information, see Appendix I.

National Lymphedema Network (NLN) A nonprofit organization that provides support and information on LYMPHEDEMA. This internationally recognized organization was founded in 1988 by Saskia R. J. Thiadens, R.N. It is supported by tax-deductible donations and is a driving force behind the movement in the United States to standardize quality of treatment of lymphedema patients nationwide. In addition, the National Lymphedema Network (NLN) supports research into the causes and possible alternative treatments for this often incapacitating, long-neglected condition. The NLN provides a toll-free recorded information line, (800) 541-3259, referrals to lymphedema treatment centers, health-care professionals, training programs, and support groups; a quarterly newsletter with information about medical and scientific developments, support groups, and pen pals/net pals; educational courses; a biennial national conference on lymphedema; and an extensive computer database. For contact information, see Appendix I.

National Marrow Donor Program A national group that maintains a registry of BONE MARROW donors, provides information about becoming a donor, and organizes donor recruitment drives. For contact information, see Appendix I.

National Patient Advocate Foundation A national network for health-care reform that supports legislation to enable cancer survivors to obtain insurance funding for medical care and participation in clinical trials. The foundation offers referrals, education, advocacy, and HEALTH INSURANCE assistance. For contact information, see Appendix I.

National Patient Air Transport Hotline   A clearinghouse used to find air transportation for patients who cannot afford to travel for medical care. For contact information, see Appendix I.

Native Americans/Alaska Natives   Native Americans/Alaska Natives experience some of the lowest cancer rates among all groups; they have the lowest PROSTATE CANCER incidence rates in the United States.

As of 1999 the rate of new cases of prostate cancer in the Native American and Alaska Native population was 107.2 per 100,000, compared to 275.3 for African Americans, 172.9 for whites, and 127.6 for Hispanics. Native Americans and Alaska Natives had a prostate cancer death rate of 18.8 per 100,000, compared to 75.1 for African Americans, 32.9 for white Americans, and 22.6 for Hispanics.

Native Americans and men's reproductive cancer
See NATIVE AMERICANS/ALASKA NATIVES.

nausea   Feelings of nausea may start within one to four hours of receiving CHEMOTHERAPY for cancer; the most intense nausea occurs during the first 12 to 24 hours. After that, there may be occasional or unexpected episodes of mild nausea or vomiting. Fortunately, since the mid-1990s several very strong antinausea medicines that reduce or eliminate this side effect have become available.

A few chemotherapy drugs—vincristine, carboplatin, BLEOMYCIN, FLUOROURACIL (5-FU), methotrexate, and VP-16—do not usually cause nausea. However, if a patient's drug regimen is likely to cause significant nausea, intravenous drugs are given with chemotherapy to prevent this side effect.

Preventing Nausea
Patients should eat lightly before and for one to two days after chemotherapy, avoiding fried food, fruit juice, spicy foods, and meat such as hamburger, steak, or hot dogs.

Patients who receive chemotherapy deemed likely to cause nausea are given medicine to prevent this symptom before treatment, together with prescriptions for medicines to prevent nausea at home. Typical antinausea medications include prochlorperazine (Compazine), lorazepam (Ativan), dexamethasone (DECADRON), ondansatron (Zofran), granisetron (Kytril), and dolasetron (Anzemet). All of these medications work well for nausea; certain drugs may work better for one person than another.

Tips to Ease Nausea
Certain dietary choices can help ease nausea, such as crackers, toast, oatmeal, soft bland vegetables and fruits, clear liquids, and skinned baked chicken. Foods to be avoided include fatty, greasy, or fried foods; sweets; and hot or spicy foods. Patients should not force themselves to eat during periods of nausea, because this practice may trigger aversions to favorite foods.

Patients who have nausea should drink liquids between meals, not during meals. They also may find it helpful to eat in a room other than a kitchen if cooking odors worsen nausea.

nerve-sparing radical prostatectomy   A surgical technique used during a radical PROSTATECTOMY in which one or both of the nerve bundles controlling erections are spared. The use of this procedure is governed by the extent of the cancer.

Because the nerves responsible for penis erections run along each side of the prostate and the urethra, damage during a prostatectomy may cause ERECTILE DYSFUNCTION—the inability to have an erection.

In a nerve-sparing prostatectomy, the urologist tries to push aside these nerves while removing the prostate. The surgeon may perform either a bilateral nerve-sparing radical prostatectomy, in which the nerves on each side are spared, or a unilateral nerve-sparing prostatectomy, in which one group of nerves from one side are removed with the prostate.

The decision to try to spare at least some of the nerves is based on a variety of factors, including the patient's original erectile function. (A man who already has erectile dysfunction would not benefit from the nerve-sparing technique.) Other factors in the decision include the amount of tumor in the biopsy sample, the location of the tumor and whether it affects both sides of the prostate, and the grade of the cancer as measured by the Gleason score. Men at high risk for cancer at the edge of the prostate are better off if the nerves and tissue on that side are all removed, since this provides a better chance of removing all the cancer.

Even after a bilateral nerve-sparing prostatectomy, a man may still experience erectile dysfunction.

neutropenia   A blood condition in which there are too few of a type of white blood cells called neutrophils, which are important in fighting infection. About 60 percent of all white blood cells are neutrophils. Because neutrophils are very important in fighting infection, low levels of neutrophils make a person much more likely to contract infections.

Neutropenia can be caused by chemotherapy or radiation therapy or by cancer cells that directly infiltrate the BONE MARROW, interfering with the production of blood cells. Neutropenia also may be caused by BONE MARROW TRANSPLANT.

People who have neutropenia contract infections readily and often, usually in the lungs, mouth and throat, sinuses, and skin. Painful mouth ulcers, gum infections, ear infections, and periodontal disease are common. Severe, life-threatening infections may occur.

In general, the blood of healthy adults contains about 1,500 to 7,000 neutrophils per cubic millimeter (children younger than age six may have a lower neutrophil count). The severity of neutropenia generally depends on the absolute neutrophil count (ANC):

- Mild neutropenia: An ANC between 1,500/mm^3 and 1,000/mm^3

- Moderate neutropenia: An ANC between 500/mm^3 and 1,000/mm^3

- Severe neutropenia: An ANC below 500/mm^3

Treatment

Often the patient must be hospitalized and receive intravenous antibiotics. Neutropenia caused by chemotherapy is treated by stopping the drugs until the white blood cell count increases (usually within a week).

noncancerous prostate disorder   See BENIGN PROSTATIC HYPERPLASIA.

nonseminoma   A type of TESTICULAR CANCER that begins in specialized sex cells called GERM CELLS. These germ cell cancers tend to develop fairly early in life, usually occurring in men who are between their late teens and early 40s. Germ cell tumors that do not contain any elements of a cell type called SEMINOMA are broadly classified as nonseminomas.

Types of Nonseminomas

Nonseminomas include EMBRYONAL CARCINOMA, TERATOMA, CHORIOCARCINOMA, and YOLK SAC CARCINOMA. Most nonseminomas have more than one cell type and are known as mixed GERM CELL TUMORS; treatment of them is the same. Because all nonseminoma germ cell cancers are treated the same way, the exact type of nonseminoma is not important. The cell type of these tumors is important for estimating the risk of cancer cell spread and the patient's response to chemotherapy.

Embryonal Carcinoma

The embryonal cell type is most common in this type of nonseminoma germ cell cancer. This type is found in about 40 percent of testicular tumors. Pure embryonal carcinomas occur in only 3 to 4 percent of patients. Seen under a microscope, these tumors can resemble tissues of very early embryos, with a diffuse pattern of disorganized and irregular, small rounded cells that do not have specific organization into organlike structures. This type of nonseminoma is more likely to grow rapidly and spread outside the testicle.

Yolk Sac Carcinomas

Yolk sac tumors are named for the resemblance of their cells to the yolk sac of an early human embryo. Other names for these cancers include *endodermal sinus tumors, infantile embryonal carcinomas,* and *orchidoblastomas.* Yolk sac carcinoma is the most common form of testicular cancer in children and is usually successfully treated in this age group.

When yolk sac tumors develop in adults, however, they are more dangerous, especially if they are pure (that is, they do not contain other types of nonseminoma cells), although they still respond very well to chemotherapy if they have spread. This type of tumor releases a protein known as ALPHA-FETOPROTEIN (AFP), whose presence can help confirm the diagnosis.

Choriocarcinomas

Choriocarcinomas are very rare and aggressive testicular cancers that occur in adults and often spread rapidly to distant organs of the body, including the lungs, bone, and brain. Pure choriocarcinoma does not often occur in the testicles. More often, choriocarcinoma cells are present with other types of nonseminoma cells in a mixed germ cell tumor. This type of tumor is classically associated with the production of a protein called HUMAN CHORIONIC GONADOTROPIN (hCG).

Teratomas

Teratomas are germ cell tumors that have areas that, when viewed under the microscope, resemble each of the three layers of a developing embryo. The three main types are mature teratoma, immature teratoma, and teratoma with malignant transformation.

Mature teratomas These tumors are formed by cells similar to cells of adult tissues and rarely spread to nearby tissues or distant areas of the body. Although a mature teratoma rarely spreads, sometimes deposits of mature teratoma are found in other parts of the body after chemotherapy is finished. Experts believe that these deposits represent elements of a tumor that are left behind after chemotherapy; they can usually be cured by surgical removal after chemotherapy.

Immature teratomas These less well-developed cancers have cells that resemble those of an early embryo and may spread to other organs. Unlike mature teratomas, this type has a greater potential to invade and occasionally to metastasize, and it is this type that sometimes recurs years after treatment.

Teratomas with malignant transformation These very rare cancers contain some areas that resemble mature teratomas and other areas that resemble types of cancers that develop outside the testicle, in tissues such as muscles, glands of the lungs or intestines, or the brain.

Treatment

After removal of the testicle with RADICAL ORCHIECTOMY, the stage of the tumor is then determined to decide appropriate therapy. Nonseminomas can be treated with additional surgery, chemotherapy, or surveillance. Standard therapy for patients with widespread disease would generally be considered to be four chemotherapy courses of bleomycin, etoposide, and Platinol (cisplatin) (BEP). Those patients who still have traces of a tumor remaining after chemotherapy should then have surgery to remove remaining cancerous tissue. Patients with nonseminomatous extragonadal germ cell tumors who experience relapse after front-line chemotherapy generally have a poor prognosis with a poor response to future chemotherapy regimens, including autologous bone marrow transplantation. These tumors are much more resistant than seminomas to the effects of radiation treatment.

nutrition and cancer treatment Although good nutrition may not cure cancer, dietary factors play an important role in cancer treatment. A person who is battling severe disease needs adequate nutrition to maintain strength and overall well-being, keep the immune system functioning, prevent the breakdown of body tissue, and help the body heal. A well-nourished person is better able to tolerate treatment side effects and may be able to handle more aggressive treatments. Good nutrition also may increase the odds of survival for people battling cancer. In general, a patient with cancer should eat the best possible mix of nutrients.

Cancer treatments such as radiation therapy and chemotherapy can cause NAUSEA, vomiting, swallowing problems, painful mouth sores and sore throat, and dry mouth. Surgery also can make eating difficult. Treatment may alter a patient's ability to taste or smell. Depression and lack of energy may affect appetite, and metabolism may change.

CACHEXIA is the medical term for the wasting and dramatic weight loss seen in many cancer patients. Patients who have cachexia exhibit body organs that starve and waste along with muscle and fat. About two-thirds of all cancer patients, and nearly all patients whose cancer has spread, experience weight loss due to appetite loss or cachexia. Although these effects may not be preventable, attention to eating and good nutrition allows better quality of life, helps the body tolerate treatment, and can contribute to resistance to infection.

Improving Nutrition

There are a number of lifestyle changes that cancer patients can make to improve their nutrition:

- *Relaxation:* Patients should choose a quiet place to eat, listening to soothing music and trying to lessen distractions.
- *Presentation:* Patients can try to make eating a more pleasurable experience by preparing and presenting food in appetizing, attractive ways.
- *Flexible mealtimes:* Patients should eat when they are hungry and not wait for mealtime. Because nausea or lack of appetite may occur intermittently, patients should eat whenever they feel they can.
- *Small meals:* It is often better to eat many small meals throughout the day than to load the stomach with three big meals.
- *Snack:* Patients should keep snacks nearby and eat between meals.
- *Favorite foods:* Cancer patients should concentrate on having favorite foods available, because availability sometimes helps improve appetite.

- *Change of diet:* Sometimes eating a different type of food can stimulate appetite.
- *Attention to temperature:* Cancer patients should pay attention to the temperature of the food they eat and notice which temperature they prefer. Some find that warm or room-temperature food is better tolerated; others find that cold foods are more soothing. In general, hot and spicy foods are not well tolerated by most patients.
- *Avoidance of strong smells:* Patients should avoid cooking foods that have unpleasant odors. It may be better to eat food with little or no smell, such as cottage cheese or crackers.
- *Loading of calories:* Patients can get extra calories by adding dry milk, honey, jam, or brown sugar to food whenever possible.

Physical Eating Problems

Some men may have eating problems that are due to physical problems related to treatment. If this is the case, patients should:

- Avoid foods that may irritate the mouth, such as spicy, acidic, citrus, or salty foods;
- Take very small bites of food instead of full mouthfuls;
- Cook foods until they are very tender;
- Puree foods in a blender or food processor;
- Mix foods with broth, sauces, or thin gravies to make them easier to swallow; and
- Drink through a straw.

obesity A number of factors increase a man's risk of developing reproductive cancer, including obesity. People who are overweight weigh too much, whereas people who are obese have an abnormally high, unhealthy proportion of body fat.

More than 65 percent of all American adults are overweight to some extent, and almost 25 percent are obese; moreover, the number of obese people has increased steadily since late 1970s and early 1980s. The obesity epidemic continued into the 1990s; from 1991 to 1998, obesity rates increased in every state of the United States, in both sexes, among smokers and nonsmokers, and across race and ethnicity, age, and educational levels. Because of this dramatic rise, even a minor link between cancer risk and obesity is cause for concern.

Researchers have found a consistent relationship between obesity and a number of diseases, including diabetes, heart disease, high blood pressure, and stroke. Although study results related to cancer have been conflicting, as some have shown an increased risk and others have shown no association, obesity does appear to be linked to PROSTATE CANCER, among other cancers.

Although there are many theories about how obesity increases prostate cancer risk, the exact mechanisms are not known. Also, because obesity develops through a complex interaction of heredity and lifestyle factors, it is not easy to determine whether obesity or another factor led to the development of cancer.

Making conclusions from studies of obesity more difficult is the fact that definitions and measurements of *overweight* and *obese* vary from study to study, which has affected earlier study results and made comparison of data across studies difficult.

Most researchers currently use a formula based on weight and height known as the body mass index (BMI) to study obesity. According to a U.S. government panel, which is consistent with the recommendations of many other countries and the World Health Organization, *overweight* is a BMI of 25 to 30, and *obese* is a BMI of 30 or more.

Health risks increase gradually with increasing BMI. BMI is useful in tracking trends in the population because it provides a more accurate measure of overweight and obesity than weight alone. By itself, however, this measurement does not provide direct specific information about a person's health.

Physical inactivity may also be associated with prostate cancer. However, because physical activity level is difficult to measure, its impact on cancer may be underestimated because of misclassification.

In the future, researchers may measure physical fitness, rather than level of physical activity. Physical fitness appears to predict heart disease better than measures of physical activity; the same may be true for cancer. The complex relationship between physical activity and obesity makes it important for researchers to include both factors in future epidemiological investigations.

occupation A man's job may affect his risk of contracting certain types of cancer. A 1996 study found that NONSEMINOMA GERM CELL TUMORS occur more frequently among men in certain occupations (miners, oil and gas workers, leather workers, food and beverage processing workers, janitors, and utility workers). It may be that exposure to certain chemicals contributes to development of the disease. Studies have not yet identified any specific chemicals as being responsible.

There appears to be no association between a man's occupation and his risk of development of SEMINOMA TUMORS. One study found a slightly higher risk of germ cell tumors among men who had prolonged occupational exposure to extremely hot or cold temperatures, but these occupational associations need to be confirmed in other studies before it can be concluded they represent a significant component of TESTICULAR CANCER risk.

oncogene A gene that may trigger cancer or allow it to grow. Normally these genes—when not damaged—are responsible for helping healthy, normal cells grow and spread. When damaged in some way, these genes can cause cells to become malignant. Cancer-susceptibility genes that may increase a man's risk of reproductive cancers include the breast cancer genes *BRCA1* and *BRCA2* and *HPC-1* on chromosome 1, all of which are linked to a higher risk of PROSTATE CANCER, and *LKB1* (also known as *STK11*), which is linked to TESTICULAR CANCER (among others).

oncologist A physician whose primary specialization is cancer. Clinical oncologists are the physicians who treat cancer patients. In most cases, when a person is diagnosed with cancer, a clinical oncologist takes charge of the patient's overall care through all phases of the disease. Within the field of clinical oncology there are three primary disciplines: medical oncology, surgical oncology, and radiation oncology.

- *Medical oncologists* are physicians who specialize in treating cancer with medicine (chemotherapy).
- *Surgical oncologists* are physicians who specialize in surgical aspects of cancer, including biopsy, staging, and surgical resection of tumors.
- *Radiation oncologists* are physicians who specialize in treating cancer with therapeutic radiation.

Education and Training

Clinical oncologists complete four to seven years of postgraduate medical education, depending on their primary discipline. In the United States, medical, radiation, and pediatric oncology are recognized as medical specialties by the American Board of Medical Specialties.

In order to become practicing cancer specialists, medical oncologists usually take board exams administered by the American Board of Internal Medicine (ABIM), and radiation oncologists usually take board exams administered by the American Board of Radiology. Surgical oncologists do not have an equivalent specialty board. General surgeons are certified by the American Board of Surgery; those surgeons who choose to specialize further in oncology receive a certificate of special competence after they complete the oncology training program.

Regardless of their own discipline, medical, radiation, and surgical oncologists are broadly trained in all three areas of oncology and are knowledgeable about the appropriate use of each treatment approach. Within the three disciplines, oncologists may further specialize in specific types of cancer such as PROSTATE CANCER or TESTICULAR CANCER.

oncology The branch of medicine related to the study of cancerous tumors.

oncology clinical nurse specialist An advanced practice nurse with a master's degree who has received extensive education in the needs of cancer patients. Clinical nurse specialists (CNSs) specialize in oncology work primarily in hospitals to provide and supervise care for cancer patients who are either chronically or critically ill. Oncology CNSs monitor their patients' physical condition, prescribe medication, and manage symptoms. They are trained to apply nursing theory and research to clinical practice and may work as researchers, administrators, consultants, and educators in this field.

The CNS can help patients who are trying to deal with their diagnosis and/or treatment regimen. Symptom management, maintaining health and wellness during treatment, and providing information about cancer and its treatment are all areas of expertise that the clinical nurse specialist can share with patients and families. The oncology CNS works closely with the entire health-care team to ensure that a patient's plan of care is comprehensive, identifies the patient's needs, and is clear and manageable for the patient and family. The CNS can help the patient and family understand and cope with a cancer diagnosis.

orchiectomy Surgical removal of a testicle. When a malignancy is suspected, a BIOPSY is generally not performed if the other testicle is normal. In nearly all cases of suspected cancer, the entire affected testicle and spermatic cord are removed to check for malignancy. This is because the only way to tell if it is malignant is by looking at the dissected testicle under a microscope. Surgeons cannot simply perform a biopsy on the testicle lump, because if it is cancer a biopsy would risk disturbing or spreading the cancer while it is still in the body. If a lump in a testicle is found, statistics indicate that it is very likely cancerous, since more than 95 percent of testicular tumors are malignant.

During an orchiectomy, the entire testicle is removed through a four-inch incision along the "bikini line" in the groin (to the right or left of the pubic bone and a few inches below the belt line); this is called an inguinal orchiectomy. Cancerous testicles should be removed through an inguinal incision and not through the scrotum. During the operation, the surgeon tries to remove the entire tumor together with the testicle and spermatic cord, because the spermatic cord contains blood and lymph vessels that may provide a pathway for TESTICULAR CANCER spread to the rest of the body. To minimize the risk that cancer cells will spread, these vessels are tied off early in the operation. An orchiectomy requires about 45 minutes to an hour. When only one testicle is removed, there is no effect on male hormone production, sexual function, or fertility.

A few days after surgery, the pathology report reveals the findings of the testicle examination, by identifying the type of cancer (if the tumor was mixed, there should be an estimate of the percentage of each type of cancer present in the tumor). The report should also indicate whether invasion of the lymphatic system or bloodstream appears to have occurred.

orchitis Inflammation or infection of a testis, characterized by pain, swelling, and a feeling of heaviness. The cause of orchitis may not be known, but could be due to bacterial or viral infection as well as syphilis, or tuberculosis.

pain control Controlling cancer pain is a key component of any overall treatment plan; the most successful methods combine multiple therapies to prevent pain. When pain does break through, the proper dose of pain reliever should be taken immediately. Many patients have a tendency to wait until the pain is excruciating before seeking relief, but waiting too long often requires the use of more painkillers and produces less effective pain control.

Estimates of the incidence of persistent pain among cancer patients range from about 14 percent to almost 100 percent. The most common estimates found that pain was poorly controlled in 26 to 41 percent of all cancer patients. One obstacle to measuring the scope of the problem is that patients themselves often give their doctors poor insight into their pain; some believe that pain is part of the cancer experience and must be tolerated. Other patients have an unrealistic fear of opiates and often choose to suffer instead of requesting painkillers.

The best pain treatment depends on the level of pain and its cause. Mild pain often can be treated with acetaminophen, aspirin, or a nonsteroidal anti-inflammatory drug (NSAID). Ibuprofen and naproxen are two NSAIDs frequently used for mild cancer pain. Moderate to severe pain usually requires an opioid, usually beginning with codeine and progressing to other options, such as oxycodone, morphine, and hydromorphone.

Long-acting narcotics such as methadone and sustained-release morphine sulfate are used when BREAKTHROUGH PAIN is a problem. For patients who have swallowing problems, options include liquid morphine and a fentanyl skin patch.

Although pain is not always a prominent feature of cancer, it is one of the most feared symptoms. Today there is no reason why most patients with cancer pain cannot be made comfortable.

The first step in managing cancer pain is proper evaluation. There are various types of pain in cancer, whether it is caused by injury of tissues around the tumor (nociceptive pain), the tumor's stimulation of nerves (neuropathic pain), or individual mental responses to sensation from the tumor (psychogenic pain). Not surprisingly, patient self-reports are the most useful way to assess pain. A full history, physical exam, and appropriate lab and imaging studies (X-ray, computed tomography [CT], magnetic resonance imaging [MRI]) should reveal how the disease process is producing pain. But the pain's intensity, features, and factors that influence it are all important in helping patients decide the best strategy for treatment.

Acute Pain

Certain procedures involved in cancer diagnosis or treatment can sometimes produce acute pain; these include BONE MARROW BIOPSY, CHEMOTHERAPY (especially by injection), immunotherapy (pain in the joints or muscles), and RADIATION THERAPY (inflammation of the mucous membranes). Such pain can usually be managed with adequate dosages of nonmorphine painkillers.

Chronic Pain

The most common chronic cancer pain is caused by bone pain. Experts do not know why some bone metastases are painless and others are painful. If the spine is involved, there may be damage to the spinal cord or nerve roots. Chemotherapy can sometimes cause persistent nerve pain, which stops when the drug is discontinued.

Opioid Drugs

The most typical method of easing pain in cancer patients involves the relatives of morphine called opioid derivatives. The choice of drug depends on the patient's age, the presence of liver or kidney disease, and possible interactions with other medications. Although taking drugs orally is usually preferred, other methods (such as the transdermal skin patch) can be used if the patient has trouble swallowing or experiences any severe gastrointestinal upset.

For continuous or frequently recurring pain, it is usually best to follow a fixed dosage schedule (such as every four hours) rather than giving the drug "as needed." Starting at a low dose, the dosage is increased until pain stops or side effects prevent an increase. If pain breaks through the schedule, a rescue dose can be added immediately; rescue dose levels are typically 5 to 15 percent of the total daily dosage of the drug.

Oral doses can be given more often, if necessary, with as little as two hours between doses; the minimal interval between intravenous (IV) administrations can be as short as 10 to 15 minutes. It is important that everyone know that there is no correct or maximum dosage for cancer patients, short of overdose—the correct dosage is whatever prevents pain. Addiction should not be a concern for patients with cancer.

In many cases, the development of side effects does not prevent further increase in dosages; the treating physician can prescribe medications or other therapies to counteract the most common problems seen with opioids, such as nausea, vomiting, and constipation.

Nonopioid Analgesics

Acetaminophen and nonsteroidal anti-inflammatory drugs (NSAIDs) are good painkillers, but they have a maximum dose level above which no more benefit can be expected. These medications are most useful for people who have bone pain or inflammatory pain in which the affected area is warm, red, and swollen. The newer cyclooxygenase-2 (COX-2) inhibitors may be superior types of NSAIDs in preventing stomach or kidney toxicity.

In addition, certain types of cancer may do well with a particular drug directed at the tissue involved, such as treating bone pain with bisphosphonates (Fosamax) or calcitonin.

Adjuvant Drugs

Adjuvant medications are drugs that help analgesics work more effectively. Some drugs that are not primarily painkillers may have pain-relieving activity as well as their main effect. For instance, steroids, antidepressants, some anesthetics, antiepilepsy drugs, and major tranquilizers may be helpful in various cases of nerve pain. They are usually given after opioid therapy has been stabilized. Adjuvant drugs include the following:

- *Tricyclic antidepressants* such as amitriptyline and doxepin can improve the action of opioids.
- *Benzodiazepines* such as lorazepam and diazepam control anxiety to help reduce dosage of pain pills.
- *Selective serotonin reuptake inhibitors (SSRIs)* and other antidepressants improve mood.
- *Nerve-pain modulators* such as gabapentin control pain through a mechanism that does not affect opioid brain receptors.

Radiation Therapy and Chemotherapy

In addition to its main use as a way of destroying cancer cells, radiation therapy is often used to control pain, chiefly in managing the spread of cancer to the bone from the prostate. Chemotherapy can provide pain relief in PROSTATE CANCER due to tumor shrinkage; however, this improvement should be balanced with the toxic effects that chemotherapy can produce.

Nondrug Therapy

There are many alternative treatments for cancer patients whose pain is not adequately controlled by medication, primarily provided by specialists in hospital settings. A cancer treatment center or pain clinic is the best place to obtain information and advice about these therapeutic approaches, if the patient's cancer management team does not offer them. The following are most common:

- Acupuncture
- Exercise
- Heat or cold treatment
- Massage
- Breathing exercises
- Relaxation techniques
- Hypnosis
- Individual, group, or family psychological therapy

palliative treatment Medical treatment used to treat pain and symptoms of cancer patients and to improve their quality of life when a cure is not possible. Treatment may include medications, RADIATION THERAPY, or surgery.

See also HOSPICE.

Patient Advocate Foundation A national network for health care reform that supports legislation to enable cancer survivors to obtain insurance funding for medical care and participation in clinical trials. The group serves as an active liaison between the patient and the insurer, employer, and/or creditor to resolve insurance, job retention, and/or debt crisis matters related to the diagnosis through case managers, doctors, and attorneys. The Patient Advocate Foundation seeks to safeguard patients through effective mediation that ensures access to care, maintenance of employment, and preservation of financial stability. Services include referrals, information, advocacy, and health insurance assistance. For contact information, see Appendix I.

pelvic lymph node dissection Removal of some lymph nodes in the pelvis to determine whether PROSTATE CANCER or PENILE CANCER has spread. The first location to which prostate cancer tends to spread once outside the prostate gland is the pelvic lymph nodes. Because the success rates of certain treatments are lower if prostate cancer has spread to the lymph nodes, it is important to discover whether they are affected. Penile cancer generally first spreads to the nodes in the groin but can then advance to deeper pelvic nodes.

The most accurate way to assess the lymph nodes is to remove them either during surgery. The nodes can be removed and examined immediately before PROSTATECTOMY; the findings are reported to the surgeon in the operating room. The surgeon can then decide whether to remove the prostate, depending on whether cancer has spread into the lymph nodes.

The chance of the presence of cancer in these lymph nodes varies and may depend on the state of the prostate cancer, the PROSTATE-SPECIFIC ANTIGEN (PSA) level, and the cells' Gleason score.

Risks

The most serious risks of lymph node removal are excess bleeding, nerve injury, and lymphocele. The pelvic lymph nodes are located near large pelvic veins; occasionally, excess bleeding may occur when the nodes are removed. The pelvic lymph nodes also surround some of the nerves that control the leg muscles. If these nerves are damaged during surgery, they can be sewn back together; if the injury is not recognized, the patient may never again be able to cross the leg on the side of the injury.

A lymphocele is a collection of lymph fluid in the pelvis that may be caused by injury to lymph vessels. The lymphatic vessels are clipped or tied during lymph node removal. If a lymphocele develops after the surgery, it may enlarge and exert pressure on other tissues, causing abdominal pain. An infected lymphocele can trigger fever, chills, and abdominal pain. Lymphoceles occur in one or two of every 100 men who have a radical prostatectomy.

See also LYMPHADENECTOMY.

pelvic node dissection See PELVIC LYMPH NODE DISSECTION.

penectomy Removal of part or all of the penis to treat PENILE CANCER or cancer of the lower end of the urethra. These operations are rare, but they can have a devastating effect on a man's self-image and his sex life.

If penile cancer is diagnosed early, RADIATION THERAPY or CHEMOTHERAPY creams can sometimes be used to treat it. More commonly, however, the only way to stop the cancer is to remove part or all of the penis.

A partial penectomy removes only the end of the penis, so that enough of the shaft is left to allow the man to direct his stream of urine away from his body. A satisfying sex life is still possible after partial penectomy, because the remaining shaft of the penis can still become erect with excitement and is usually long enough to achieve penetration. Although the most sensitive area of the penis (the glans or head) is gone, a man can still reach orgasm and have normal ejaculation. His partner also can still enjoy intercourse and often reach orgasm.

However, if the shaft cannot be saved, the man must have a total penectomy, in which the entire penis, including the roots that extend into the pelvis, are removed. The surgeon creates a new opening for the urethra between the scrotum and the anus. The man can still control urination, because the "on–off" valve in the urethra is above the level of the penis.

Since cancer of the penis is most common in elderly men, many have already stopped sexual activity because of other health problems. If a man is willing to put some effort into his sex life, however, pleasure is possible after total penectomy. He can learn to reach orgasm when sensitive areas such as the scrotum, skin behind the scrotum, and area surrounding the surgical scars are caressed. The activity some couples enjoy after total penectomy can give hope to those coping with lesser changes in their sex lives.

penile cancer   Cancer of the tissues in the penis, a rare kind of cancer in the United States. About 1,400 new cases of penile cancer are diagnosed in the United States each year, and an estimated 200 men die. Penile cancer occurs in about one American man in 100,000, accounting for just about 0.2 percent of cancers in men and 0.1 percent of cancer deaths in men in the United States.

Penile cancer is much more common in some parts of Africa and South America, where it accounts for up to 10 percent of cancers in men. Many scientists currently believe that some penile tumors are caused by cancer-producing effects of substances that become trapped within the foreskin if they are not washed away on a regular basis. This may be why this type of malignancy is extremely common in Third World countries, where public health and personal hygiene often are limited. The low incidence in North America and Europe could be due to improved sanitary and hygienic conditions in addition to commonly practiced circumcision.

Types of Penile Cancer

The penis contains several types of cells, and different types of penile cancer can develop in each kind of cell. These include epidermoid carcinoma, verrucous carcinoma, SQUAMOUS CELL CARCINOMA, ADENOCARCINOMA, MELANOMA, BASAL CELL CARCINOMA, and SARCOMA.

Epidermoid carcinoma   About 95 percent of penile cancers develop from flat skin cells that tend to grow slowly; when found early, these tumors usually can be cured, but most develop on the glans or on the foreskin in men who have not been circumcised.

Verrucous carcinoma   An uncommon benign but aggressive tumor that resembles a benign genital wart; when it appears on the genitals, it is sometimes also called a Buschke-Löwenstein tumor. It can spread deeply into surrounding tissue but rarely spreads to other parts of the body.

Adenocarcinoma   This very rare type of penile cancer can develop from sweat glands in the skin of the penis. Paget's disease of the penis is a condition in which adenocarcinoma cells are found in the penile skin. Although the cancer cells at first spread within the skin, they may eventually invade the area below the skin and spread to lymph nodes. Paget's disease can affect skin anywhere in the body, but it most often affects skin around the anus. (This condition should not be confused with Paget's disease of the bone, an entirely different disease.)

The earliest stage of squamous cell cancer is called squamous cell carcinoma in situ (CIS). Penile CIS is contained entirely within the skin of the penis and has not spread to deeper tissues of the penis. CIS of the glans is sometimes called erythroplasia of Queyrat. The same condition, when it occurs on the shaft of the penis, is called Bowen's disease.

Melanoma   About 2 percent of penile cancers are melanomas, which develop from pigment-producing skin cells called melanocytes. This type of cancer is more dangerous because it spreads more quickly. Melanomas usually develop from sun-exposed areas of skin, but some of these cancers can develop on the penis or other areas not likely to become sunburned.

Basal cell penile cancer   This slow-growing uncommon type of cancer represents less than 2 percent of penile cancers. It rarely spreads to other parts of the body.

Sarcomas   The remaining 1 percent of penile cancers are sarcomas—cancers that develop from blood vessels, smooth muscle, and other connective tissue cells of the penis.

Benign and Precancerous Conditions

Sometimes abnormal but benign growths develop on the penis, some of which may eventually evolve into invasive cancer if they are not treated. These precancerous conditions can resemble warts or irritated patches of skin and may develop on the glans, the foreskin, or along the shaft. Some of these benign conditions include condylomas—wartlike growths that resemble tiny cauliflowers, ranging from microscopic to more than an inch or more in diameter.

Symptoms

In most cases, the first sign of penile cancer is a painless ulcer on the glans, foreskin, or shaft of the penis. Other symptoms include changes in color, skin thickening, or tissue buildup. Most penile cancers are not painful, although there may be some bleeding. Penile cancers may be red, blue, or brown and appear as velvety, small and crusty bumps or flat. Swelling at the end of the penis (especially when the foreskin is constricted) is a common sign of penile cancer. There may be a persistent foul-smelling discharge below the foreskin. If cancer has progressed to a more advanced stage, the lymph nodes in the groin may be swollen.

Most lesions on the penis are caused by viral, bacterial, or fungal infections or by allergic reactions, all of which respond readily to antibacterial or antifungal ointments and creams. But growths or areas that do not heal should be considered malignant until proved otherwise.

Risk Factors

The exact cause of most penile cancers is not known, but the disease is associated with a number of risk factors.

Human papillomavirus Many researchers believe that infection by human papillomavirus (HPV) is the most important preventable risk factor for penile cancer. HPVs are a group of more than 100 types of viruses called papillomaviruses because they can cause warts (papillomas). Different HPV types cause different types of warts; some types cause common warts on the hands and feet; others cause warts on the lips or tongue.

Other HPV types, which are transferred sexually, can infect the genital organs and the anal area. A person's risk of sexually transmitted HPV infection increases with beginning sexual activity at an early age, having many sexual partners or having sex with a partner who has had many partners, and having unprotected sex. When HPV infects the skin of the external genital organs and anal area (around the opening of the intestinal tract), it often causes raised, bumpy warts. HPV types HPV-6 and HPV-11 cause most genital warts, but these warts rarely develop into cancer. However, other sexually transmitted HPVs have been linked with genital or anal cancers in both men and women. These high-risk HPV types and include HPV-16, HPV-18, HPV-33, HPV-35, and HPV-45.

HPVs can also cause flat warts on the penis that are not visible and cause no symptoms. Flat warts caused by low-risk HPV types have little or no effect on cancer risk, but flat warts caused by high-risk HPV types can become malignant.

There is currently no cure for HPV infection, but the warts and abnormal cell growth these viruses cause can be effectively treated. These treatments can destroy warts and prevent them from developing into cancers.

New tests are now available that can identify the type of DNA in an HPV and identify the exact HPV type that is causing an infection. At this time, it is not clear how treatment will be affected by this information. HPV testing and typing are not presently routinely recommended, and most health-care professionals do not use this testing. However, scientists are trying to determine how this test can help prevent genital cancers.

Smoking People who smoke are exposing themselves to many cancer-causing chemicals that affect more than the lungs. These harmful substances are absorbed into the bloodstream throughout the body, especially in men who also have HPV infections.

Smegma Oily secretions from the skin, dead skin cells, and bacteria can accumulate under the foreskin, creating a thick, odorous substance called smegma. Some studies have suggested that smegma may contain cancer-causing substances, but most recent studies disagree. Smegma is unlikely to have a significant impact on the risk of development of penile cancer. However, if uncircumcised men do not retract the foreskin and thoroughly wash the entire penis, the presence of smegma may irritate and inflame the penis.

Phimosis This condition that makes the foreskin difficult to retract, so that men are less likely to clean the penis routinely and effectively; this can lead to a buildup of smegma.

Psoriasis treatment Men who have psoriasis and who have been treated with a combination involving of a drug psoralen with exposure to ultraviolet light have a higher rate of penile cancer.

Age Most cases of the disease are diagnosed in men older than age 50, but about 20 percent occur in men younger than 40.

AIDS Men who have acquired immunodeficiency syndrome (AIDS) may have a higher risk of penile cancer, which could be due to lowered immune response.

Circumcision Some experts have suggested that removing part of or all of the foreskin provides some protection against cancer of the penis by helping to improve hygiene. Whether lack of circumcision is a risk factor is a controversial issue. Penile cancer risk is low in some uncircumcised populations, and circumcision is strongly associated with other socioethnic practices that are also associated with lower risk. Most studies have concluded that circumcision alone is not the major factor preventing cancer of the penis.

Diagnosis

When penile cancer is detected early, treatment is simplest, more likely to result in a cure, and less likely to cause significant side effects or complications. Unfortunately, penile cancer is usually not diagnosed early because it is so rare in the United States that many physicians may only see two or three cancers in a lifetime.

Because several harmless conditions (such as genital warts) may produce similar symptoms, a doctor should visually examine any suspicious signs on the penile surface. If cancer is suspected, a biopsy and other tests may be recommended.

Biopsy In a biopsy procedure, a small piece of the skin tissue is removed so a pathologist can check the tissue under a microscope for cancer cells.

An incision biopsy removes only a portion of the affected tissue and is performed on lesions that are larger, ulcerated, or that appear to grow deeply into the tissue. These biopsies are usually done in a doctor's office, clinic, or outpatient surgical center with the patient under local anesthesia. Results are usually available within three to four days.

Fine needle biopsy In this procedure, the biopsy can be done in a doctor's office with only local anesthesia. A doctor places a thin needle directly into the mass for about 10 seconds, withdrawing cells and a few drops of fluid to be viewed under a microscope. If the mass is deep inside the body and the doctor cannot feel it, imaging methods such as ultrasound or computed tomography (CT) scan can be used to guide the needle into the enlarged lymph node. Needle biopsy may sometimes be used instead of a lymph node dissection for some patients.

Sentinel node biopsy Sentinel node biopsy is an alternative to total lymph node dissection that has been used successfully for some patients with breast cancer or malignant melanoma; some doctors recommend its use for some men who have penile cancer.

In this procedure, a radioactive tracer and/or a blue dye is injected into the region of the tumor, where it is carried to a sentinel node (the first lymph node that receives lymph from the tumor and the one most likely to contain a metastasis if the cancer has spread). The surgeon finds this node during the operation either visually (by the blue dye) or with a Geiger counter (radioactive tracer) and removes it. If the sentinel node contains cancer, more lymph nodes are removed. If the sentinel node does not have cancer cells, additional lymph node surgery is unnecessary. Through this approach, fewer patients need to have many lymph nodes removed.

Removal of lymph nodes carries a risk of side effects such as LYMPHEDEMA (fluid accumulation in tissues) and wound healing problems.

Computed tomography (CT) The CT test can help determine whether penile cancer has spread into the liver, lungs, or other organs. CT scans can also be used to guide a biopsy needle precisely into a suspected metastasis.

Chest X-ray X-ray may be used to determine whether penile cancer has spread to the lungs.

Staging

Stage 0: Cancer has not invaded below the superficial layer of skin and has not spread to lymph nodes or distant sites.

Stage I: Cancer cells are found only on the surface of the glans (the head of the penis) and on the foreskin (the loose skin that covers the head of the penis). It has not spread to lymph nodes or distant sites.

Stage II: Cancer cells are found in the deeper tissues of the glans and have spread to the shaft of the penis (the long, slender cylinders of tissue inside the penis that contain spongy tissue and expand to produce erections).

Stage III: The cancer has

- Invaded the penis, but not the urethra or prostate, and has spread to many superficial groin lymph nodes but not to distant sites *or*
- Invaded the urethra or prostate and may or may not have spread to single or multiple superficial groin lymph nodes, but not to distant sites

Stage IV: The cancer has

- Invaded nearby tissues and may or may not have spread to groin lymph nodes, but not to distant sites
- Invaded and spread to lymph nodes deep in the groin, but not to distant sites
- Invaded tissue, may or may not have spread to lymph nodes, and has spread to distant sites

Recurrent: Cancer has recurred after treatment has ended (recurrent penile cancer may return to the same location or to any other part of the body)

Treatment

Treatment of cancer of the penis depends on the stage of the disease, the type of disease, and the patient's age and overall condition. Standard treatment may be considered because of its effectiveness in patients in past studies, or participation in a clinical trial may be considered. Not all patients are cured with standard therapy, and some standard treatments may have excessive side effects. Treatments for cancer of the penis include surgery, radiation therapy, chemotherapy, and biological therapy.

Surgery Surgery is the most common treatment for all stages of penile cancer. If the lesion is limited, a doctor may recommend small local excision or Mohs's technique or surgery (a procedure in which layers of abnormal tissue are shaved off until normal tissue is reached). These procedures are not very disfiguring, but careful follow-up is critical to identify early recurrence. When these small lesions are removed, it is very unlikely that cancer has spread to lymph, and, therefore, removal of the lymph nodes is usually not necessary.

If the lesion is larger, more tissue must be removed, along with lymph nodes in the groin. In these circumstances, combinations of surgery, radiation therapy, and chemotherapy may be necessary.

Wide local excision removes only the cancer and some normal tissue on each side. If the cancer is limited to the foreskin, treatment is probably wide local excision with circumcision. Microsurgery is an operation that removes the cancer and as little normal tissue as possible, with the aid of a microscope to make sure all the cancer cells are removed. If the cancer begins in the glans and does not involve other tissues, treatment may involve microsurgery plus topical chemotherapy (fluorouracil cream). Laser surgery also can be used to remove cancer cells.

Amputation of the penis (either partial or total) is the most common and effective treatment. Lymph nodes in the groin may be taken out during surgery.

Radiation therapy and chemotherapy Radiation may be used alone or after surgery. Topical chemotherapy with fluorouracil cream is sometimes used for very small surface cancers, but otherwise chemotherapy is not a common treatment for penile cancer.

Biological therapy Biological therapy uses the immune system to prompt the body to fight its own cancer by using material made by the body or a lab to boost, direct, or restore the body's natural defenses against disease. Biological treatment is sometimes called biological response modifier (BRM) therapy.

Prognosis

About 67 percent of men are likely to live five years or longer after the diagnosis and treatment of penile cancer. The earlier the cancer is detected and the lower its stage, the better the chance of a complete cure and long-term survival. About 80 percent of men who have stage I or stage II cancer that has not spread to lymph nodes can expect to live at least five years, but the five-year survival rate drops to 50 percent for men who have stage III disease and to 20 percent for men who have stage IV penile cancer.

Prevention

Experts believe that the large variations in penile cancer rates around the world strongly suggest that it is a preventable disease. The best way to reduce the risk of penile cancer is to avoid known risk factors whenever possible. Of course, some men who have penile cancer have no known risk factors, so it is not possible to completely prevent this disease.

Circumcision   In the past, many experts considered circumcision a good way to prevent penile cancer because studies reported much lower penile cancer rates among circumcised men. However, most researchers now believe those studies were flawed because they failed to consider other factors that are now known to affect penile cancer risk.

For example, some studies suggest that circumcised men tend to have other lifestyle factors associated with lower penile cancer risk—they are less likely to smoke or have multiple sexual partners and more likely to have better personal hygiene. Most researchers believe that the penile cancer risk among uncircumcised men without known risk factors living in the United States is extremely low. The current consensus of most experts is that circumcision should not be recommended as a prevention strategy for penile cancer.

Sexual practices   On the other hand, avoiding sexual practices likely to result in HPV infection may lower penile cancer risk. Until recently, experts thought that the use of condoms could prevent HPV infection, but recent research shows that condoms do not protect against HPV infection very well because the virus can be transmitted by skin-to-skin contact with any HPV-infected area of the body, such as skin of the genital or anal area not covered by the condom.

Moreover, HPV can be passed on to another person even when warts or other symptoms are not visible and can be present for years with no symptoms. The longer a person remains infected with any type of HPV that can cause cancer, the greater the risk that infection will lead to cancer. For these reasons, postponing the beginning of sexual activity and limiting the number of sexual partners are two ways to reduce the risk of developing penile cancer.

Quitting smoking   Quitting smoking or never smoking is an excellent recommendation for preventing many diseases, including penile cancer.

Good hygiene   Because some studies suggest that smegma below the foreskin may contain cancer-causing substances, many public health experts recommend that uncircumcised men retract the foreskin to clean the entire penis.

penile prosthetic implant   A permanent device inserted into the penis that allows for an erection in cases of impotence (ERECTILE DYSFUNCTION), which often occurs in the wake of treatment for some types of male reproductive cancers. When other therapies for erectile dysfunction fail, men can choose from a variety of other options.

Surgical implantation of penile prosthetic devices is still an accepted means of restoring erectile capability in impotent men. In 1989 U.S. surgeons implanted an estimated 27,500 penile prostheses. That number has declined only somewhat since the advent of penile injection, alprostadil (MUSE) therapy, and Viagra. Since about 30 to 35 percent of impotent men who try Viagra or other medications do not respond well enough to resume sex, some impotent men will probably continue to have penile prosthesis surgery or other erection assistance to help them resume sexual activity.

The primary risk of the penile implant is infection; if this occurs, the entire device must be removed. Moreover, once a prosthesis has been implanted and then removed, other forms of treatment usually are not effective. This is why other treatment methods should be tried before choosing surgical prosthesis.

Types of Devices

There are more than 15 different varieties of implants, ranging from one-piece rigid structures to self-contained unit implants, which cost an average of between $8,000 and $15,000. Most involve synthetic cylinders surgically placed inside the penis; after four to six weeks, the patient is ready to engage in sex. Because erection is achieved through the implant parts and not the flow of blood into the penis, the erect penis is generally cooler to the touch than it would be otherwise.

The semirigid device does not increase penis width but bends up for intercourse and down at other times. This type of prosthesis is the easiest to insert and involves the fewest mechanical problems, but is also the least natural-looking.

Inflatable prosthesis look quite natural, since when deflated the penis is flaccid, and when inflated the penis is erect. The two-piece inflatable unit includes two cylinders, one in each side of the penis, with a small pump in the scrotum. Squeezing the pump pushes fluid into the cylinders, making the penis erect. The three-piece unit includes a reservoir inside the abdominal wall near the bladder that contains additional fluid; this allows for a more rigid penis.

However, the more complex the device, the more likely are mechanical problems. Today the failure rate is about 10 percent at 10 years. This treatment is irreversible and should be considered a last resort. Still, although the method is expensive and requires surgery, up to 90 percent of patients are satisfied with the inflatable prosthesis.

perineal prostatectomy See PROSTATECTOMY, RADICAL.

personality and cancer Although the idea has been popular for a long time, there is no scientific evidence for the belief that there is a "cancer personality." It is possible that men who have been diagnosed with reproductive cancer are anxious and depressed, but it does not follow that these uncomfortable emotions caused the malignancy.

Most recently, a June 2003 Japanese study found that personality type does not appear to be associated with the risk of cancer. In this study, researchers examined the incidence of cancer among 30,000 people in Japan who had completed personality questionnaires with four personality subscales: extroversion (sociability, liveliness), neuroticism (emotional instability, anxiousness), psychoticism (tough-mindedness, aggressiveness, coldness), and social naïveté or conformity. During seven years of follow-up, there were 986 cases of cancer but no association between any personality subscales and risk of breast cancer. Although higher levels of neuroticism were associated with cancers diagnosed in the first three years of follow-up, this result could be attributable to neuroticism's being a consequence of cancer rather than a cause.

In the 2003 Japanese study, scientists gave personality tests to 30,277 people living in northern Japan; seven years later, they studied which people had cancer and which did not. The researchers used a test called the Eysenck Personality Questionnaire, which uses four measures to analyze personality:

Extroversion–introversion Extroverts are very social people who have many friends and must constantly talk with others. They like excitement, take risks, and act on the spur of the moment. Introverts are quiet and studious people who plan ahead, do not readily lose their temper, and value ethical standards.

Neuroticism People who have high "N" scores tend to be very emotional and overactive and have problems calming down. They complain about vague physical problems and tend to be worried, anxious, and irritated.

Psychoticism (tough-mindedness) People who have high "P" scores are not necessarily insane but tend to be cruel, intolerant, and aggressive and tend to make trouble for other people and to lack empathy.

Liars People who score high on the liar scale are conformists who pretend to be better than they are in order to please others.

After seven years, the researchers saw no link between cancer and any personality trait. However, people who already had cancer tended to score higher on the neuroticism scale. But since high "N" scores were not linked to cancer in the long run, the researchers suggest that an "N" personality do not cause cancer—cancer, or early symptoms of cancer, make a person anxious and emotional.

Phase I trials   A study in which researchers test a new drug or treatment in a small group of people (between 20 to 80 subjects) for the first time to evaluate its safety, determine a safe dosage range, and identify side effects.

See also CLINICAL TRIALS; PHASE IV TRIALS; PHASE III TRIALS; PHASE II TRIALS.

Phase II trials   A clinical study in which researchers test a drug or treatment with a larger group of people than are included in PHASE I TRIALS (100 to 300 subjects) to see whether the drug or treatment is effective and to evaluate safety further.

See also CLINICAL TRIALS; PHASE IV TRIALS; PHASE I TRIALS; PHASE III TRIALS.

Phase III trials   A clinical study in which researchers test a drug or treatment with a larger group of people than are included in a Phase I or II trial (1,000 to 3,000 subjects) to confirm effectiveness, monitor side effects, compare the treatment to commonly used methods, and collect safety information.

See also CLINICAL TRIALS; PHASE I TRIALS; PHASE IV TRIALS; PHASE II TRIALS.

Phase IV trials   Postmarketing studies that provide more information about a drug or treatment, including the treatment's risks, benefits, and optimal use.

See also CLINICAL TRIALS; PHASE I TRIALS; PHASE III TRIALS; PHASE II TRIALS.

phenolics   A very large category of more than 2,000 PHYTOCHEMICALS. The term *phenol* is derived from the chemical structure of these phytochemicals, which have one to several phenol groups, with the ability to mop up many FREE RADICALS as they circulate through the bloodstream. For this reason, phenolics are considered to be among the most powerful antioxidants and are studied for their ability to interfere with tumors.

Physician's Data Query (PDQ)   A comprehensive cancer database maintained by the NATIONAL CANCER INSTITUTE (NCI). It has been distributed since 1984 to physicians and the public and is now available in multiple forms including fax, e-mail, conventional mail, and the Internet, in both English and Spanish. The Physician's Data Query (PDQ) contains peer-reviewed summaries of cancer treatment, screening, prevention, genetics, and supportive care and directories of physicians, professionals who provide genetic services, and organizations that provide cancer care.

PDQ also contains the world's most comprehensive cancer clinical trials database with about 1,800 abstracts of trials that are open and accepting patients, including trials for cancer treatment, genetics, diagnosis, supportive care, screening, and prevention. In addition, there is access to about 12,000 abstracts of clinical trials that have been completed or are no longer accepting patients.

The PDQ cancer information summaries are peer reviewed and updated monthly by six editorial boards comprised of specialists in adult treatment, pediatric treatment, complementary and alternative medicine, supportive care, screening and prevention, and genetics. The boards review current literature in more than 70 biomedical journals, evaluate its relevance, and synthesize it into clear summaries.

phytochemicals   Substances found only in plants that provide health benefits in addition to those provided by vitamins and minerals alone. Phytochemicals are natural compounds that protect plants from the ravages of sunlight and other environmental threats. Many of these compounds are currently under investigation for their roles in blocking the formation of some cancers. They may also protect against some forms of heart disease, arthritis, and other degenerative diseases.

Phytochemicals can be found in varying amounts in all fruits, vegetables, grains, oils, nuts, and seeds, some have higher levels of phytochemicals, which make them a better choice for a health diet. Among the thousands of phytochemicals in plants, each may potentially have some benefit to humans. Some of these phytochemicals are currently being studied for their potential to prevent certain cancers. Many studies already have provided evidence that eating more fruits and vegetables decreases the risk of several different types of cancer. In fact, phytochemical research helped prompt the National Cancer Institute to initiate its "5-a-Day" program for healthy eating, in which consumers are urged to eat more foods such as garlic, broccoli, onions, and soy products.

Phytochemicals, which represent thousands of different components in plant foods, differ from vitamins and minerals in that they are not considered essential nutrients. A diet that includes phytochemicals from a wide range of fruits and vegetables has been associated with the prevention and treatment of cancer. Since different phytochemicals are present in different foods, eating a varied diet is important to ensure that a person obtains all the cancer protection possible.

The specific phytochemical content of different fruits and vegetables tends to vary by color, and each has unique functions. Some phytochemicals act as ANTIOXIDANTS, some protect and regenerate essential nutrients, and others work to deactivate cancer-causing substances. Phytochemicals include allium compounds, carotenoids, glucosinolates, polyphenols, and flavonoids.

Allium compounds Allium compounds such as allyl sulfides may help detoxify and rid the body of some carcinogenic compounds. Food sources include onions, garlic, scallions, and chives.

Carotenoids Carotenoids such as alpha-carotene, beta-carotene, cryptoxanthin, lycopene, and LUTEIN work as antioxidants, helping to offset harm caused by environmental pollutants such as pesticides and smoke. Food sources include dark green, orange, or red fruits and vegetables, especially carrots, sweet potatoes, tomatoes, spinach, broccoli, cantaloupe, and apricots.

Glucosinolates Glucosinolates such as glucobrassicin are metabolized to produce two other phytochemicals, isothiocyanates and INDOLES, which trigger production of enzymes that block cell damage due to carcinogens. Food sources include cruciferous vegetables such as broccoli, broccoli sprouts, cabbage, and brussels sprouts.

Polyphenols Polyphenols such as ellagic acid and ferulic acid are thought to prevent conversion of substances into carcinogens and to inhibit mutations. Food sources include oats, soybeans, and fruits and nuts—especially strawberries, raspberries, blackberries, walnuts, and pecans.

Flavonoids Flavonoids include more than 2,000 powerful antioxidants from sources such as coffee, tea, cola, berries, tomatoes, potatoes, broad beans, broccoli, Italian squash, onions, and citrus fruits.

In the Future

Someday, scientists may develop "superbreeds" of certain foods that have extra amounts of beneficial phytochemicals. Seed catalogs already offer home gardeners the opportunity to buy seeds for several of these supervegetables. For example, sulforaphane has been identified as a potent inducer of the action of detoxifying enzymes (broccoli is a good source). In fact, three-day-old broccoli sprouts contain 20 to 50 times more sulforaphane than does mature broccoli. In one study, rats fed sulforaphane had fewer malignant tumors, which developed at a slower rate.

In addition to high-sulforaphane broccoli sprouts, consumers can now buy high-lycopene tomatoes and high-beta-carotene cauliflower. Soon, some package labels may even list the amounts of dominant protective substances, just as food labels today list the amounts of calories and carbohydrates.

phytoestrogens Estrogen-like compounds found in plants. Many different plants produce compounds that may mimic or interact with estrogen hormones in animals. At least 20 compounds have been identified in at least 300 plants in more than 16 different plant families. These compounds are weaker than natural estrogens and can be found in herbs and seasonings such as garlic or parsley, grains such as soybeans and wheat, vegetables, fruits, and drinks such as coffee. Most consumers are exposed to many of these natural compounds by eating fruits, vegetables, and meat.

Because scientists have found phytoestrogens in human urine and blood samples, they know that these compounds can be absorbed into the human body. After being consumed, phytoestrogens can either be excreted, absorbed into the body, or broken down into other potent phytoestrogen compounds.

Phytoestrogens differ remarkably from synthetic ENVIRONMENTAL ESTROGENS in that they are easily broken down, are not stored in tissue, and are quickly excreted.

Scientists do not agree on the role that phytoestrogens play in human health. When consumed as part of an ordinary diet, phytoestrogens are probably safe and may even help protect against PROSTATE CANCER, among other types of cancer.

However, eating too many phytoestrogens may cause some health problems. Laboratory animals, farm animals, and wildlife whose entire diet was made up of phytoestrogen-rich plants developed reproductive problems. Humans rarely have an exclusive diet of phytoestrogen-rich foods, and those who eat uncooked soy or use phytoestrogen pills may be exposing themselves to some health risks. Many natural compounds, especially hormones, can be potent and can have both good and bad health effects, depending on their level in the body. These substances should always be used in moderation to prevent unintended health consequences.

Cancer Prevention

Phytoestrogens have been investigated as possible cancer preventatives. One study found that Asians who eat large amounts of soy products containing high levels of phytoestrogens have lower rates of hormone-dependent cancers than do Westerners, who do not traditionally eat these products. Asian immigrants to the West increase their risks of cancer as they include more protein and fat and reduce fiber and soy amounts in their diet.

Scientists suggest that even short-term exposure to phytoestrogens may offer some long-term protection against some prostate cancers. According to some animal studies, soy-based compounds can protect against some types of cancer and may slow tumor growth.

The health effects of phytoestrogens may depend on the kind and amount of phytoestrogens eaten and the age, gender, and health of the diner. Phytoestrogens may help reduce risk because they may lower a person's lifetime exposure to natural estrogens by competing for estrogen receptor sites in the body or by changing the process through which natural estrogens are broken down. This endocrine interference can reduce a person's exposure to natural estrogens, thus reducing cancer risk.

Health Risks

The most likely risks associated with phytoestrogens are linked to infertility and developmental problems, although very large amounts of dietary phytoestrogens would probably be needed to create these risks.

Humans have used plants for medicinal and contraceptive purposes for hundreds of years. Many plants historically used to prevent pregnancies or cause abortions contain phytoestrogens and other hormonally active substances. For instance, during the fourth century B.C.E., Hippocrates noted that Queen Anne's lace prevented pregnancies.

Phytoestrogens behave as hormones do, and as far any hormone levels that are too high or too low can alter hormone-dependent tissue functions. Using too much of any hormone may not be good for anyone. Similarly, consuming too many phytoestrogens at the wrong time may have adverse health effects.

See also ENVIRONMENTAL ESTROGENS; PHYTO-CHEMICALS.

pineal gland A small gland in the center of the brain that seems to function primarily as a melatonin-producing endocrine gland. The pineal gland is one of a number of primary sites for EXTRAGONADAL GERM CELL TUMORS, particularly in children.

placental alkaline phosphatase A tumor marker sometimes used to check for GERM CELL TUMORS (particularly SEMINOMA). However, it is not used very often and is more likely to be used by a pathologist in examination of a specimen than in blood testing.

port Also called a life port or port-a-cath, this device is surgically implanted below the skin (usually on the chest) to enter a large blood vessel. It is used to deliver medication, CHEMOTHERAPY, and blood products and to obtain blood samples. A port is usually inserted if a man has veins in his arm that are difficult to use for treatment, or if certain types of chemotherapy drugs need to be administered.

positron emission tomography scan (PET scan) A highly specialized experimental research imaging technique that uses low-dose radioactive sugar to measure metabolic activity. This technique is very sensitive in picking up active tumor tissue but cannot measure its size. It may be useful in a wide variety of cancers.

Prostascint scan   A scan introduced in 1996 that looks for PROSTATE CANCER's spread to lymph nodes elsewhere in the body. Some experts believe this scan may help identify areas of cancer spread after surgery, when PROSTATE-SPECIFIC ANTIGEN (PSA) levels increase and bone scan findings are negative. The scan also may be more sensitive than a computed tomography (CT) scan or magnetic resonance imaging (MRI) in detecting the spread of prostate cancer into the lymph nodes.

The test itself involves two scans; one within 30 minutes of starting the test and another four days later. (In some cases, patients may need to return for a third scan five days after the injection). On the first day, a radioactive tracer (Prostascint) is injected into the vein, followed 30 minutes later by a pelvic scan. The total test takes about two hours. On the fourth day, the patient returns for another, more involved scan that takes about five hours. To better view the pelvic area, a catheter will be placed in the bladder to drain urine.

It is not yet widely available in the United States because of limitations in the scan's accuracy.

prostatalgia   Pain in the prostate gland.

prostate cancer   The cancer diagnosed most often among men in the United States, striking about one of every 11 Caucasian men and one of every nine African-American men. The diagnosis is usually made at age 70 or older, but many older men will develop "silent" prostate cancer that produces few (if any) symptoms and does not affect life expectancy.

Prostate cancer incidence has been increasing rapidly in recent years, probably because of the greater use of prostate cancer screening—especially the widespread introduction of the PROSTATE-SPECIFIC ANTIGEN BLOOD TEST. As yet, however, there is little medical consensus about prostate cancer's cause, recommendations for screening, or usefulness of early detection and treatment.

Prostate cancer is the most common solid tumor among American men, and is the second leading cause of cancer deaths in the United States; about 220,000 new cases of prostate cancer are diagnosed each year in the United States. Because most prostate cancers are tiny, have not spread, and do not cause symptoms, another 9 million American men may have prostate cancer without knowing it.

The incidence rates for prostate cancer, which is rare before age 50, have been particularly high in the developed areas of the world, such as North America, Europe, Australia, and New Zealand. These high incidence rates may, in part, reflect better cancer detection strategies.

Prostate cancer develops from cells inside the prostate gland, found near the neck of the bladder, which produces part of the fluid of semen. When cells in the prostate become malignant, they remain within the gland in about a third of all men as they grow older. In many cases, decades pass before this limited type of cancer spreads beyond the prostate gland's tough outer shell. Before they spread, up to 90 percent of these cancers can be cured with local treatment, such as radical prostatectomy (surgical removal of the prostate gland) or radiation therapy.

However, if cancer grows beyond the prostate gland, it may invade surrounding parts of the bladder and urethra, causing urinary problems. The cancer also may spread to nearby lymph nodes, or to the bones, liver, or rectum. Cancers that have spread to lymph nodes or other organs generally are not curable, although they often can be controlled for a number of years with proper treatment.

Cause

Experts do not know what causes prostate cancer; theoretically all men are at risk for developing this disease. Experts do know that this type of cancer—like breast cancer—is stimulated by hormones. Prostate cancer and normal prostate tissue are stimulated by the male hormones TESTOSTERONE and dihydrotestosterone (a chemical that the body makes from testosterone).

Another chemical, called transferrin, which is stored in the bones, also appears to stimulate the growth of prostate cancer cells. As prostate cancer develops, it secretes chemicals that make blood vessels grow into the cancer and introduce nutrients to nourish the malignant cells.

The prevalence of prostate cancer rises with age, and the increase with age is more significant for prostate cancer than for any other type of cancer. A number of risk factors are known to be linked to the development of prostate cancer.

Age   The remarkably sharp increase in incidence with age is a hallmark of this type of cancer. A man's risk of development of prostate cancer before age 39 is only one in 100,000; this drops to one in 103 between ages 40 and 59 and plummets to one in eight in men between 60 and 79. Microscopic traces of prostate cancer can be identified in about 30 percent of men at age 60, and in 50 percent to 70 percent at age 80. For every 10 years after age 40, the incidence of prostate cancer doubles.

Sixty percent of all newly diagnosed prostate cancer cases and almost 80 percent of all deaths occur in men 70 years of age and older. In most older men, the prostate cancer does not grow, and many die of other causes and are not identified as having prostate cancer before they die. Mortality rates for prostate cancer are much lower than incidence rates, because the survival rate of men who have this cancer is generally quite high.

Race   Prostate cancer is directly related to a man's race. African-American men are 60 percent more likely to have prostate cancer than other men and are twice as likely to die of it than Caucasian men, perhaps because they also tend to have prostate cancers that are more advanced at the time of diagnosis. Only 66 percent of African-American men who have prostate cancer survive at least five years after diagnosis, versus 81 percent of Caucasian men. In addition, African-American men have the highest rates of this cancer in the world. Higher rates of prostate cancer have been observed in temperate and tropical South America (especially Brazil), where substantial numbers of men of African descent live. Among African countries, those with higher incidences of prostate cancer also have relatively higher per capita incomes and life expectancies.

Although the incidence of prostate cancer among Caucasians is quite high, it is distinctly lower than among African Americans; Asian and Native American men have the lowest rates. The incidence rate among African-American men (180.6 per 100,000) is more than seven times that among Koreans (24.2 per 100,000). Men of Asian descent living in the United States have lower rates of prostate cancer than do Caucasian Americans; however, they have higher rates than Asian men in their native countries. Japan has the lowest prostate cancer death rate in the world; Switzerland has the highest.

Researchers suspect that genetic differences, diet, or lifestyle factors may help to explain the higher rates of prostate cancer among African-American men, who also are more likely to develop an aggressive form of prostate cancer.

In addition to having higher rates of prostate cancer, African-American men may be less likely to seek or receive treatment and so are more likely to die of this disease. When they do receive adequate treatment, African-American men who have prostate cancer appear to live as long as Caucasian Americans men after diagnosis.

Family history   Men who have a first-degree relative who has prostate cancer may be more than twice as likely to have this malignancy than men with no family history, according to a major 2003 review of medical literature published in *Cancer.* Having more than one first-degree relative with this type of cancer increases the risk even further. Whether this is due to genetic characteristics or to shared environmental influences (or both) is unclear.

Between 5 percent and 10 percent of all cases of prostate cancer are considered to be hereditary. Genetic factors may be responsible for about half the rare early-onset prostate cancers that develop in men before the age of 55. The younger the family member is when diagnosed with prostate cancer, the higher the risk for other male relatives of being diagnosed at a younger age as well. The risk also increases with the number of relatives who have prostate cancer. However, the son of a man who is diagnosed with prostate cancer after age 70 probably has no higher risk than any other man in the general population.

Prostate cancer genes   Some genes do appear to increase the risk of prostate cancer. These include the *HPC1* gene, the *BRCA1* and *BRCA2* genes, and the p53 chromosome. *HPC1* appears to cause about a third of all inherited cases of prostate cancer, and has been identified on the long (q) arm of chromosome 1 in region 1q24-q25. The gene encodes an enzyme that acts as a tumor suppressor. Inherited mutations in this gene result in hereditary prostate cancer.

Another hereditary prostate cancer gene is called *HPCX* (hereditary prostate cancer on the X), located on the X chromosome in region Xq27-q28.

Together, HPC1 and HPCX together account for just a fraction of all prostate cancer.

In addition, a number of other genes play a role in prostate cancer. These include the KAI1 antimetastasis gene on chromosome 11p11.2 and a gene predisposing to early-onset prostate cancer (PCAP) which has been mapped to chromosome 1 at some distance from the HPC1 gene.

The *BRCA1* and *BRCA2* genes are primarily linked to breast cancer; however, there is a suggestion that *BRCA1* and possibly *BRCA2* are also linked to prostate cancer risk in men. Men who have inherited an abnormal *BRCA1* gene have a threefold higher risk of developing prostate cancer than other men.

Changes in the p53 chromosome also have been associated with high-grade aggressive prostate cancer.

Hormones The development of prostate cancer is related to hormones, since men who have had their testicles removed (castrated) rarely have this malignancy. There is also a link between prostate cancer and high levels of testosterone.

Diet There is a growing body of evidence that suggests that diet may be related to prostate cancer. A high-fat (especially of animal fat and high-fat dairy products) diet is associated with an increased risk for prostate cancer, and a diet low in selenium and vitamin E may contribute to the risk. Research has shown that tumors grown in the lab grew faster when the amount of fat in the diet was 40.5 percent and grew more slowly with a 21 percent fat content. The average North American diet contains 40 percent fat, which is significantly higher than the percentage consumed in Asian countries. There is also current interest in the possibility that the low risk of prostate cancer in certain Asian populations may result from their high intake of soy products.

Obesity Although there does not seem to be a clear link between body size and prostate cancer risk, men who gained weight in early adulthood and who then develop prostate cancer seem to have more aggressive cancers.

Smoking Although smoking does not seem to trigger the development of prostate cancer, smokers tend to have more aggressive forms of prostate cancer than do nonsmokers.

Vasectomy The effects of vasectomy on the risk of prostate cancer are not clear, but at present most experts believe that having a vasectomy does not increase a man's risk of prostate cancer. Although some studies suggest that there may be a higher risk among men who have had vasectomy, these men tend to have lower-grade, earlier-stage prostate cancer that is associated with a better prognosis. Other studies have not found any link between the procedure and prostate cancer.

Symptoms

In early stages, prostate cancer rarely causes symptoms. Typically it grows very slowly, and some of the symptoms linked to enlargement of the prostate are also the same as for BENIGN PROSTATIC HYPERPLASIA (BPH). If the prostate cancer spreads into the urethra or bladder neck, it can cause the following problems:

- Urinary problems
- Decreased force of the urine stream
- Frequent urination and intense need to urinate
- Inability to urinate
- Repeated urinary tract infections
- Presence of blood in the urine or semen
- Fatigue
- Weight loss
- Aches and pains

If prostate cancer spreads to the bones, it may cause continual or intermittent bone pain that may be located in just one area or may move around the body. More common sites for spread of prostate cancer to the bones include the ribs, hips, back, and shoulders. Because some of these sites are also common areas for the development of arthritis, determining the cause of the pain can be difficult. Significant weakening of the bones may lead to fractures.

Prostate cancer also may spread to the lymph nodes or other organs; it can cause swollen glands, weight loss, anemia, and shortness of breath. Cancer that has spread to the spine may cause paralysis if the nerves become compressed. If the cancer grows into the bladder or affects most of the pelvic lymph nodes, it may obstruct one or both of the ureters that drain urine from the kidneys into the bladder. This obstruction may cause a drop in urine volume (or total absence of urine if both ureters are blocked), back pain, nausea and vomiting, and sometimes fever.

Screening

The goal of prostate cancer screening is to find this malignancy while it is still at the early, curable stage. However, experts disagree about whether all men should be screened routinely for prostate cancer, since prostate abnormalities are common and because in many cases prostate cancer never threatens a man's life. Nevertheless, regular screening does greatly increase the chance that prostate cancer will be detected at an early stage; for this reason, many experts recommend that prostate screening be performed once a year for all men except those who have a very low baseline prostate-specific antigen (PSA) level (below 2), who may want to consider screening every other year. The American Cancer Society recommends that all men be offered routine screening for prostate cancer starting at age 50 and that African-American men consider screening at age 45.

The best way to screen for prostate cancer is a combination of a DIGITAL RECTAL EXAM (DRE) of the prostate and a blood test known as the prostate-specific antigen blood test (PSA test). PSA is a protein produced by the prostate and normally secreted into the semen; in prostate cancer (and some other prostate disorders) large amounts of PSA can leak out of the prostate, raising PSA level in the blood. In the DRE test, a doctor inserts an index finger into the rectum and gently feels the surface of the prostate through the rectal wall to check for lumps, hardness, and enlargement.

The combination PSA–DRE is important because men who have a normal PSA level may have prostate cancer; if a rectal exam reveals a firm area, a biopsy should be performed. Only about 10 percent of prostate cancers are found by a DRE (in the setting of a normal PSA finding). Most healthcare providers and Medicare cover annual DREs and PSA tests for qualified Medicare patients older than age 50.

Patients should tell the doctor if they are using any prescription or over-the-counter medication to treat an enlarged prostate. Certain prostate medications, such as finasteride (Proscar) or saw palmetto, can affect the results of the PSA test.

In addition, a doctor usually takes a personal medical history, including a history of any noncancerous condition of the prostate, such as inflammation or enlargement, and any history of prostate cancer in first-degree relatives.

Diagnosis

If a man's PSA level is high or the DRE result is abnormal, the doctor orders a biopsy of the prostate, usually performed while guided by a transrectal ultrasound. In the biopsy, tissue is removed from the top, middle, and bottom of the gland on both sides or from any suspicious areas identified by DRE or ultrasound. In order to lessen the pain and discomfort associated with performing prostate biopsies dramatically, the surgeon uses a nerve block identical to that injected by dentists. After the nerve block is performed, a thumb-sized probe is placed into the rectum and the ultrasound measures the size of the prostate and locates the areas for biopsy. Eight to 12 biopsy specimens are taken, depending on the size of the prostate, and sent to a pathologist. The results are sent to the urologist within a week.

Depending on the biopsy results, PSA level, physical findings, and family history of prostate cancer, a doctor may order additional tests to determine whether the cancer has spread to the lymph nodes, bones, or other sites. These tests may include a computed tomography scan, magnetic resonance imaging scan, or bone scan. However, if a patient has a PSA level less than 10 and a Gleason score of 6 or less, there appears to be no need for a bone scan, CT scan, or an MRI, since spread of the cancer is virtually never observed in those circumstances. For all other patients, the urologist decides on the appropriate test as indicated by the PSA level and Gleason score.

Sometimes, prostate cancer may be discovered when a pathologist examines tissue removed during a TRANSURETHRAL PROSTATECTOMY (TURP) for an enlarged prostate (BENIGN PROSTATE HYPERPLASIA). This is becoming more rare as TURP is less common due to the success of medical therapy for BPH.

Grading

The most common way to determine how likely the prostate cancer is to grow and spread quickly is to grade the cancer by using the GLEASON GRADING SYSTEM.

If prostate cancer is diagnosed, the laboratory assesses how abnormal the cancer cells look and assigns a Gleason score to the tumor; the score ranges from 1 (low grade) to 5 (high grade). The grade of prostate cancer cells describes the appearance of the cells, whether they are aggressive and very abnormal (high grade) or not aggressive or barely abnormal (low grade). The grade of the cancer is an important factor in predicting long-term results of treatment and survival.

Prostate cancer may have cells of different grades, so the pathologist assigns numbers to the two most common types present, ranging from 1 to 5. A Gleason score is the total of these two numbers; for example, a man who has a Gleason grade of 3 and 4 has a Gleason score of 7. Low-score cancers are those with a Gleason score of 2, 3, or 4; intermediate-score cancers are those with a Gleason score of 5, 6, or 7; high-score cancers have a Gleason score of 8, 9 or 10.

Stage E

Classifying the tumor by using the TNM system indicates whether—or how far—the cancer has spread. In the TNM system, the *T* stands for *tumor;* it classifies a growth on the basis of its size, its location on one or both sides of the prostate, and its spread beyond the gland into other parts of the body. The tumor is given a numerical score ranging from the least dangerous (T1) through the most dangerous (T4). The classifications are further divided into (a), (b), and (c) categories. T1, T1a, T1b, T1c, T2, T2a, T2b, or T2c is considered a "local" cancer: It has not spread beyond the prostate. T3, T3a, or T3b refers to cancer that has spread just slightly beyond the prostate, but not into other organs or throughout the body. T4 (there are no initialed subcategories) describes the most advanced type of prostate cancer, which has spread to other organs or throughout the body.

The *N* part of the TNM system is an assessment of whether the tumor has spread to the lymph nodes in the pelvis. This classification is either N0 (no contamination of the lymph nodes) to N1 (has spread into the lymph nodes). The last part of the TNM staging system is used to assess whether the tumor has spread (metastasized) beyond the lymph nodes in the pelvis. There are four categories, ranging from M0 (has not spread) to M1a (has spread into lymph nodes beyond the pelvis), M1b (has spread to the bones), to M1c (has spread to other parts of the body besides bones and lymph nodes).

Treatment

One of the problems facing prostate cancer patients is the uncertainty of many issues surrounding the management of the disease. It is not known, for instance, whether surgery is better than radiation therapy or whether treatment is better than no treatment in some cases. This means that making decisions about treatment is not easy.

This uncertainty is related to the fact that it is difficult for a physician to predict whether a prostate tumor will grow slowly and cause no health problems or will grow quickly and become life threatening. Until recently, there were no randomized trials that compared the relative benefits of treating early-stage patients with radiation therapy, radical prostatectomy (surgical removal of the entire prostate gland along with nearby tissues), or watchful waiting (following the patient closely and postponing aggressive therapy unless symptoms of the disease progress).

Added to this problem is that it is not at all clear that aggressive treatment is indicated in all cases. Although prostate cancer is the most frequently diagnosed cancer aside from skin cancer in men, the fact remains that as much as 80 percent of the time, *not* treating prostate cancers does not decrease survival rate or quality of life. Nevertheless, most cases of prostate cancer are treated because a few men clearly do benefit from early diagnosis and aggressive treatment of the cancer and, in fact, may die without it. Unfortunately, doctors cannot predict in general who will benefit and who will not. For this reason, treatment is usually recommended for most men who have prostrate cancer though many men experience negative side effects as a result of treatment and most of them would not be harmed if the cancer were not treated.

However, studies have found that on average, men treated for prostate cancer can expect the same general quality of life two years after diagnosis regardless of the treatment they choose. Men who are more bothered by urination or impotence are more likely to report worse quality of life. Individual patients must weigh the unique and significant risks of urinary, bowel, and sexual dysfunction association with the different prostate cancer treatments before making a decision about therapy choice.

The specific type of treatment chosen for prostate cancer varies a great deal, depending on the extent of cancer, its chance of spreading, and the man's age, life expectancy, willingness to risk side effects, and underlying health conditions.

If the cancer is confined to the prostate gland and has not spread, there are at least three treatment options—WATCHFUL WAITING, RADIATION TREATMENT, and surgery to remove the prostate (PROSTATECTOMY).

Watchful waiting In watchful waiting, the patient receives no immediate medical or surgical treatment, but a doctor monitors regular PSA level testing and DRE results. This strategy generally is reserved for men who have a low-grade or intermediate tumor as evidenced by their Gleason score or for elderly men who are too weak to tolerate radiation therapy or surgery or who also have serious medical conditions that limit life expectancy to less than 10 years.

Radiation therapy External beam radiation therapy entails five to seven weeks of treatment given by machine aimed at the prostate. Alternatively, the radiation can be administered internally (BRACHYTHERAPY) by implanting radioactive seeds or pellets directly inside the prostate with a sterile needle guided by either ultrasound or magnetic resonance imaging (MRI). Side effects of radiation therapy may include impotence (in up to 50 percent of patients), diarrhea, rectal bleeding, and incontinence.

In general, more men experience side effects from external beam radiation than from brachy-

therapy. Sexual dysfunction is the most common problem after external beam radiation therapy; problems continue to increase 12 to 24 months after radiation. Bowel function problems often increase at six months but improve after 24 months.

Earlier studies have reported adverse effects of radiation therapy on sexual, bowel, and urinary function, but most of these studies were small and conducted in referral centers or academic institutions. In comparison, the PROSTATE CANCER OUTCOMES STUDY (PCOS) examined long-term complications of external beam radiation therapy for prostate cancer in a large random sample of men who had clinically localized prostate cancer from six population-based cancer registries in the United States. The study population included 497 white, Hispanic, and African-American men who had localized prostate cancer diagnosed between October 1, 1994, and October 31, 1995, and were treated initially with external beam radiotherapy. The study authors found that sexual function was the most adversely affected aspect of quality of life. A total of 43 percent of men who were potent before diagnosis became impotent after 24 months, while the urinary function score was relatively unchanged. Bowel function problems increased at six months but were somewhat better by 24 months. Despite these side effects, the men were very satisfied with therapy: More than two-thirds said they would make the same decision again.

Surgery A radical prostatectomy entails the removal of the prostate gland, the seminal vesicles, and sometimes the nearby pelvic lymph nodes. Side effects of this procedure can include incontinence and impotence, both of which are more common after radical prostatectomy than after radiation therapy. Recently, a new nerve-sparing surgical technique has helped preserve sexual potency in many men who undergo radical prostatectomy.

Men with clinically localized prostate cancer who are treated with radical prostatectomy are more likely to experience urinary and sexual dysfunction than those treated with radiation, according to the PCOS study. Bowel dysfunction, on the other hand, is more common among men receiving external radiation therapy. In general, prostatectomy had very little effect on bowel function, whereas radiation therapy produced bowel function problems within the first four months of treatment, with recovery of some function over two years. No clear difference in emotional and mental health or overall physical health status was seen between the two groups.

Of the 1,591 men aged 55 to 74 who were treated for localized prostate cancer and followed for two years in the PCOS study, the 1,156 men who had a radical prostatectomy reported more urinary incontinence (9.6 percent versus 3.5 percent) and were more affected by this side effect (11.2 percent versus 2.3 percent) than the 435 men receiving radiation. More men treated with prostatectomy also reported being impotent (79.6 percent versus 62.5 percent), and among men ages 55 to 59 years, the prostatectomy patients were more affected by the loss of sexual function than were the radiation therapy patients (59.4 percent versus 25.3 percent).

In general, men in the radical prostatectomy group recovered some urinary and sexual function during the second year after treatment; men in the radiation group remained the same or became slightly worse. Two years after treatment, men who had radiation reported more diarrhea (37.2 percent versus 20.9 percent) and bowel urgency (35.7 percent versus 14.5 percent) than did men who had a radical prostatectomy.

On the other hand, radical prostatectomy causes significant sexual dysfunction and some decline in urinary function, according to the PCOS study. At 18 months or more after surgery, at least 8.4 percent of the patients were incontinent and at least 59.9 percent were unable to achieve an erection. At 24 months, 8.7 percent of men were bothered by the lack of urinary control; 41.9 percent reported that sexual function was a moderate to major problem. Nevertheless, most men were satisfied with their treatment choice.

Hormonal therapy and radiation therapy   For men whose prostate cancer has grown beyond the prostate capsule but has not spread to other locations in the body, radiation therapy combined with hormonal therapy (androgen deprivation therapy) is usually the preferred treatment. Androgens are male sex hormones (such as testosterone); androgen deprivation therapy reduces levels of testosterone and other androgens that stimulate the prostate cancer to grow. Today, doctors most commonly use drugs either to block the effects of testosterone or to stop its production by the testicles. An alternative way of blocking the androgens is to remove the testicles surgically (ORCHIECTOMY).

Side effects of androgen deprivation therapy include impotence, weight gain, decreased sex drive, and osteoporosis. Some men experience hot flashes, which often can be controlled by medication.

However, men who are considering androgen deprivation therapy as an initial treatment should be aware that sexual function and some aspects of physical well-being are likely to be affected in the first year after treatment. In the ongoing PCOS study, 245 patients received androgen deprivation therapy (ADT) and the remaining 416 patients received no therapy. Among men who were sexually potent before diagnosis, 80 percent of those on ADT reported being impotent after one year, compared with 30 percent of those receiving no treatment. Patients who had ADT reported more physical discomfort one year after diagnosis than did men who had received no therapy. Men who had ADT also experienced a statistically significant decline in vitality, but not in physical function. However, patients who received ADT were more likely to be satisfied with their treatment decision than those who received no therapy.

Side Effects of Treatment

Men who undergo treatment for prostate cancer must be prepared for the possibility of urinary incontinence or a decline in their ability to have an erection. Urinary problems may result after damage to the urethra during treatment for prostate cancer, because the urethra runs through the prostate. This incontinence may be temporary or permanent.

Impotence may be caused by damage to the bundle of nerves responsible for erection that run along each side of the prostate. Eventually, a man's sexual potency may return to normal, depending on his health and age. Fortunately there are several treatments from which to choose that may help restore erections, including medications such as sildenafil (VIAGRA), vacuum devices, and PENILE PROSTHETIC IMPLANTS.

However, recent studies have found that most men who are treated for early prostate cancer are satisfied with their treatment decision. After radical prostatectomy or androgen deprivation therapy (ADT), Hispanic men are less satisfied than non-Hispanic white men. Men who after treatment were cancer free, had urinary and bowel control, could have erectile function (65.9 percent), had good general health (71.3 percent), and preserved social relationships (68.1 percent) were significantly associated with being satisfied with treatment choice. Men who received no active treatment were less satisfied (50.5 percent) than actively treated men, and Hispanic men were less satisfied than non-Hispanic Caucasian men after undergoing radical prostatectomy (50.1 percent versus 58.0 percent) or androgen deprivation therapy (29.7 percent versus 71.8 percent). The majority of men were satisfied with their treatment selection for clinically localized prostate carcinoma. Receiving an active treatment, believing oneself to be free of cancer, having no treatment complications, and having good overall health and social support were positively associated with satisfaction.

Prevention

The AMERICAN CANCER SOCIETY recommends that men limit intake of high-fat foods from animal sources and eat five or more servings of fruits and vegetables each day. Several factors may help prevent the development of prostate cancer, including eating a low-fat diet, getting lots of exercise, and taking certain medications. A man may be able to decrease the risk for prostate cancer by eating a low-fat diet high in vitamin E, selenium, and natural antioxidants such as LYCOPENE. Helpful foods include tofu and soy milk, tomatoes, green tea, strawberries, raspberries, blueberries, red grapes, peas, watermelon, rosemary, garlic, and citrus fruits.

Vitamin E may reduce prostate cancer risk, according to a recent study of more than 29,000 men in Finland. About half of the men took 50 mg of vitamin E daily, and this group experienced 32 percent fewer cases of prostate cancer than men who did not take vitamin E supplements. Foods rich in vitamin E include vegetable oils, particularly those from safflower, sunflower, and cotton seeds; wheat germ and whole grains; and whole nuts, such as almonds. Currently, however, doctors do not recommend vitamin E or selenium supplements to decrease prostate cancer risk.

Getting lots of exercise appears to lower risk of developing prostate cancer.

The drug finasteride (Proscar) reduced the risk of prostate cancer by nearly 25 percent, according to a June 2003 report that represented the culmination of three decades of research that began in the early 1970s at University of Texas Southwestern Medical Center. The study, reported in *The New England Journal of Medicine*, showed that finasteride, which is already proved effective as a therapy for enlarged prostate, also delays or prevents prostate cancer and reduces the risk of urinary problems. However, the drug has significant sexual side effects and may increase the risk of high-grade prostate cancer in some patients, the study reports.

Finasteride inhibits the conversion of testosterone to dihydrotestosterone by the enzyme 5-alpha-reductase. By doing so, it reduces by 90 percent the level of dihydrotestosterone (the primary androgen in the prostate that is involved in the development of prostate cancer). The findings are the result of the Prostate Cancer Prevention Trial, a seven-year study of 9,457 men.

Prostate Cancer Outcomes Study (PCOS) A large research studied begun in 1994 by the NATIONAL CANCER INSTITUTE (NCI) to assess the impact of PROSTATE CANCER treatments on patient quality of life. The study is a collaboration among six cancer registries that are part of the NCI's Surveillance, Epidemiology, and End Results (SEER) Program. (The SEER Program was established by the NCI in 1973 to collect cancer data on a routine basis from designated population-based cancer registries in various areas of the United States.)

The Prostate Cancer Outcomes Study (PCOS) is the first systematic evaluation of quality-of-life issues for prostate cancer patients conducted in different health care settings and provides a model for similar large follow-up studies with other cancers. It is expected that better knowledge of the effects of treatment will help patients, families, and doctors make more informed choices about treatment alternatives. PCOS will also provide some of the most detailed data collected to date on the patterns of prostate cancer care. The results of this study will be published in various medical journals over the next few years.

The study is important because one of the problems facing prostate cancer patients is the uncertainty of many issues surrounding the management of the disease. Experts do not know whether the potential benefits of prostate cancer screening outweigh the risks, whether surgery is better than radiation therapy, or whether treatment is better than no treatment. Making treatment decisions is not easy because predicting whether a tumor will grow slowly or quickly is difficult. There are no studies that compare the relative benefits of treating early-stage patients with RADIATION TREATMENT, radical PROSTATECTOMY (surgical removal of the entire prostate gland along with nearby tissues), or WATCHFUL WAITING (following the patient closely and postponing aggressive therapy unless symptoms of the disease progress). About 80 percent of men diagnosed with prostate cancer have early-stage disease. In spite of all of these uncertainties, doctors do know that radiation therapy, radical prostatectomy, or HORMONAL THERAPY can harm urinary, bowel, and sexual functions. By collecting comprehensive data on the health outcomes of various treatments for prostate cancer, the PCOS can help patients, families, and physicians make decisions about treatment options.

Several ongoing analyses are examining the effects of treatments on quality of life five years after diagnosis, the use of complementary and alternative therapies among prostate cancer survivors, the risk of recurrence and use of secondary therapies for prostate cancer, and treatments for sexual dysfunction after therapy.

Prostate Cancer Prevention Trial A study designed to determine whether the drug finasteride (Proscar) can prevent PROSTATE CANCER in men ages 55 and older that was stopped early (in June 2003) because of a clear finding that finasteride reduced the incidence of prostate cancer. However, participants who did had prostate cancer while taking finasteride experienced a slightly higher incidence of high-grade tumors. Researchers are continuing to analyze the data to find out whether finasteride actually caused high-grade tumors.

The study found that men who took finasteride, a drug that affects male hormone levels, reduced their risk of having prostate cancer by nearly 25 percent compared to the risk of men who had a placebo. These findings resulted in the early closing of the study, which was funded by the National Cancer Institute (NCI). The 10-year trial, involving nearly 19,000 participants nationwide, was scheduled to end in May 2004.

Finasteride is the first drug found to reduce the risk of prostate cancer, according to study authors. The drug worked for men at low risk for prostate cancer, as well as those at high risk. Age, PROSTATE-SPECIFIC ANTIGEN (PSA) level at enrollment, family history of prostate cancer, and race or ethnicity did not affect the drug's ability to prevent the disease. Although men in the study who had prostate cancer while taking finasteride were more likely to have high-grade cancers, more than 97 percent of men who did have prostate cancer during this study had early-stage cancers, which are most often curable. Scientists do not know why men who used finasteride had more high-grade tumors and are studying several possibilities.

The drug affects the appearance of prostate cancer cells, and this effect may lead to a false estimate of tumor grade, which is determined visually by a pathologist. Another possible explanation being examined is whether finasteride truly causes development of more aggressive tumors—either by preventing only low-grade tumors or by making the prostate gland more favorable to aggressive tumors.

Finasteride was approved in 1992 at a five-milligram (mg) dosage for treating BENIGN PROSTATIC HYPERPLASIA (BPH), a noncancerous enlargement of the prostate that can cause problems with urine flow. A few years later, the drug was approved at a one-milligram dosage to treat male-pattern baldness. In the PCPT test, healthy men age 55 and older were randomly assigned to take either five milligrams of finasteride or placebo daily for seven years. Men chosen for PCPT showed no evidence of prostate cancer at the start of the trial. To enter the study, men needed to have a normal digital rectal exam (DRE) result and a prostate-specific antigen (PSA) level of three or less. These tests were repeated annually. The participants also agreed to have a prostate biopsy after they had participated for seven years. At the time the trial ended, about 9,000 men had had biopsies.

On March 3, 2003, the Data and Safety Monitoring Committee, an independent body that periodically examined the study, advised that the trial be closed early. The recommendation was made because data already collected were sound and the conclusions were extremely unlikely to change with the addition of more data.

By the end of the study, prostate cancer had been found in about 18 percent of the men who took finasteride, or 803 men of 4,368. About 24 percent of men who took placebo, or 1,147 men of 4,692, also had been diagnosed with prostate cancer. Many of the men who had cancer had normal DRE results and PSA levels, and the disease was found only because the trial required an end-of-study biopsy.

The researchers regularly monitored participants for side effects. Compared to men on placebo, more men who took finasteride experienced sexual side effects at some point during the study. On the other hand, urinary symptoms were reported by more men who took placebo.

Finasteride is just one agent to prevent prostate cancer that the NCI has been studying. Another large prevention study currently under way, the Selenium and Vitamin E Cancer Prevention Trial, or SELECT, is determining whether these two dietary supplements can protect against prostate cancer.

prostatectomy   Surgery to remove the prostate, the most commonly used treatment to cure PROSTATE CANCER. There are several different types of prostate removal surgery. A radical prostatectomy includes the removal of the entire PROSTATE GLAND, the seminal vesicles, a section of the urethra, the ends of the vas deferens, and a portion of the bladder neck, through an incision from the navel to the pubic bone, an incision between the scrotum and the anus (perineal incision), or laparoscopically.

After the prostate and other structures are removed, the bladder is then reattached to the rest of the urethra and a catheter is inserted into the penis and bladder, to allow urine to drain while the bladder and urethra heal. A small drain is often placed through the abdomen into the pelvis to help remove mild bleeding, lymph drainage, and urine drainage. The drain is removed as the fluid level decreases. During a radical prostatectomy, the pelvic lymph nodes are often removed as well, since they are a common location of prostate cancer cell migration.

The best candidates for a radical prostatectomy are men whose prostate cancer is confined to the prostate, who are healthy enough to withstand surgery, and who are expected to live for at least seven to 10 years. However, it is sometimes difficult to estimate correctly whose disease is really confined to the prostate; between 20 and 60 percent of men who have a radical prostatectomy have a more advanced stage of prostate cancer than previously believed.

The decision to perform surgery depends not just on the stage of cancer, but on the man's lifestyle and the potential impact of the surgery on his life.

More than 70 percent of men whose cancer was confined to the prostate remain free of tumor more than seven to 10 years after radical prostatectomy.

Types of Radical Prostatectomy

There are three different ways to perform a radical prostatectomy: the retropubic, the perineal, and the laparoscopic prostatectomy. The choice of approach depends on the urologist's preferences, the patient's body characteristics, and whether or not a PELVIC LYMPH NODE DISSECTION is planned.

Retropubic prostatectomy   The most common type is the retropubic prostatectomy, in which the surgeon removes the entire prostate gland and seminal vesicles through the lower abdomen, making an incision from the navel to the pubic bone. The benefit of this option is that it allows the doctor easy access to the pelvic lymph nodes. Moreover, the blood vessels and nerves controlling the patient's sexual potency are easily seen.

The disadvantage of this approach is that it requires an abdominal incision, which can lead to a longer recovery time and more discomfort.

Laparoscopic radical prostatectomy   A radical prostatectomy also may be performed by using a laparoscope and several small incisions in the abdomen. This relatively new procedure is similar to the retropubic method, but because of the smaller incision there is less discomfort and quicker recovery. Early reports of this technique were criticized due to high rate of positive margins and the steep learning curve associated with the procedure.

Perineal prostatectomy Alternatively, the perineal approach utilizes an incision in the area between the scrotum and anus. The benefit of this method is that it does not require an abdominal incision and is therefore less uncomfortable and has a shorter recovery period. Although this method allows the surgeon to see the outlet of the bladder and the urethra clearly, nerves that control potency are less easily visualized than in the retropubic approach. In addition, the pelvic lymph nodes cannot be removed through the perineal incision. Removal of these lymph nodes requires a separate incision. The perineal method is best suited for overweight men or men with pre-existing erectile dysfunction and low probability of spread to pelvic lymph nodes.

Nerve-Sparing Radical Prostatectomy

Because the nerves responsible for penis erections thread along each side of the prostate and the urethra, damage during a prostatectomy may cause erectile dysfunction—the inability to have an erection. If the nerves are not preserved, the chance of retaining the ability to have an erection is small. If both nerves are preserved, the chance of maintaining erections with or without the use of sildenafil (Viagra) is about 50 percent, depending on the patient's age. (Men younger than age 50 are much more likely to recover erections than those older than 65.) However, even after a bilateral nerve-sparing prostatectomy, a man may still experience erectile dysfunction.

In a nerve-sparing prostatectomy, the urologist tries to push aside the nerves while removing the prostrate. The surgeon may perform a bilateral nerve-sparing radical prostatectomy, in which the nerves on each side are spared, or a unilateral nerve-sparing prostatectomy, in which one group of nerves from one side are removed with the prostate.

It is critical to decide who is best suited for a nerve-sparing procedure. The decision as to whether or not to preserve the nerves near the prostate depends on the patient's age, his potency before surgery, the location and extent of the tumor determined by the biopsy information, and the Gleason score. If these factors suggest that the cancer is confined to the prostate and the patient is potent, then a nerve-sparing procedure is performed.

Men at high risk for having cancer at the edge of the prostate are better off if the nerves and tissue on that side are all removed, since this provides a better chance of removing all the cancer.

Preparing for Surgery

Before the surgery, the patient is given a physical examination, blood tests, and a chest X-ray or electrocardiogram to make sure he is healthy enough to undergo surgery. The urologist may prescribe a bowel preparation to clean out the lower intestines.

After Surgery

Men who have laparoscopic radical prostatectomy usually go home the day following the surgery; other methods usually require at least one- or two-day hospital stay. Men are usually discharged with a Foley catheter to drain urine for 10 days to three weeks, which, allows the area where the bladder has been reattached to the urethra to heal. Full recovery may take up to a month. Once the catheter is removed, KEGEL EXERCISES strengthen the pelvic muscles to help control urine flow. Most men regain control of their urine within a month of catheter removal.

Complications

Any surgery may include complications such as infection or anesthesia problems; complications of radical prostatectomy also include hernia, impotence, urinary incontinence, bladder neck contracture, blood clots, lymphoceles, and rectal injury. Bleeding is also a risk, since there are several large blood vessels in the pelvis and around the prostate. In order to remove the prostate, these large veins must be tied off and cut. Although the amount of blood lost is usually less than a pint, a transfusion is required for 5 to 10 percent of patients. Death after radical prostatectomy occurs in less than 0.1 percent of cases; the older the patient, the higher the risk of complications and death.

In general, the retropubic approach has a higher risk of heart, breathing, and gastrointestinal complications than the perineal approach.

However, the perineal approach has a higher risk of a variety of surgical complications such as rectal injury (discussed later), stool incontinence, and infection.

Impotence   Erectile dysfunction is a common risk of radical prostatectomy, because the nerves of the penis lie along each side of the prostate and urethra. These nerves may be removed deliberately by the surgeon in a non-nerve-sparing prostatectomy, or they may be avoided in a nerve-sparing prostatectomy. The decision to spare the nerves is based on a combination of factors, including the surgeon's experience, the tumor's Gleason score and stage, the PSA level, and the extent of the tumor.

The incidence of erectile dysfunction after this surgery is as low as 25 percent in men younger than age 60 who have a bilateral nerve-sparing radical prostatectomy to as high as 60 to 80 percent in men older than age 70 who have unilateral nerve-sparing surgery.

Factors that affect the likelihood of erectile dysfunction include the penis function before surgery, patient's age, tumor stage, and extent of nerve preservation.

Erectile dysfunction after a prostatectomy may improve up to a year or two after surgery. After a radical prostatectomy the patient has no ejaculate, since the source of the fluid (prostate and seminal vesicles) has been removed, but men may still reach an orgasm.

Different treatments are available for erectile dysfunction, including medications and injections, a vacuum device, and a PENILE PROSTHESIS (a device surgically inserted into the penis that allows impotent men to have an erection). Nerve grafting is also being studied as a possible treatment.

Urinary incontinence   Fortunately with the technical improvements in performing the radical prostatectomy, the risk of significant urinary incontinence is less than 1 percent, and very few patients have required surgery for urinary incontinence. About 20 percent of patients wear a small pad in case a few drops of urine leak with physical stress, such as heavy exercise or sports. About half have excellent urinary control when the catheter is removed 10 days after surgery; the remainder gain control over the next several weeks.

Incontinence may improve over time. The older the man, the higher the risk of incontinence after prostatectomy.

Bladder neck contracture   After a radical prostatectomy, scar tissue can form in the area where the bladder and urethra are sewn together (the anastomosis) in one of every 20 to 30 cases. Signs of a bladder contracture include weaker urine stream and straining to urinate. The problem can be diagnosed by inserting a cystoscope through the urethra to the bladder neck. If the opening is very small, a wire can be inserted to help dilate the area. Once the bladder neck is dilated, it usually remains open, although a few patients require a second dilation. Although these procedures can be done in the office, occasionally an incision into the scar with anesthesia may be required.

Blood clots   After radical prostatectomy patients are at higher risk for development of blood clots in the veins of the leg or pelvis (deep venous thrombosis). Lack of movement after surgery increases the risk of a blood clot; therefore, special inflatable stockings are often used. The biggest problem created by these clots is that a piece can break off and move into the heart or lungs, which can be fatal. Although rare, these clots are among the causes of sudden death after surgery and may occur weeks afterward. Because these clots occur most often after discharge from the hospital, patients should report any acute swelling in the leg, pain in the calf, or shortness of breath.

Rectal injury   Less than 2 percent of men experience rectal injury after a radical prostatectomy. The perineal approach carries a slightly higher risk of this damage (1.73 percent) when compared to the retropubic approach (.68 percent). In most cases, small injuries can be closed and should heal; larger injuries may require a temporary colostomy to lessen the chance of stool leakage; the colostomy can be later removed.

prostate gland   A collection of glands covered by a capsule located below the bladder, encircling the urethra in front of the rectum. Because this walnut-sized gland is found close to the rectum, the back of this gland can be checked during a rectal examination.

The prostate is divided into three different zones: the transition, peripheral, and central zones. Most prostate cancers are found in the peripheral zone. Occasionally, a tumor appears in the transition zone around the urethra. About 85 percent of the time, prostate cancer is found in more than one spot in the gland, and about 70 percent of the time a patient whose tumor can be felt during a rectal exam also has cancer on the other side of the gland as well.

The prostate also can be divided into five separate lobes—two lateral lobes, a middle lobe, an anterior lobe, and a posterior lobe. Nonmalignant enlargements of the prostate typically affect the lateral lobes and sometimes may include the middle lobe.

Function

The prostate gland adds substances to a man's ejaculate, helping to nourish sperm. The prostate also produces a protein called PROSTATE-SPECIFIC ANTIGEN (PSA). This protein liquifies the semen after ejaculation. Levels of PSA tend to rise as prostate cancer develops, presumably due to obstruction or increased leakage from prostate glands. PSA can be elevated in many other conditions besides cancer. Although women do not have a prostate gland, they also have some PSA in their tissues and body fluids; however, these are at very low levels and are not important.

Enlargements

A typical prostate is about the size of a walnut in an adult male. As the years pass, the prostate may enlarge, either as part of a harmless process called BENIGN PROSTATIC HYPERPLASIA or as the result of prostate cancer.

Prostate, Lung, Colorectal, and Ovarian Screening Trial (PLCO)

A large-scale study designed to determine whether certain tests reduce the number of deaths of these cancers. Sponsored by the NATIONAL CANCER INSTITUTE (NCI), the study involves nearly 155,000 men and women ages 55 through 74 at medical facilities in 10 geographic areas across the United States. Although enrollment is complete, the PLCO Trial will continue to collect and analyze essential health data from participants for up to 14 years from the time they enrolled.

Together, prostate, lung, colorectal, and ovarian cancers account for nearly half of all cancers diagnosed as well as half of cancer deaths in the United States each year. The tests being studied may detect these cancers before symptoms develop, but whether treatment at this stage reduces the chance of dying from the diseases is unknown. Experts believe that the earlier prostate, lung, colorectal, and ovarian cancers are detected, the better the chance that treatment will extend or save lives. However, early detection with the available screening tests does not necessarily guarantee that a patient's life is extended. The PLCO Trial is designed to help answer this question.

Different tests are being studied for each type of cancer. For prostate cancer, men have a digital rectal exam (DRE) and a blood test for prostate-specific antigen (PSA) level. A DRE is a physical exam in which a doctor feels for abnormalities in a man's prostate gland by inserting a gloved finger into the rectum. PSA is a protein produced by both normal and cancerous prostate cells. Blood PSA levels are frequently higher in men who have prostate cancer and certain noncancerous conditions.

The men and women who participate in the PLCO Trial are randomized either to have the tests being studied (intervention group) or to have usual health care their doctors provide (control group). The intervention group has the tests at the first visit and once every year for the next three years. PSA screening is also offered during the fourth and fifth years of participation. The researchers maintain contact with the participants for at least 10 years from the time they enter the study.

prostate needle biopsy A surgical procedure in which a small sample of tissue is removed from the prostate gland and examined under the microscope by a pathologist for signs of PROSTATE CANCER. The procedure takes about 15 minutes and is usually performed in a urologist's office in conjunction with TRANSRECTAL ULTRASOUND (TRUS), a procedure that uses sound waves to create a video image of the prostate gland. No anesthetic is required. With the help of TRUS, a doctor guides a handheld device with a spring-loaded slender needle through the wall of the rectum into the area of the prostate gland that appears abnormal. The rectal wall is so thin the needle can be placed accurately with less injury to other tissues.

Once it is in place, a sliding sheath opens and quickly removes a core of sliver tissue (about one-half inch by one-sixteenth inch). An 8-12 biopsy is the most common prostate biopsy procedure: An average of eight cores are taken from the top, middle, and bottom and right and left sides of the prostate to get a representative sample of the gland and determine the extent of cancer.

Preparation

As with TRUS, the patient may need to have an enema before the procedure to remove feces and gas from the rectum, which might impede the progress of the rectal probe. In addition, patients may take oral antibiotics beginning the night before the biopsy and for 24 to 48 hours afterward to protect against possible infection. To limit the risks of bleeding, patients are advised to stop using aspirin seven to 10 days before the biopsy and to stop using anti-inflammatory medications such as ibuprofen three days before the biopsy.

Risks and Complications

Minor bleeding after needle biopsy is normal because the needle has entered areas that contain small veins. Blood may appear in the urine, semen, and bowel movements intermittently for a few days to a few weeks. However, very rarely is there more severe bleeding or infection of the prostate gland or urinary tract. These effects occur in less than 1 percent of patients.

Transurethral Resection of the Prostate (TURP)

Prostate tissue also can be examined after a TRANSURETHRAL RESECTION OF THE PROSTATE (TURP), a surgical procedure used most often to treat a noncancerous condition known as BENIGN PROSTATIC HYPERPLASIA (BPH). In this procedure, the surgeon removes part of the prostate gland surrounding and constricting the urethra by using a tool with a wire loop that is passed into the penis and through the urethra to the prostate gland. Electricity then heats the wire, which is used to cut the tissue. A pathologist then examines the tissue sample to determine whether it is malignant. Although BPH is not cancer, BPH and prostate cancer can exist within the same prostate gland at the same time.

prostate nodule A hard area in the prostate; although not all nodules are cancerous, this type of growth can be malignant and therefore should be biopsied.

Other causes of a prostate nodule include a prostate infection or inflammation (PROSTATITIS), PROSTATE STONES, an old area of dead tissue, or an abnormality in the rectum such as a hemorrhoid.

prostate-specific antigen (PSA) A protein made by the PROSTATE GLAND and found in the blood that at higher levels may indicate cancer in the prostate gland.

PSA is produced in both normal and malignant prostate glands, but it is not found in significant amounts elsewhere in the body. Normally, only a small amount of PSA can be detected in a man's blood. However, when the prostate gland becomes damaged or inflamed for a variety of reasons, PSA leaks into the blood more readily, raising the blood level of this chemical.

A man's normal PSA level should range between one and four, although some experts suspect that the level varies with race and age. The baseline measurement of a man's PSA is less important than tracking of the change over time. Age-adjusted normal ranges for a man between age 40 and 49 is 0 to 2.5. For men between ages 50 and 59 the upper level increases to 3.5; for men between 60 and 69, the upper level increases to 4.5; for men age 70 to 79 the upper level increases to 6.5. Although women do not have a prostate, PSA is also found in women in small amounts in breast tissue and fluid, and in breast cancer tissue.

PSA can occur in two forms in the blood, either as bound PSA, in which the PSA is attached to proteins, or as free PSA, in which it is not attached. The amount of both bound and free PSA is measured and the total is then calculated. In cases of a mildly elevated PSA level (between four and 10), the free-to-bound PSA ratio may help a doctor decide whether or not to perform a biopsy. The higher this ratio, the less likely that there is prostate cancer. A free PSA value above 14 to 25 percent suggests that prostate cancer is less likely.

prostate-specific antigen blood test The PROSTATE-SPECIFIC ANTIGEN blood test measures the level of prostate-specific antigen (PSA) in a man's blood. A PSA blood test is part of routine prostate cancer screening for most men older than 50. If the test result shows a moderately elevated PSA level, a referral for a BIOPSY is usually recommended. However, evidence now suggests that biopsy should not be performed until the test is repeated, because PSA levels commonly fluctuate above and below the normal range.

Although the PSA test is a sensitive diagnostic assessment of prostate cancer, it is not flawless; high PSA levels can be caused by other conditions than malignancy. Although it is not perfect, and many flag a high number of men who do not have prostate cancer, recent studies have found that prostate cancer screening has increased survival rates.

PSA was discovered in the 1970s by Japanese and American scientists; it was named in 1979 by Dr. Ming Wang. The next year, Dr. Wang and his colleague Lawrence Papsidero created a blood test to assess PSA levels, which was approved by the U.S. Food and Drug Administration in 1985. The test was first used simply to figure out whether treatments for prostate cancer were effective: If the PSA level dropped, the treatment was considered to be successful. Today its use has been broadened to detect cases of early prostate cancer as well as assess treatment success.

Free PSA Test

PSA can occur in two forms in the blood: as bound PSA, in which the PSA is attached to proteins, or free PSA, in which it is not attached. In addition to the regular PSA test, a doctor can use the newer free PSA test, which measures the inactive form of the antigen. The free PSA test is about twice as expensive as the standard PSA test. A free PSA value above 25 percent suggests that prostate cancer is less likely; a score of 15 percent or below means the chance of cancer is higher.

In cases of a mildly elevated PSA level (between four and 10), the free-to-bound PSA ratio may help a doctor decide whether or not to perform a biopsy. The higher this ratio number, the less likely that there is prostate cancer; the lower the percentage score, the worse the outlook.

High PSA Levels

A number of factors can increase the PSA level, including anything that irritates the prostate gland, such as a urinary tract infection, recent use of a urinary catheter, prostate stones, a recent prostate biopsy, a vigorous rectal exam, urinary retention, prostatic massage, or prostate surgery. Even sexual ejaculation can increase the level by up to 10 percent.

BENIGN PROSTATIC HYPERPLASIA (BPH) may increase the PSA level because in a larger prostate more prostate cells are present to produce more PSA. However, the condition of BPH tends to produce lower levels of PSA than does prostate cancer. And because the prostate continues to grow as men age, the PSA level may continue to increase slightly from year to year. However, some experts believe that normal enlargement with aging should still not increase a man's PSA level by more than 0.75 ng/ml a year or by more than 20 percent of the previous level.

Fluctuating Levels

The PSA test is very sensitive, and because any inflammation or irritation of the prostate can affect PSA level, the PSA test result may fluctuate in men who do not have prostate cancer. In a 2003 study published in the *Journal of the American Medical Association*, researchers at Memorial Sloan-Kettering Cancer Center and colleagues studied nearly 1,000 men who had five consecutive PSA tests over a four-year period. Up to one-third of these men had an elevated PSA level, a finding that usually prompts a referral for a prostate biopsy. However, subsequent testing of the same men a year or more later indicated that the PSA level of half of the men had returned to normal. Had a biopsy been performed, it might have been unnecessary.

Researchers concluded that a single elevated PSA level does not automatically warrant a prostate biopsy. Instead, experts recommend having the findings confirmed by repeating the PSA test after waiting at least six weeks. Even if the repeat test shows an elevated level, prostate cancer is discovered in only about one-quarter of men who have a biopsy. A policy of confirming newly elevated PSA levels several weeks later may reduce the number of unnecessary procedures as well as the number of men diagnosed with a small incidental tumor that poses no threat to life or health. Waiting to confirm the diagnosis does not have a negative effect on those men who actually have prostate cancer, experts note, because a delay in diagnosis of a few weeks or months is unlikely to alter treatment outcome.

Frequency of PSA Screening

The AMERICAN UROLOGIC ASSOCIATION and the American College of Surgeons recommend that most men start prostate cancer screening at the age of 50. However, these experts suggest that African Americans and men who have a family history of prostate cancer start screening at age 40. Not every expert agrees with these recommendations. The American Academy of Family Physicians questions the wisdom of annual testing, concerned that it may lead to excessive biopsy procedures among men who do not have prostate cancer. They point to the fact that a mild elevation (up to four) in level is not cancer about 70 percent of the time.

In addition, some doctors determine the frequency of required screenings by comparing the PSA level to the size of a man's prostate gland (PSA density). Usually a high PSA level in a man who has a small prostate gland is more of a concern than the same PSA level in a man who has a larger prostate. The higher the PSA density, the more concern there is for prostate cancer.

Those Who Do Not Need PSA Testing

Study results suggest that not all men, specifically those who have a PSA level less than two, benefit from annual PSA screenings. Older men with limited life expectancy are also unlikely to benefit from screening.

Drugs and PSA Levels

Any drug that affects the size of the prostate or the amount of testosterone produced by the testicles affects PSA level. Finasteride (Proscar), a medication used to help shrink a prostate enlarged as a result of BPH, decreases the PSA level by up to 50 percent. This decrease occurs when a man uses this drug, regardless of the baseline. Any steady increase of PSA that occurs while taking this medication must be evaluated immediately. The percentage of free PSA should not decrease while taking this drug.

Medications that decrease the testosterone level may cause prostate tissue to shrink and therefore also lower PSA level. Alternatively, boosting testosterone level may stimulate the growth of both normal and malignant prostate cells. Although testosterone therapy has not been shown to trigger the development of prostate cancer, it is known that prostate cancer is composed of cells, some of which are and some of which are not sensitive to hormones. The cells not sensitive to hormones grow regardless of the testosterone level, but the hormone-sensitive cells may be affected by testosterone level.

Therefore, men who are having testosterone therapy have a theoretical risk that the testosterone may cause an undetected prostate cancer to grow. For this reason, men who use this drug treatment should have a digital rectal exam and a PSA level test every six months (instead of yearly). Any significant increase in PSA level or change in rectal exam results during testosterone therapy requires evaluation.

Having the Test

A PSA test should ideally be performed by the same lab each time, since different labs may use different forms of PSA tests.

prostate stones   Mineral buildups in the prostate that are extremely common among men older than age 50 but infrequent among men younger than 40 and rare in children. Prostate stones grow within the prostate, probably as a result of infection; they do not migrate or pass.

There are usually no symptoms produced by prostate stones; when they do occur, they may include a reduced urine stream, lower back pain and leg pain, or recurrent passage of stones after TRANSURETHRAL URINARY RESECTION OF THE PROSTATE or ORCHITIS (testicular inflammation). Treatment is not usually needed.

prostatic acid phosphatase (PAP)   An enzyme produced by the PROSTATE GLAND that may be found at a higher level in men who have PROSTATE CANCER. A blood test that measures prostatic acid phosphatase (PAP) can determine the health of the prostate gland. However, this test is no longer used routinely, because it has been replaced by the more sensitive and specific PROSTATE-SPECIFIC ANTIGEN (PSA) BLOOD TEST. Cancer that has not spread beyond the prostate gland may not produce high enough levels to indicate a problem. A normal PAP test result does not preclude the possibility of prostate cancer.

prostatic intraepithelial neoplasia (PIN) An abnormal area in a prostate BIOPSY specimen that is not malignant but that may be precancerous or be associated with cancer elsewhere in the prostate. Prostatic intraepithelial neoplasia (PIN) is divided into two types, low grade and high grade, depending on the appearance of the prostate cells. Low-grade PIN does not appear to be linked to PROSTATE CANCER, but high-grade PIN is often linked to this type of malignancy. In some studies prostate cancer cells are found in as many as 35 to 45 percent of men who have a repeat biopsy for high-grade PIN. These men also may be at risk for future development of prostate cancer. Men with PIN are often targeted as candidates for clinical trials that test new drugs with potential to prevent or slow development of prostate cancer.

prostatism Any condition of the prostate that causes interference with the flow of urine from the bladder.

prostatitis An inflammation of the PROSTATE GLAND that may be accompanied by discomfort, pain, frequent urination, infrequent urination, or, sometimes, fever.

PSA test See PROSTATE-SPECIFIC ANTIGEN BLOOD TEST.

pyelogram, intravenous X-ray study of the kidneys and urinary tract using an injectable substance that highlights the urinary duct. It is used most often when a detailed outline of the renal collecting system and ureters is required.

R. A. Bloch Cancer Foundation, Incorporated A nonprofit foundation that offers a cancer hotline, home volunteers with diagnosis similar to that of clients, support groups, educational and special interest presentations, and a free list of medical multidisciplinary second-opinion boards. The foundation's toll-free hotline matches newly diagnosed patients with people who have survived the same cancer. For contact information, see Appendix 1.

race A man's race has an effect on the development of several types of reproductive cancers. African-American men are 60 percent more likely to have PROSTATE CANCER than other men and are twice as likely to die of it than are Caucasian men, perhaps because they also tend to have prostate cancer that is more advanced at the time of diagnosis. Only 66 percent of African-American men who have prostate cancer survive at least five years after diagnosis versus 81 percent of Caucasian men. In addition, African-American men have the highest rate of this cancer in the world.

Although the incidence of prostate cancer among Caucasians is quite high, it is distinctly lower than among African Americans; Asian Americans and Native American men have the lowest rates. The incidence rate among African-American men (180.6 per 100,000) is more than seven times that among Koreans (24.2). Whereas men of Asian descent living in the United States have lower rates of prostate cancer than do Caucasian Americans, they have higher rates than Asian men in their native countries. Japan has the lowest prostate cancer death rate in the world; Switzerland has the highest.

Researchers suspect that genetic differences, diet, or lifestyle factors may help to explain the higher rates of prostate cancer among African-American men, who also are more likely to have an aggressive form of prostate cancer. This characteristic is particularly interesting in light of the fact that Africans have one of the lowest rates of prostate cancer in the world.

In addition to having higher rates of prostate cancer, African-American men may be less likely to seek or receive treatment and so are more likely to die of this disease. When they do receive adequate treatment, African-American men who have prostate cancer appear to live as long as Caucasian men after diagnosis.

radiation oncologist See ONCOLOGIST.

radiation therapy The treatment of cancer by using penetrating beams of high-energy waves or streams of particles to kill cancer cells in a specific area of the body. The radiation used for cancer treatment is generated by specialized machines or radioactive substances that aim specific amounts of radiation at tumors. Radiation at these high dosages kills malignant cells or prevents them from growing and dividing. Because cancer cells grow and divide more rapidly than most of the normal cells around them, radiation therapy can successfully treat many kinds of cancer.

Although normal cells are also affected by radiation, unlike cancer cells, most of them recover from the effects of radiation. To protect normal cells, doctors carefully limit the dosage of radiation and spread out the treatment over time. They also shield as much normal tissue as possible while they aim the radiation at the site of the cancer. The goal of radiation therapy is to kill the cancer cells with as little risk as possible to normal cells.

A radiation ONCOLOGIST prescribes the type and amount of radiation treatment. The radiation team may include a radiation physicist, who makes sure that the equipment is working properly and that the machines deliver the correct dosage of radiation. The physicist also works closely with the doctor to plan treatment. The dosimetrist works under the direction of a doctor and the radiation physicist in administering the treatment plan by calculating the amount of radiation to be delivered to the cancer and normal nearby tissues. The radiation therapist positions patients for treatments and runs the equipment that delivers the radiation. The radiation nurse coordinates patient care and helps patients learn about treatment and side effects.

The radiation health care team also may include a physician assistant, radiologist, dietician, radiation oncologist, physical therapist, social worker or other health care professional, and radiation nurse.

Radiation Alone

For early cases of prostate cancer that has not spread, radiation treatment may be offered as an alternative to surgery. External beam radiation treatment is commonly used to treat prostate cancer that has spread too widely in the pelvis to be removed surgically but has not spread to the lymph nodes.

Types of Radiation Treatment

Radiation therapy can be given in one of two ways: externally or internally. Some patients have both, one after the other. Most people have external radiation for the treatment of male reproductive cancer, usually during outpatient visits to a hospital or treatment center. In external radiation therapy, a machine directs high-energy rays at the cancer and a small marginal of normal tissue surrounding it.

The various machines used for external radiation work in slightly different ways. Some are better for treating cancers near the skin surface; others work best on cancers deeper in the body. The most common type of machine used for radiation therapy is called a linear accelerator. Some radiation machines use a variety of radioactive substances (such as cobalt 60) as the source of high-energy rays.

When internal radiation therapy (BRACHYTHERAPY) is used, the radiation source is placed inside the body to target cancer cells without harming the surrounding tissues. This type of treatment is not often recommended when the cancer has spread beyond the prostate gland. The source of the radiation (such as radioactive iodine) sealed in a small holder is called an implant, which may be thin wires, plastic catheters, capsules, or seeds. An implant may be placed directly into a tumor or inserted into a body cavity; sometimes after a tumor has been removed by surgery, the implant is placed in the area from which the tumor was removed to kill any tumor cells that may remain.

Another type of internal radiation therapy uses unsealed radioactive materials, which may be swallowed or injected into the body. This type of treatment may require a hospital stay of several days. Brachytherapy may be used alone or combined with hormonal therapy or external beam radiation therapy.

Radiation before, during, and after Surgery

Radiation therapy can be used to treat many kinds of male reproductive cancers. Doctors may use radiation before surgery to shrink a tumor, making removal of cancerous tissue easier and allowing the surgeon to perform less radical surgery.

Alternatively, a doctor may choose to combine radiation therapy and surgery at the same time in a procedure known as intraoperative radiation.

Most typically, radiation therapy is used after surgery to stop the growth of cancer cells that may remain.

In some cases, instead of surgery doctors use radiation with chemotherapy to destroy cancer. Radiation may be administered before, during, or after chemotherapy. Doctors carefully tailor this combination treatment to each patient's needs, depending on the type of cancer, its location, and its size. The purpose of radiation treatment before or during chemotherapy is to make the tumor smaller and thus improve the effectiveness of the anticancer drugs. Doctors sometimes recommend that a patient complete chemotherapy and then have radiation treatment to kill any cancer cells that remain.

Palliative Treatment

In advanced prostate cancer, radiation can help to shrink tumors and relieve pain when curing cancer is not possible. Many cancer patients find that they have a better quality of life when radiation is used for this purpose.

Side Effects

The brief high dosages of radiation that damage or destroy cancer cells can also injure or kill normal cells, producing uncomfortable side effects. Most side effects of radiation treatment are well known and are easily treated; their risk is usually less important than the benefit of killing cancer cells.

Diarrhea and fatigue are common problems, which usually end after treatment is completed. Some men may experience continuing problems such as urinary incontinence and impotence after external radiation; treatments that can help alleviate these problems are available.

Long-term complications are uncommon with brachytherapy. Most men experience some discomfort and temporary urinary incontinence after the implant, and some may experience temporary problems with impotence.

radical prostatectomy See PROSTATECTOMY, RADICAL.

radiologist A medical doctor who has specialized in radiology and who diagnoses diseases of the human body by using X-rays, ultrasound, radiowaves, and radioactive materials. Some radiologists may perform minimally invasive procedures such as needle biopsies if they have specialized training. To become a radiologist, a student must complete four years of premedical college studies, followed by four years of medical school and usually four additional years as an intern and resident in radiology.

radiotherapy See RADIATION THERAPY.

Rb2/p130 A tumor suppressor gene located on chromosome 16, in a region that is damaged in many forms of cancer, including those affecting the prostate as well as the lung, ovaries, and breast. Temple University researchers found that *Rb2* can be used to monitor the progress of prostate cancer, since *Rb2* becomes progressively less active as disease progresses. Although such a test could be applied to biopsy samples, it would be simpler and more convenient to adapt it to a blood test. This means that gene therapy might someday be used to treat some types of prostate cancer. If Rb/p130 were introduced into a prostate tumor, the normal tumor suppressor function could be restored, and the tumor might shrink.

rectal exam Because the PROSTATE GLAND lies directly in front of the rectum, a doctor can feel the back wall of the prostate by inserting a gloved, lubricated finger into the rectum and pressing on the back wall of the rectum. This procedure is the only physically noninvasive way to examine the prostate called a DIGITAL RECTAL EXAM (DRE), this test is commonly used to check for PROSTATE CANCER.

However, this exam only allows a doctor to feel the back of the prostate. The exam can be performed either by an experienced primary care provider or by a urologist.

red blood cells Blood cells that carry oxygen from the lungs to other parts of the body. Red blood cells contain hemoglobin, an iron-rich protein that is responsible for absorbing oxygen in the lungs and later releasing it to the body's tissues. CHEMOTHERAPY drugs kill rapidly dividing cells, including red blood cells. This is why more than 60 percent of chemotherapy patients eventually have the deficiency of red blood cells known as ANEMIA, which leads to FATIGUE, dizziness, headaches, and shortness of breath.

During chemotherapy treatment patients have regular blood tests to check the number of red cells in the blood; the next chemotherapy treatment may be postponed, and a blood transfusion given, if the count is very low. Other treatments for anemia include injections of ERYTHROPOIETIN (EPO), which can boost red blood cell count.

Erythropoietin is the major blood growth factor that encourages the bone marrow to produce more red blood cells. Although it is a naturally occurring substance, it can now be made in the laboratory in much larger quantities than the body normally produces. EPO is often used near the end of chemotherapy treatment for patients who are anemic, very tired, or breathless. EPO has side effects, including flu-like symptoms, rashes, and high blood pressure.

red clover supplement (Trinovin) A supplement that, according to one study, causes early-stage PROSTATE CANCER cells to die in numbers five times greater than those in an untreated control group. The study, which was described in December 2002 in *Cancer Epidemiology Biomarkers and Prevention,* was conducted at Monash University, Victoria, Canada.

Researchers suggest that the findings may explain the fact that precancerous prostate cells in Asian men become malignant far less often. One previously reported study, for example, found that 1.8 percent of men in China have prostate cancer compared to 53.4 percent of U.S. men. These findings led researchers to study dietary differences between the cultures.

In the Canadian study, 20 patients who had confirmed prostate cancer were given 160 mg of Trinovin, which has similar isoflavone content to that of the Asian diet over a range of one to eight weeks. The men then underwent prostate surgery. The data were compared to a random sample of data from 18 patients who received no treatment.

Before and after treatment, investigators measured the blood levels of prostate-specific antigen (PSA) and testosterone, the grade of cancer, incidence of cancer cell death, and excreted isoflavone levels.

The incidence of cancer cell death was an average of five times higher (0.25 percent versus 1.5 percent) among patients who received Trinovin than among the untreated men. No adverse side effects were reported in the treatment group.

Trinovin contains four isoflavones common in the Asian diet: biochanin, genistein, formononetin, and daidzein. (Soy isoflavones, contained in common American supplements, do not contain all four of these isoflavones known to show beneficial activity in humans and commonly consumed in Asia.)

Scientists already know that there is a link between diet and cancer because when Asian men move to Western countries, they have same cancer rate as the Western population. This Canadian study further supports the link between dietary isoflavones and prostate disease.

Relief Band Explorer A patented watchlike electronic motion sickness device that provides drug-free, noninvasive relief of NAUSEA and vomiting by gently stimulating nerves on the underside of the wrist. When activated, the device emits a low-level electrical current across two small electrodes on its underside. It is available by prescription for the treatment of nausea and vomiting caused by chemotherapy. The band is the only medical device approved by the U.S. Food and Drug Administration (FDA) for use in hospitals and doctors' offices for the treatment of severe forms of nausea and vomiting caused by CHEMOTHERAPY.

resveratrol An organic compound produced by many plants during times of environmental stress, such as adverse weather or insect, animal, or pathogenic attack, which may protect against cancer.

Resveratrol has been identified in more than 70 species of plants, including mulberries and peanuts; grapes and wine are particularly good sources. Resveratrol is found in the skin (not the flesh) of grapes; fresh grape skin contains about 50 to 100 micrograms of resveratrol per gram, whereas red wine concentrations range from one and a half to three milligrams per liter.

Research indicates that this chemical acts as an ANTIOXIDANT and damps down the cellular processes involved in the promotion and growth of cancerous cells.

The concentrations of resveratrol in fruits vary considerably. One large study found about five parts per million of resveratrol in French red wines; Muscadine grapes and products contain higher levels of resveratrol. In 1996 Muscadine wines made in North Carolina were found by researchers at Campbell School of Pharmacy to average 50 parts per million.

Researchers at the University of Illinois have found that resveratrol inhibited the development of lesions and reduced the number of skin tumors in cancer-prone mice by up to 90 percent. Scientists at the University of California at Davis found that similar cancer-prone mice fed a diet that included resveratrol avoided cancerous tumors 40 percent longer than sibling mice that had no resveratrol in their diet. This compound is also thought to be partly responsible for the cholesterol-lowering effects of red wine and may explain the "French paradox"—that is, why those who consume a Mediterranean-type diet of high fat and plenty of red wine appear to have a low risk of heart disease.

retrograde ejaculation   Movement of the sperm backward into the bladder instead of out the opening of the penis during ejaculation. Retrograde ejaculation may be caused by the severing of the sympathetic nerves during RETROPERITONEAL LYMPH GLAND DISSECTION surgery. The presence of semen in the bladder is harmless; it mixes into the urine and leaves the body during normal urination.

retroperitoneal lymph gland dissection (RLND) A surgical operation in which the lymph nodes surrounding the aorta on the back wall of the abdomen are removed in order to determine whether cancer has spread outside the testicle and to remove any cancerous cells in the glands. This major operation involves an incision from the sternum to the pubic bone.

A full bilateral lymphadenectomy involves the removal of all lymphatic tissue from the back of the abdomen, where the kidneys lie; modified versions of the operation remove only nodes on the left or right side. A possible side effect of the bilateral procedure is RETROGRADE EJACULATION (movement of the sperm back into the bladder instead of out the penis during ejaculation). A nerve-sparing technique used in a modified procedure may prevent this problem.

See also TESTICULAR CANCER.

retropubic prostatectomy   See PROSTATECTOMY, RADICAL.

risk factors   There are a number of factors that may increase the risk that a man may develop a male reproductive cancer. Some of these risk factors are typically linked to many forms of cancer in addition to cancers of the male reproductive organs. These common cancer-causing factors include age, diet or weight, heredity, and race. Other risk factors are unique to a specific type of cancer.

Prostate Cancer Risk Factors

A number of risk factors are known to be linked to the development of prostate cancer, including age, race, family history, genetic mutations, hormones, diet, obesity, and smoking. Having a vasectomy is not related to the development of prostate cancer.

Age   The remarkably sharp increase in incidence with age is a hallmark of PROSTATE CANCER. A man's risk of developing prostate cancer before age 39 is only one in 100,000; this risk drops to one in 103 between age 40 and age 59 and plummets to one in eight for men between 60 and 79. Microscopic traces of prostate cancer can be identified in about 30 percent of men at age 60, and in 50 percent to 70 percent at age 80. For every 10 years after age 40, the incidence of prostate cancer doubles.

Sixty percent of all newly diagnosed prostate cancer cases and almost 80 percent of all deaths occur in men 70 years of age and older. In most older men, the prostate cancer does not grow, and many die of other causes and are not identified as having prostate cancer before they die. Mortality rates for prostate cancer are much lower than incidence rates, because the survival rate of men who have this cancer is generally quite high.

Race   Prostate cancer is directly related to race. African-American men are 60 percent more likely to have prostate cancer than other men and are twice as likely to die as Caucasian men, perhaps because they also tend to have prostate cancers that are more advanced at the time of diagnosis. Only 66 percent of African-American men who have prostate cancer survive at least five years after diagnosis, versus 81 percent of white men. In addition, African-American men have the highest rate of this cancer in the world. Elevated rates of prostate cancer have been observed in temperate and tropical South America (especially Brazil), where substantial numbers of men of African descent live. Among African countries, those with higher incidences of prostate cancer also have relatively higher per capita income and life expectancy.

Although the incidence of prostate cancer among Caucasians is quite high, it is distinctly lower than among African Americans; Asian Americans and Native American men have the lowest rates. The incidence rate among African American men (180.6 per 100,000) is more than seven times that among Koreans (24.2). Whereas men of Asian descent living in the United States have lower rates of prostate cancer than do Caucasian Americans, they have higher rates than Asian men in their native countries. Japan has the lowest prostate cancer death rate in the world; Switzerland has the highest.

Researchers suspect that genetic differences, diet, or lifestyle factors may help to explain the higher rates of prostate cancer among African-American men, who also are more likely to develop an aggressive form of prostate cancer. This tendency is particularly interesting in light of the fact that Africans have one of the lowest rates of prostate cancer in the world.

In addition to having higher rates of prostate cancer, African-American men may be less likely to seek or receive treatment and so are more likely to die of this disease. When they do receive adequate treatment, African-American men who have prostate cancer appear to live as long as Caucasian men after diagnosis.

Family history Men who have a first-degree relative who has prostate cancer may be more than twice as likely to have this malignancy than men who have no family history, according to a major 2003 review of medical literature published in *Cancer*. Having more than one first-degree relative with this type of cancer increases the risk even further. Whether this risk is related to genetic or shared environmental influences (or to both) is unclear.

Between 5 percent and 10 percent of all cases of prostate cancers are considered to be hereditary. Genetic factors may be responsible for about half the rare early-onset prostate cancers that develop in men before the age of 55. The younger the family member is when diagnosed with prostate cancer, the higher the risk for other male relatives of having the diagnosis at a younger age as well. The risk also increases with the number of relatives affected by prostate cancer. However, sons of a man diagnosed with prostate cancer after age 70 probably have no higher risk than does any other man in the general population.

Prostate cancer genes Some genes do appear to increase the risk of prostate cancer. These include the *HPC1* gene, the *BRCA1* and *BRCA2* genes, and the *P53* chromosome. *HPC1* appears to cause about a third of all inherited cases of prostate cancer. The *BRCA1* and *BRCA2* genes are primarily linked to breast cancer; however, there is a suggestion that *BRCA1* and possibly *BRCA2* are also linked to prostate cancer risk in men: Men who have inherited an abnormal *BRCA1* gene have a threefold higher risk of developing prostate cancer than other men.

Changes in the p53 chromosome are associated with high-grade aggressive prostate cancer.

Hormones The development of prostate cancer is related to hormones, since men who have had their testicles removed (have been castrated) rarely have this malignancy. There is also a link between prostate cancer and high levels of testosterone.

Diet There is a growing body of evidence that suggests diet may be related to prostate cancer. A high-fat (especially animal fat and high-fat dairy products) diet is associated with an increased risk for prostate cancer, and a diet low in selenium and vitamin E may contribute to the risk. Research has shown that tumors grown in the lab grew faster when the amount of fat in the diet was 40.5 percent and grew more slowly with a 21 percent fat content. The average North American diet contains 40 percent fat, which is a significantly higher percentage than that in Asian countries. There is also current interest in the possibility that the low risk of prostate cancer in certain Asian populations may result from their high intake of soy products.

Obesity Although there does not seem to be a clear link between body size and prostate cancer risk, men who gained weight in early adulthood and who then have prostate cancer seem to have more aggressive cancers.

Smoking Although smoking does not seem to trigger the development of prostate cancer, smokers tend to have more aggressive forms of prostate cancer than do nonsmokers.

Vasectomy The effect of vasectomy on the risk of prostate cancer is not clear, but at present most experts believe that having a vasectomy does not increase a man's risk of prostate cancer. Although some studies suggest that there may be a higher risk among men who have had vasectomy, these men tend to have lower-grade, earlier-stage prostate cancer associated with a better prognosis. Other studies have not found any link between the procedure and prostate cancer.

Testicular Cancer Risks

While the causes of testicular cancer are not known, studies show that several factors increase a man's risk of development of testicular cancer, including an undescended testicle or testicle problems, Klinefelter syndrome, abnormal genes, personal or family history of testicular cancer, and race. Accumulated data have convincingly demonstrated that having a vasectomy is not a risk factor for testicular cancer.

Undescended testicle (cryptorchidism) Normally, the testicles descend into the scrotum before birth, but occasionally they remain inside the abdomen. Men who have had a testicle that did not move down into the scrotum are at greater risk for developing testicular cancer, even if surgery was performed during the child's infancy to place the testicle into the scrotum. (However, most men who develop testicular cancer do not have a history of undescended testicles.)

Abnormal testicular development Men whose testicles did not develop normally are at increased risk for testicular cancer.

Klinefelter syndrome Klinefelter syndrome, a sex chromosome disorder characterized by low levels of male hormones, sterility, breast enlargement, and small testicles, has been linked to a higher risk of developing testicular cancer.

Personal history Men who have had testicular cancer are at increased risk of developing cancer in the other testicle.

Genes and family history Genetic abnormality of chromosome 12 has been linked to testicular cancer, as has a family history of the disease.

Age Testicular cancer affects younger men, particularly those between ages 15 and 35; it is uncommon in children and in men older than age 40.

Race Testicular cancer is more common among Caucasians than men of other races. Incidence rates in Switzerland and Denmark—about eight new cases per 100,000 men per year—are among the world's highest.

Penile Cancer Risks

The exact cause of most penile cancers is not known, but the disease is associated with a number of risk factors, including sexually transmitted HUMAN PAPILLOMAVIRUS (wart virus), SMOKING, smegma, tightening of the foreskin (phimosis), psoriasis treatments, advanced age, AIDS, and lack of circumcision.

Human papillomavirus Many researchers believe that infection by human papillomavirus (HPV) is the most important preventable risk factor for penile cancer. HPVs are a group of more than 100 types of viruses called papillomaviruses because they can cause warts (papillomas). Different HPV types cause different types of warts; some types cause common warts on the hands and feet; others cause warts on the lips or tongue.

Other HPV types, which are transferred sexually, can infect the genital organs and the anal area. A person's risk of sexually transmitted HPV infection increases with beginning sex at an early age, having many sexual partners or having sex with a partner who has had many other partners, and having unprotected sex. When HPV infects the skin of the external genital organs and anal area (around the opening of the intestinal tract), it often causes raised, bumpy warts. HPV types HPV-6 and HPV-11 cause most genital warts, but these warts rarely develop into cancer. However, other sexually transmitted HPVs have been linked with genital or anal cancers in both men and women. These high-risk HPV types include HPV-16, HPV-18, HPV-33, HPV-35, and HPV-45.

HPVs can also cause flat warts on the penis that are not visible and cause no symptoms. Flat warts caused by low-risk HPV types have little or no effect on cancer risk, but flat warts caused by high-risk HPV types can become malignant.

There is currently no cure for HPV infection, but the warts and abnormal cell growth these viruses cause can be effectively treated. These treatments can destroy warts and prevent them from developing into cancers.

Tests that are now available identify the type of DNA in an HPV infection. At this time, it is not clear how treatment will be affected by this information. HPV testing and typing are not presently routinely recommended, and most health-care professionals do not use this testing. However, scientists are studying ways to find out how testing can help prevent genital cancers.

Smoking People who smoke are exposing themselves to many cancer-causing chemicals that affect more than the lungs. These harmful substances are absorbed into the bloodstream throughout the body, especially in men who also have HPV infections.

Smegma Oily secretions from the skin, dead skin cells, and bacteria can accumulate under the foreskin, creating a thick, odorous substance called smegma. Some studies suggested that smegma may contain cancer-causing substances, but most recent studies disagree. Smegma is unlikely to have a significant impact on the risk of developing penile cancer. However, if uncircumcised men do not retract the foreskin and thoroughly wash the entire penis, the presence of smegma may irritate and inflame the penis.

Phimosis Phimosis is a condition that makes the foreskin hard to retract, so that men are less likely to clean the penis routinely and effectively. This can lead to a buildup of smegma.

Psoriasis treatment Men with psoriasis who have had combination therapy with the drug psoralen and exposure to ultraviolet light have a higher rate of penile cancer.

Age Most cases of the disease are diagnosed in men older than age 50, but about 20 percent occur in men younger than 40.

AIDS Men who have AIDS may have a higher risk of penile cancer, which could be due to lowered immune response.

Lack of circumcision Some experts have suggested that removing part of or the entire foreskin provides some protection against cancer of the penis by helping to improve hygiene. Whether circumcision is a risk factor is a controversial issue. However, penile cancer risk is low in some uncircumcised populations, and circumcision is strongly associated with other socioethnic practices associated with lower risk. Most studies have concluded that circumcision alone is not the major factor preventing cancer of the penis.

Urethral Cancer Risk

The cause of urethral cancer is unknown, but there are a number of risk factors, including bladder cancer, human papillomavirus (wart) infection, advanced age, chronic irritation of the urethra, and smoking.

Bladder cancer The primary risk factor for urethral cancer is a history of bladder cancer.

HPV Infection with human papillomavirus (HPV) or other sexually transmitted diseases is also a risk factor. HPV is a group of more than 70 viruses that are transmitted sexually and cause genital warts. Two types of HPV are associated with warts that appear on the urethra. Having unprotected sexual intercourse with multiple partners increases the risk for HPV infection.

Age People older than age 60 are at higher risk of development of urethral cancer.

Chronic irritation Irritation of the urethra that results from sexual intercourse or chronic urinary tract infection (UTI) may lead to urethral cancer.

Smoking Smoking cigarettes increases the risk for bladder cancer, which in turn is a risk factor for urethral cancer.

screening tests   There are a number of screening tests for PROSTATE CANCER but none for testicular or PENILE CANCER. The goal of prostate cancer screening is to find this malignancy while it is still at the early, curable stage. The best way to screen for prostate cancer is a combination of the PROSTATE SPECIFIC ANTIGEN (PSA) TEST and DIGITAL RECTAL EXAMINATION (DRE).

Prostate screening should be performed once a year for all men except those who have a very low baseline PSA level, who may want to consider screening every other year. Most health care providers and MEDICARE cover annual DREs and PSAs for qualified Medicare patients older than age 50.

Prostate-Specific Antigen Blood Test

The PSA screening test measures the level of PSA in a man's blood. A PSA blood test is part of routine prostate cancer screening for most men after age 50. If the test result shows a moderately elevated PSA level, a biopsy is usually recommended. However, there is now evidence that suggests that biopsy should not be performed until the test is repeated because PSA levels commonly fluctuate above and below the normal range.

Digital Rectal Exam

In the DRE procedure a physician inserts a gloved finger into the rectum to examine the area as well as the prostate gland for signs of cancer. If a rectal exam reveals a firm area, a biopsy should be performed. Only about 10 to 15 percent of prostate cancers are detected by a DRE only in presence of normal PSA (more are detected by an abnormal PSA level finding).

scrotum   The pouch of skin and thin muscles that contains the testicles.

selenium   A little-known trace element that may help protect against PROSTATE CANCER, one of the most common cancers of men. Selenium is found to a varying extent in soil and enters the human diet through plants such as corn and through the meat of animals that graze on vegetation containing selenium. Products from selenium-rich soils of the western plains carry proportionately more selenium than those from the upper Midwest, Northeast, and Florida, where selenium soil concentration is low. Grains (especially from the Great Plains), fish, organ meats, and Brazil nuts tend to be high in selenium. This element is often included in broad-spectrum nutritional supplements. Although there is no official U.S. government nutritional guideline related to selenium, typical dietary intake recommendations range from 70 to 200 micrograms a day.

Scientists first became aware of the potential importance of this element when researchers at the University of Arizona showed in preliminary studies that daily selenium supplements cut the rate of prostate cancer by more than half. Now, new research is under way to determine whether selenium may also help those who already have prostate cancer.

The same study that showed selenium users had a much lower incidence of prostate cancer also showed a much lower incidence of lung and colorectal cancer as well. More than a thousand men volunteered for the trial, which was published in December 1996. Almost immediately it caught the attention of many cancer researchers interested in the potential role of diet and nutrition in prevention of cancer.

Since then, scientists have been looking for possible explanations for selenium's benefits; one possibility is a specific type of protein within the prostate that is very responsive to selenium intake. Scientists suspect this protein may help protect against oxidative damage in the prostate.

The human body needs selenium, which is an antioxidant that may help control the cell damage that can lead to cancer. In one animal study, dogs fed a diet supplemented with selenium showed a lower level of DNA damage in their prostate when compared with dogs fed a normal (unsupplemented) diet. The finding suggests that dietary selenium supplementation decreases cellular changes that may lead to prostate cancer.

self-injection therapy A method of artificially producing an erect penis rigid enough to have sex, by injecting a medication into the penis itself. In this method, the patient uses a half-inch needle to inject alprostadil (Caverject) into the base of the penis about 10 to 20 minutes before sexual activity. The medication relaxes the smooth muscle cells and allows more blood to enter the penis, thus causing an erection.

Of all the types of treatment for ERECTILE DYSFUNCTION, the injection method is reported to be the most successful among users: erections lasting 30 to 60 minutes may be achieved on demand.

Side Effects
Some men experience discomfort from the injection. Occasionally an erection may last longer than wanted (a condition known as priapism). Unfortunately, the injection method cannot be used every day, and some men find the injection uncomfortable.

semen The fluid portion of the ejaculate, consisting of secretions from the seminal vesicles, PROSTATE GLAND, and several other glands in the male reproductive tract. *Semen* may also refer to the entire ejaculate, including the sperm.

semen analysis A laboratory test used to assess semen quality: sperm quantity, concentration, morphology (form), and motility (movement). In addition, the test measures semen volume and presence of white blood cells, which may indicate an infection.

seminal vesicles Glands in the male reproductive system that produce much of the semen volume.

seminoma The most common type of malignant tumor of the testicle, formed from sperm-producing tissue, usually diagnosed about age 40. A seminoma is one of the GERM CELL TUMORS (the other type is a NONSEMINOMA). About half of all testicular cancers are seminomas. The condition is usually limited to the testicles, although in about 25 percent of cases it has spread to the lymph nodes. Almost all men recover from this type of cancer if it is treated early.

Symptoms
Symptoms usually begin with testicular swelling and pain. Testicular tumors trigger high blood levels of HUMAN CHORIONIC GONADOTROPIN (hCG) in 10 percent of patients and of PLACENTAL ALKALINE PHOSPHATASE (PLAP) in half of all cases.

Diagnosis
All patients who have a suspected seminoma should have full blood count, creatinine, electrolyte, and liver function tests. A doctor should recommend that the patient be tested for TUMOR MARKERS (ALPHA-FETOPROTEIN [AFP], beta-hCG, and LACTATE DEHYDROGENASE [LDH]) before and after the removal of the testicles (ORCHIECTOMY). A computed tomography (CT) scan of the chest, abdomen, and pelvis is mandatory, and a bone scan should be done in patients whose cancer may have spread.

Treatment
Standard treatment for all patients who have early-stage seminoma includes radical inguinal orchiectomy. In the past, radiation treatment also has been a standard adjuvant treatment for early-stage seminoma, but today the trend in managing patients with early seminoma should focus on reduced radiation treatment fields. Some patients may be managed without additional treatment but this should only be done in patients who are reliable and who

understand the importance of close followup. See also TESTICULAR CANCER.

Sertoli's cell tumors Rare tumors of the testicle. Although some of these tumors are malignant, doctors are usually not able to determine whether a tumor is malignant by visual inspection alone. Sertoli's cells are responsible for nurturing the immature sperm, trapping male hormones necessary for sperm production. They also form tight junctions with other Sertoli's cells to form a blood–testis barrier, preventing sperm proteins from leaving the testes to provoke an immune response that would sterilize the male. This barrier is one reason why CHEMOTHERAPY does not kill all the GERM CELLS in the testes and why a cancerous testicle must always be removed. When a Sertoli's cell tumor is suspected, a radical ORCHIECTOMY is usually performed and cures the cancer, eliminating the need for further treatment.

See also LEYDIG'S CELL; TESTICULAR CANCER.

sexual problems Sexuality is a complex characteristic that involves a patient's physical, psychological, interpersonal, and behavioral aspects. However, it is important to recognize that "normal" sexual functioning covers a wide range. Ultimately, sexuality is defined by each patient and his partner according to sex, age, personal attitudes, and religious and cultural values.

Unfortunately, many types of male reproductive cancers and treatments can cause sexual dysfunction that interferes with a man's active sex life. Patients should talk with their doctor about possible side effects and whether they are likely to be temporary or permanent.

An individual's sexual response can be affected in many ways, and the causes of sexual problems are often both physical and psychological. The most common sexual problems of people who have cancer are loss of desire for sexual activity, problems in achieving and maintaining an erection, inability to ejaculate, backward movement of ejaculation into the bladder, and inability to reach orgasm.

Unlike many other physical side effects of cancer treatment, sexual problems may not improve within the first year or two of disease-free survival, and they can interfere with the return to a normal life. Patients who are recovering from cancer should discuss their concerns about sexual problems with a health-care professional.

In general, a wide variety of treatments are available for sexual dysfunction after cancer. Patients can learn to adapt to changes in sexual function by reading books, pamphlets, and Internet resources or listening to and watching videos and CD-ROMs. Health professionals who specialize in sexual dysfunction can provide these resources as well as information about national organizations that may provide support.

Some patients may need medical intervention such as hormone replacement, medications, or surgery. Patients who have more serious problems may need sexual counseling on an individual basis, with a partner, or in a group.

Sources of the Problem

Both physical and psychological factors contribute to the development of sexual dysfunction. Physical factors include loss of function due to the effects of cancer treatments, fatigue, and pain. Surgery, chemotherapy, and radiation therapy may have a direct physical impact on sexual function. Other factors that may contribute to sexual dysfunction include pain medications, depression, feelings of guilt, changes in body image after surgery, and stress in personal relationships. Increasing age is often associated with a decrease in sexual desire and performance; however, sex may be important to the older person's quality of life and the loss of sexual function can be distressing.

Surgery Surgery to male reproductive organs or in the pelvic area can directly affect sexual function. Surgeries that may affect sexual function include procedures for prostate cancer, TESTICULAR CANCER, and other pelvic tumors. For example, a radical PROSTATECTOMY damages nerves that make blood vessels open wider to allow more blood into the penis. Factors that help predict a patient's sexual function after surgery include age, sexual and bladder function before surgery, tumor location and size, and extent of tissue removed during surgery.

After a radical prostatectomy, a man may have a problem having or maintaining an erection because the nerves that control erections may be damaged, weakening or interrupting blood flow. However, these nerves do not control orgasm, ejaculation, or sensation. This means that the desire and ability to enjoy sexual touching usually remain intact, and a man who has had this operation still has the ability to experience orgasm. Although they may not have experienced it before, men are physically able to have an orgasm without an erection or ejaculation of fluid.

Nerve-sparing prostatectomy was designed to avoid the nerve pathways involved in erection. Depending on the location and size of the prostate tumor, sparing of the nerves on both sides of the prostate may not be possible. Recovery of erections after nerve-sparing surgery is gradual; it can take several months to a year and sometimes continue into a second year. Younger, healthier men are most likely to recover the ability to have strong erections.

Newer nerve-sparing techniques for radical prostatectomy are being studied as a more successful approach for preserving potency than radiation treatment for prostate cancer. Long-term follow-up is needed to compare the effects of surgery with the effects of radiation therapy. Recovery of erectile function usually occurs within a year after a radical prostatectomy.

Radiation treatment RADIATION THERAPY to the pelvic area can cause direct physical problems with having and maintaining an erection. External beam radiation can cause gradual changes in sexual functioning. The exact cause of sexual problems after radiation therapy is unknown. Most physicians believe that it is related to accumulating damage to small arteries bringing blood to the penis or decreased levels of TESTOSTERONE. Between 25 and 50 percent of men have new erection problems after radiation therapy. Internal radiation (seed implantation or BRACHYTHERAPY) has a much lower rate of impeding sexual functioning.

Just as chemotherapy can, radiation can cause side effects such as fatigue, nausea and vomiting, diarrhea, and other symptoms that can decrease feelings of sexuality.

Sexual changes occur very slowly over a period of six months to one year after radiation therapy. Men who had problems with erectile dysfunction before having cancer have a greater risk of developing sexual problems after cancer diagnosis and

treatment. Other risk factors that can contribute to a greater risk of sexual problems in men are cigarette smoking, history of heart disease, high blood pressure, and diabetes.

Chemotherapy Chemotherapy is associated with a loss of desire and decreased frequency of intercourse for both men and women. The common side effects of chemotherapy, such as NAUSEA, vomiting, DIARRHEA, CONSTIPATION, weight loss or gain, and HAIR LOSS, can affect a man's sexual self-image and make him feel unattractive. It is important to remember that an interest in sex often returns when normal energy levels return. Occasionally chemotherapy may interfere with testosterone production in the testicles. Testosterone replacement may be necessary to restore sexual function.

Sexual problems such as loss of desire and erectile dysfunction are more common after bone marrow transplant because of graft-versus-host disease or nerve damage.

Prescription medications Medications for pain, depression, and anxiety also may interfere with a man's sex life. Patients should ask the doctor for information on possible side effects of all medications. If medications are causing sexual problems, a change in medications or a lower dosage may help.

Hormonal changes HORMONE THERAPY for male reproductive cancers can lower normal hormone levels and cause a decrease in sexual desire, impotence, and problems reaching orgasm. However, younger men do not always experience the same degree of sexual dysfunction.

There are several situations that may produce a lower hormone level. Surgical testicle removal to treat testicular cancer may interfere with sexual desire if both testicles are removed or if the remaining testicle is not producing enough testosterone. BONE MARROW TRANSPLANTS and radiation therapy can sometimes temporarily or permanently interfere with the production of testosterone as well.

Hormone therapy for PROSTATE CANCER is based on the fact that prostate cancer cells require testosterone for growth. By preventing the production of testosterone, the cancer loses its stimulus. Combination hormonal therapy affects sexual activity as long as treatment is given. Men report that having an erection during treatment may require more time and effort. Sexual desire generally decreases over the duration of the treatment because hormone treatment decreases male hormone levels in order to slow the growth of the cancer, and these same hormones are responsible for sexual drive.

Men may be given leuprolide (Lupron) or goserelin to decrease production of testosterone, of flutamide or bicalutamide (Casodex) in combination to stop testosterone production at the cell level. About 80 percent of men who have these treatments report little interest in sexual activity; 20 percent manage to remain sexually active. Erections may take longer and may be less firm. Orgasm also can take more effort and ejaculate may not contain any semen. Sex can still be enjoyed by adjusting the definition of what is satisfying and trying new ways to become aroused.

Some treatment centers are experimenting with delayed or intermittent hormone therapy to prevent sexual problems. It is not yet known whether these modified treatments affect the long-term survival of younger men.

Cryotherapy The experimental treatment cryosurgery also carries the possibility of damaging the nerves responsible for erection. About two-thirds of men report problems becoming erect after having this procedure. However, the ability to achieve an erection may improve over time.

Erections and Cancer Treatment

One of the most serious problems related to the treatment of some types of male reproductive cancers is the inability to have an erection after treatment. However, in the last 20 years, important advances have been made in treating these problems. It is still possible to enjoy a satisfying sex life after prostate cancer treatment. Most men can find solutions, either through methods that help with impotence or by discovering new ways to achieve intimacy with their partner.

There are several options available to men who are impotent and many strategies for approaching sex that can help, even before beginning cancer treatment. Before treatment begins, it is important that the patient be honest about pretreatment sexual functioning. The doctor may ask questions about frequency of sexual activity, detailed information about erections (including firmness and frequency), and current problems related to erec-

tions. A clear discussion of sexual functioning before treatment can help in identifying any problems that occur after treatment.

Before a patient makes any treatment choices to restore potency, it is important that he learn about all the treatment options first and involve the partner in decisions. Counseling may help when talking about sexuality is uncomfortable.

Treatment for sexual problems is not required; the patient and his partner may decide not to treat the problem after exploring all the issues. There is no reason that patients cannot enjoy a satisfying sex life in other ways than having intercourse. For many men and their partners, this is the best choice.

Counseling Counseling may help the patient and his partner talk about sexual issues. Counseling can help reduce a man's anxiety about sexual functioning and body image issues and help him deal with depression or sadness that results from a cancer diagnosis. Many people seek guidance from a mental health professional when cancer strikes.

When dealing with impotence, starting with the least invasive treatment method first and proceeding from there can make sense. For example, a man may wish first to try sildenafil (Viagra) and then the vacuum device, followed by injection therapy or implant if other methods prove unsatisfactory. Men also need to remember that even if a treatment restores potency, erections will probably not feel as they did before. A realistic goal is to achieve erections that are firm enough to allow penetration.

Medication Three drugs can treat impotence successfully for many patients: sildenafil (VIAGRA); TADALAFIL (Cialis); and VARDENAFIL (Levitra).

Vacuum Alternatively, vacuum erection devices (or vacuum pumps) are a noninvasive option that can be used immediately after a man recovers from radical prostate surgery. In this method, the man inserts the penis into a cylinder and activates a pump (by hand or by battery), which causes a vacuum that draws blood into the penis. After the penis becomes swollen and erect, an elastic ring is placed at the base of the penis to retain the blood. This is done each time an erection is desired, and each erection can last 20 to 30 minutes. (The elastic ring must be removed within 30 to 40 minutes to restore the normal flow of blood.)

This method tends to work best for men who still achieve some swelling in the penis with sexual stimulation. However, these devices may cost $75 to more than $200. Fortunately, the cost is often covered at least partially by insurance and Medicare.

Some men find the elastic ring uncomfortable or have difficulty coordinating the process. Using the device can be built into the sexual experience, although some partners report discomfort caused by the disruption.

Injections   Injections of medication directly into the penis also can stimulate or help maintain erections. Most men actually report little discomfort from the procedure. The medication most often used is prostaglandin E_1 (Caverject) or a combination of papaverine and phentolamine (Regitine). Combinations of all three drugs may be the best option for long-term use and decreased risk of side effects.

The erections last between 40 and 60 minutes and most men report no adverse side effects. A few men develop scar tissue at the site of the injection. Injections can be expensive, and are often not covered by insurance.

Penile implant   Also called a penile prosthesis, the implant can be surgically implanted into the penis to provide an erection rigid enough for sexual intercourse. Because an implant destroys the natural erection reflex, it is important to use this option only when erections are unlikely to improve. Complications of the procedure include mechanical failure of the device and infection (about 10 percent of men have complications).

The cost is usually between $15,000 and $20,000; insurance usually covers it when a medical problem has been documented.

Available devices include simple semirigid or malleable models that are inserted surgically, making the penis permanently semierect. The rod can be bent up into an erection or down into a relaxed position. The implant procedure is simple, and there is little risk of infection or other complications. Inflatable implants include a small reservoir, two cylinders on each side of the penis, and a pump that squirts fluid into the cylinders to create an erection. After sex, a valve releases the liquid back into the reservoir. There are several models of inflatable implants, which range from simple to more complex.

Inability to Reach Orgasm and Dry Orgasm

There are a number of changes in orgasm that can result from cancer treatments. A man may be slower to reach orgasm, need different kinds of stimulation, or have a dry orgasm in which no semen is ejaculated. Some men find reaching orgasm difficult. It is somewhat uncommon for a man to have a problem in reaching orgasm as a result of cancer treatment. Still, there are a number of reasons why cancer treatment may interfere with orgasm.

Treatment of reproductive cancer that has spread to the brain or spinal cord tumors may result in numbness or paralysis that could affect the sense of touch and pleasure in genital stimulation. In penile cancer, men who have lost their penis can learn to reach orgasm through caressing the remaining genital areas.

Cancer treatment also can decrease genital sensation. Medications such as antidepressants, tranquilizers, and pain medication may reduce the ability to have an orgasm.

To achieve orgasm despite these problems, the man should focus on increasing desire and enjoying the experience rather than focusing on the orgasm. Increasing pleasure helps the patient eventually reach climax. Men can experiment through masturbation to find out what works best. Using a vibrator to intensify stimulation either at the base or at the head of the penis may be effective.

Fortunately, premature ejaculation rarely is a problem after cancer treatments, although some men experience no ejaculations or dry orgasm. There are a number of treatments that can cause this to occur, including radical prostatectomy, radical cystectomy, radiation to the pelvis, and use of some chemotherapy drugs. The damage affects the prostate and seminal vesicles that produce semen. Erection problems may also occur but may be helped by oral and hand stimulation. Orgasm still occurs without semen; half of men report their climax as pleasurable but weaker than before, and many report no change in orgasm. Although men have worried that a dry orgasm may be less pleasurable for their partner, partners report that lack of semen can in fact increase pleasure during oral sex. Dry orgasm becomes an issue usually only for a man who wishes to father a child.

Sex after Surgical Removal of Body Parts
Cancer treatments also may cause physical changes that affect a man's attitude about his physical appearance, making him feel sexually unattractive. Surgical treatment for men who have penile cancer, testicular cancer and metastatic prostate cancer may require partial or total removal of body parts. It is important that patients discuss their feelings and concerns with a doctor, so they can learn how to deal with any problems these surgeries may cause.

Penis removal The most common form of treatment of penile cancer is surgical removal of part or all of the penis (PENECTOMY). If the tumor is limited to the tip of the penis, a partial penectomy (removal of part of penis) is performed, leaving enough of the shaft to direct the urine stream away from the body. The remaining shaft is long enough for penetration of the vagina and is able to become erect on sexual arousal.

When the shaft of the penis cannot be saved, a total penectomy (removal of the entire penis) is required. A new opening in the area between scrotum and anus called the perineal urethrostomy is created for urination. Many men who have penile cancer are elderly and adjust to the loss of the penis by simply giving up sex. However, those who wish to have a sex life can do so by deep kissing, sexual massages, and kissing and caressing of sensitive genital areas (such as the scrotum, skin behind the scrotum, and skin around the area where the penis was removed).

Testicle loss Men treated for metastatic prostate cancer or for testicular cancer may have one or both testicles removed to stop the production of testosterone and other male hormones that feed the tumor. (In men who have testicular cancer, only the testicle with cancer is removed; rarely does a man develop a cancer in the second testicle.)

Although sexual functioning and fertility often remain unimpaired, a young, single, and dating male may consider a missing testicle emotionally painful and embarrassing. Although some men are not affected by the new appearance, others may fear the reaction of a partner. In such cases, surgical implantation of a prosthesis that looks and feels like a testicle can help deal with body image issues.

Psychological Factors
One of the most important factors in adjustment after cancer treatment is the patient's feeling about his sexuality before a cancer diagnosis. Patients who felt good about themselves sexually may be more likely to resume sexual activity after treatment for cancer.

Patients recovering from male reproductive cancer often worry that previous sexual activities may have caused their cancer. Some patients believe that sexual activity may cause the cancer to recur or pass the cancer to their partner. Discussing their feelings and concerns with a physician or mental health professional is a good idea. This way, patients can be reassured that cancer is not passed on through sexual contact.

In addition, a drop in sexual desire and sexual pleasure is a common symptom of depression, which is more common in patients with cancer than in the general healthy population. It is important that patients discuss their feelings with their doctor. Treatment for depression may help relieve sexual problems.

The stress of a cancer diagnosis and treatment can worsen existing problems in relationships. Patients who do not have a committed relationship may stop dating because they fear rejection by a potential new partner who learns about their history.

Moreover, many patients are fearful or anxious about their first sexual experience after cancer treatment. Fear and anxiety can cause patients to avoid intimacy, touch, and sexual activity. The healthy partner may also worry or be afraid to initiate any activity that may be misconstrued as pressure to be intimate or may cause physical discomfort.

Patients and their partners should discuss these concerns with their doctor, because honest communication of feelings, concerns, and preferences is important.

Social Security Disability Insurance (SSDI) A U.S. government social program that pays benefits to a person who is insured: meaning the person worked long enough and paid Social Security taxes. If a person expects to be disabled for at least six months, he may be eligible for Social Security Disability Insurance (SSDI). Often the government accepts as a disability cancer that has spread.

soy products　Foods (such as tofu and miso) that contain proteins and substances called isoflavones that may help prevent PROSTATE CANCER (among others). Isoflavones are a type of PHYTOESTROGEN, a naturally-occurring plant estrogen.

Although studies have not been done on the effects of soy on a healthy human prostate, men who have prostate cancer are routinely advised to eat soy foods because soy isoflavones have been shown to reduce the growth of prostate cancer cells in test tubes. However, the effects of soy on cancer are not fully understood.

Current advice for eating soy ranges from eating none to eating soy foods (not soy pills or powder) several times a week as a low-fat replacement for animal protein. Patients should seek medical advice about soy for their individual needs. Soy can be obtained by eating the following:

- Tofu (a curd made from cooked, pureed soybeans)
- Miso (a mixture of fermented soybean paste and a grain such as rice or barley)
- Dried soybeans
- Roasted soybeans or nuts (soybeans that are soaked in water and baked)
- Edamame and natto (steamed whole green soybeans and fermented, cooked whole soybeans)
- Tempeh (a combination of whole, cooked soybeans and grains cultured with an edible mold)
- Soy milk (the liquid expressed from cooked, pureed soybeans)

The ability of the body to use the nutrients in soy foods varies with the food and its preparation. In general, soy that has been processed least (such as tofu, tempeh, and mature, green, and roasted soybeans) contains the highest level of protein and naturally occurring isoflavones. Soy germ is the source highest in isoflavone level.

spermatocytoma　Also called spermatocytic seminoma, this is a unique type of benign tumor distinct from other GERM CELL TUMORS, which occurs only in men and never outside the gonads. It is not found in conjunction with any other germ cell tumor and occurs almost exclusively in men older than age 50. Spermatocytomas constitute only 2 to 3 percent of all testicular tumors; in 10 percent of patients they occur in both testicles.

See also TESTICULAR CANCER.

sperm banking　Removal and storage of sperm before treatment for male reproductive cancer. A sperm bank is a place where sperm are kept frozen in liquid nitrogen for up to 50 years, for later use in artificial insemination. There is usually an annual fee for storage.

If a man has been diagnosed with reproductive cancer, subsequent medical treatment may affect his ability to father a child in the future; sperm banking offers a patient the chance to father his own children. Although a man's fertility may be restored after cancer treatment, there is no guarantee that it will.

The Process

Collection of enough semen samples usually takes about two weeks. If time is an issue, men who need to start treatment quickly can sometimes collect enough semen within a couple of days. If a man is planning to bank sperm, doctors request that he not ejaculate for one to two days before each sample is taken. Three to six samples are usually needed to bank enough semen to provide a reasonable chance of later conception.

The sample is collected when a man masturbates at the laboratory, since it is important to decrease the risk of bacterial contamination. Moreover, sperm may die if not quickly frozen. Once the sample has been collected, the lab tests the sample to count sperm cells and assess sperm health. The semen, which is then placed into a container and frozen at extremely low temperatures, can be safely stored in this frozen state for up to 50 years. No evidence suggests that pregnancies produced with frozen sperm have a higher chance of birth defects.

For the patient approaching cancer treatment, having even one sample of frozen sperm stored in the sperm bank increases the chance of having a biological child in the future, regardless of how his fertility is affected by treatment. With modern techniques of infertility treatment (in vitro fertilization using an injection of a single sperm cell into each egg), only a few live sperm cells need to survive the freezing and thawing process in order to create a pregnancy. If a man has good sperm quality and can freeze three to six semen samples, the couple may be able to achieve pregnancy by using simpler infertility treatments, such as artificial insemination.

Although many men have abnormal sperm counts before cancer treatment is begun, it is still worthwhile to freeze the sperm in advance.

Infertility treatments are expensive and not often covered by insurance, so a patient should be sure to check with his health insurance provider to learn about his benefits. Patients interested in exploring infertility treatments should contact a fertility clinic that specializes in male fertility issues and ask about their experience in helping cancer survivors. The American Society for Reproductive Medicine can offer more information about infertility treatments for cancer survivors.

sperm health and cancer treatment The male hormone TESTOSTERONE and sperm are both produced in the testicles. Because cancer treatments target cells that are rapidly dividing (as cancer cells do), they can also harm other rapidly dividing cells in the body, including sperm cells. Radiation to the pelvic area, some types of CHEMOTHERAPY, and surgical side effects all can harm sperm cells, with potential to cause temporary or permanent male infertility.

Chemotherapy Although chemotherapy may not affect the production of testosterone, studies have shown that chemotherapy can damage sperm production. It is quite likely that a man will experience at least some period of infertility after chemotherapy treatment. There are different estimates as to whether or when a man's sperm count will return to near-normal levels after chemotherapy. In some situations, sperm production never returns; in other cases sperm formation resumes about one to four years after treatment.

However, in some situations sperm counts remain low as long as five years after treatment has stopped. Depending on the types of anticancer drugs given, the dosage received, and the man's health, fertility potential may return, or the man may produce only a few sperm, which may not be sufficient to cause pregnancy without medical help. Permanent sterility is especially common among men who are given high doses of chemotherapy before bone marrow or stem cell transplant.

Combinations of chemotherapy with radiation to the pelvis or abdomen can be especially damaging.

Radiation treatment When RADIATION THERAPY is aimed at or near a man's testicles, it also may damage sperm production or create the potential for birth defects in the children of men who have radiation treatment. The testicles may be a direct target for radiation in TESTICULAR CANCER or metastatic PROSTATE CANCER. A dosage of 600 rad to the testicles is sufficient to destroy stem cells that produce sperm cells permanently; dosages less than 600 rad to the testicles slow or stop sperm cell production.

After radiation therapy, a man's fertility may return, depending on the dosage of radiation received by his testicles. Sperm cell counts may recover in months or years, but there is no guarantee this will occur. Higher dosages of radiation negatively affect sperm count for longer periods than lower dosages, and men younger than age 40 are less susceptible to damage than older men. Although specially molded lead sheets can be used to protect the testicles, sometimes there is an indirect effect.

In addition, because radiation can potentially damage sperm production, it may be necessary to wait one year or more before trying to conceive.

Surgery Some types of cancer require the removal of parts of the man's reproductive system, such as the prostate or testicles; the surgery may affect sperm production or may cause damage to the nerves important to normal ejaculation. Some surgeries, such as RETROPERITONEAL LYMPH NODE DISSECTION for testicular cancer, may cause ejaculatory problems as well.

Prevention

Once sperm cell production is damaged, there is currently no way to fix the damage. Therefore, the best option to protect a man's fertility is to bank sperm before surgery to the pelvis or chemotherapy and radiation therapy. It is a choice that may be difficult to make, since many men assume they will not lose their fertility or do not know whether they want to have children. Many cancer centers offer SPERM BANKING, as do most large cities. Banking sperm may not be recommended for men who have low sperm counts and motility (sperm's ability to move) problems. However with advances in fertility, any type of sperm cell can be important. Research has shown no increased risk for birth defects in babies conceived from frozen sperm.

Wanting to conceive a child and being unable to do so can cause immense heartbreak for a couple. When the reasons a couple cannot conceive are related to cancer, feelings of grief and anger can be especially intense. A man may have a feeling of being damaged or defective along with the range of burdensome emotions that a diagnosis of cancer can cause. For a couple who looked forward to having children, the loss of the dream is real and must be mourned. For these reasons, experts consider it important to find emotional support to help the couple cope with these difficult issues.

staging   A medical attempt to find out whether a patient's cancer has spread and, if so, to what parts of the body. A doctor stages cancer by studying information obtained during surgery, X-rays and other imaging procedures, and lab tests. Knowing the stage of the disease helps the doctor plan treatment.

Typically, cancer stages are numbered from I through IV (IV is the most severe); in some types of cancer the Roman numerals are subdivided into a and b subcategories.

statistics in men's reproductive cancer   Reproductive system cancers are among the most deadly because they often remain undiagnosed longer than other types of cancers. Of the three main types of male reproductive cancers, PROSTATE CANCER is the most common, followed by TESTICULAR CANCER and then PENILE CANCER.

Prostate cancer occurs more commonly than lung cancer, but early detection and treatment have led to lower death rates than in lung cancer.

However, death rates for prostate cancer are still high in African-American men, who are two to three times more likely to die of prostate cancer than are Caucasian men. According to the American Cancer Society, 220,900 new cases of prostate cancer occur each year and 28,900 deaths.

About 7,400 men in the United States are diagnosed with testicular cancer each year. Although testicular cancer accounts for only 1 percent of all cancers in men, it is the most common form of cancer in young men 15 to 35. Although any man may have testicular cancer, it is more common among Caucasians than African Americans.

Penile cancer is the most rare of the three reproductive malignancies: In a year 1,400 new cases occur and 200 men die of this type of cancer in the United States. Penile cancer occurs in one in every 100,000 men.

Usefulness of Statistics

The usefulness of cancer statistics depends on their interpretation and use. Cancer statistics are often cited in medical stories and can be helpful for a broad perspective, but they are less helpful in understanding one person's specific outlook. For example, the lifetime risk of development of a type of cancer is not a man's risk at any moment. The *actual* chance of development of many types of men's reproductive cancer changes throughout a man's life, increasing with age, so that a man's *current* risk of developing the disease this year is quite different from the risk of developing the disease some time in his life, or after age 70 or 80. Moreover, heredity, ethnicity, lifestyle, and other risk factors all contribute to a person's overall cancer risk.

Incidence

Incidence describes the number of new cases of cancer that occur in a specific population group within a set period—usually one year. For example, the total 2001 incidence of testicular cancer was about 7,200 men. *Incidence rate* is the number of new cases in a population, usually expressed in terms of the number of cases per 100,000 people. For example, the *incidence rate* for testicular cancer in the United States is about four new cases per 100,000 men, often stated simply as four per 100,000.

Prevalence

Prevalence refers to the total number of people with cancer or with a particular risk factor for cancer at a particular moment in time in the entire population. For large groups of people, prevalence is estimated by collecting information from a smaller subset of people and then extrapolating that information to the general population.

Morbidity and Mortality

Morbidity is a term that means a state of illness. For instance, experts may comment that smoking is a major cause of morbidity in the United States. *Mortality* pertains to death; the cancer *mortality rate* is the number of people in a population group who die of cancer within a set period (usually one year). The cancer mortality rate usually is expressed in terms of deaths per 100,000 people.

Prognosis

Prognosis is the prediction of the outcome of a disease, usually including the chance of recovery. Physicians may base a prognosis on statistical precedents; however, each patient's individual prognosis is affected by many factors, including age and general health, type and stage of cancer, and effectiveness of the particular treatment used. Therefore, although a prognosis may help explain the severity of a disorder or guide treatment decisions, it cannot predict disease outcomes for an individual.

Survival Rate

Survival rate refers to the number of people who develop cancer and survive over a period. Scientists commonly use five-year survival rate as the standard statistical basis for defining when a cancer has been successfully treated.

The five-year survival rate includes anyone who is living five years after a cancer diagnosis, including those who are cured, those who are in remission, and those who still have cancer and are undergoing treatment. For example, when colorectal cancers are detected early, the five-year survival rate is 92 percent, meaning that 92 percent of all colorectal cancer patients live at least five years after diagnosis if the cancer is detected early.

The *overall five-year survival rate* measures everyone who has ever been diagnosed with a particular cancer equally; such a measurement can produce distorted statistics. For example, a 90-year-old man and a 30-year-old man who have the same cancer are grouped together. The 90-year-old may die of other causes within the five-year period because of normal life expectancy, and his death can skew the data. A more statistically accurate view of survival is the *relative five-year survival rate*, which compares a cancer patient's survival rate with the survival rate of the general population, taking into account differences in age, gender, race, and other factors. In this case, the 30-year-old and the 90-year-old are treated as statistically different.

Risk

Risk is the chance that an individual will develop a disease. *High-risk* indicates a chance of having cancer that is higher than the chance of the general population.

A *risk factor* is anything that has been identified as increasing a person's chance of having disease. It may be controllable or uncontrollable, personal or environmental. For example, risk factors for development of prostate cancer include having a hereditary predisposition to the disease (uncontrollable) and being obese (controllable).

Relative risk is a measure of the extent to which a particular risk factor increases the risk of development of a specific cancer. *Attributable risk* is a measure of the part of the total incidence of disease that is caused by that risk factor. *Lifetime risk* is the probability of developing or dying of cancer sometime during one's lifetime. A person has a lifetime risk of two in five of developing cancer, meaning that for every five people in the population, two eventually will develop cancer. The lifetime risk of dying of cancer in one in five.

(See also individual cancers for more information on specific cancer statistics.)

stem cells Cells that are able to produce other cells when they divide. Usually the term *stem cells* refers to blood cells. Most stem cells are found in the BONE MARROW; some stem cells, called peripheral blood stem cells, can be found in the bloodstream. Umbilical cord blood also contains stem cells. Stem cells can divide to form more stem cells, or they can mature into white blood cells, red blood cells, or platelets.

Stem Cell Transplant

High-dose CHEMOTHERAPY can severely damage or destroy a patient's bone marrow so that the body is no longer able to produce needed blood cells. In the case of TESTICULAR CANCER, this may simply be a side effect of treatment.

A stem cell transplant allows stem cells that are damaged by treatment to be replaced with healthy stem cells that can produce the blood cells the patient needs. A stem cell transplant allows a patient who has testicular cancer to be treated with high dosages of drugs, radiation, or both. The high dosages destroy both leukemia cells and normal blood cells in the bone marrow so that later the patient can be given healthy stem cells. New blood cells develop from the transplanted stem cells.

Stem cells may be taken from the patient (autologous transplant) or from a donor (allogeneic transplant). In an autologous stem cell transplantation, the patient's own stem cells are removed and the cells treated to kill leukemia cells. The stem cells are then frozen and stored. After the patient receives high-dose chemotherapy or RADIATION THERAPY, the stored stem cells are thawed and returned to the patient. In an allogeneic stem cell transplantation, the patient is given healthy stem cells from a donor (such as a brother, sister, or parent); sometimes stem cells are from an unrelated donor. Doctors use blood tests to be sure the donor's cells match the patient's cells. In a syngeneic stem cell transplantation, the patient is given stem cells from the patient's healthy identical twin.

Types of Stem Cell Transplants

There are several types of stem cell transplantation:

- *Bone marrow transplantation:* The stem cells are taken from bone marrow.
- *Peripheral stem cell transplantation:* The stem cells are taken from peripheral blood.

stereotactic radiosurgery A new technique that focuses high dosages of radiation at a tumor while minimizing radiation delivered to normal tissue. After the location of the tumor is precisely measured by computed tomography (CT) or MAGNETIC RESONANCE IMAGING (MRI) scans, radiation beams are aimed from several directions to meet at the tumor. Photon beams from a linear accelerator or X-rays from cobalt 60 are often used; proton beams can also be used. This treatment may be useful for tumors that are in locations where conventional surgery would damage essential tissues or in situations in which a patient's condition does not permit conventional surgery.

St. John's wort An herb widely used for the treatment of mild depression that may significantly interfere with the action of irinotecan (Camptosar), a common cancer drug, reducing its effectiveness for weeks after people stop taking the herbal supplement. St. John's wort is often used as an over-the-counter remedy for mild depression. In a small study, doctors showed that St. John's wort decreases blood levels of one chemotherapy drug by about 40 percent. This effect lingered for more than three weeks after people stopped taking the supplement. Despite the small size of the study, experts said the findings are believable because they fit with earlier reports showing that St. John's wort can disrupt drug treatment. St. John's wort interferes with an enzyme called P450 that the body uses to break down many drugs. Because of this, St. John's wort is believed to inhibit the action of many of the most widely prescribed medicines.

stomatitis Inflammation of the soft tissues of the mouth that often occurs as a side effect in CHEMOTHERAPY, RADIATION THERAPY, and some types of BIOLOGICAL THERAPY drugs, such as interleukin-2. Stomatitis can cause dry mouth, soreness, burning feelings, soreness, swelling, redness, and taste changes. In a cancer patient, this condition can lead to serious problems of malnutrition, which can further lead to infections.

In addition to using medication to ease symptoms, patients should avoid the following:

- Hot, spicy food
- Highly acidic fruits and juices such as tomato or orange

- Carbonated drinks
- Salty food
- Toothpaste or mouthwash that contains salt or alcohol

Patients should eat soft unseasoned food, rinse the mouth and teeth with warm water or a rinse of baking soda and warm water; and use lip balm on lips.

stress and cancer The complex relationship between physical health and psychological health is not completely understood. Scientists do know that many types of stress activate the body's endocrine system, which can affect the immune system, although it has not been shown that stress-induced changes in the immune system directly cause cancer.

Some studies have indicated an increased incidence of early cancer death among people who have experienced the recent loss of a spouse or other loved one. However, most cancers have been developing for many years and are diagnosed only after they have been growing in the body for a long time. This fact suggests there cannot always be a link between the death of a loved one and the onset of cancer.

stromal tumors, gonadal Malignant growths that begin in the testicles' supportive and hormone-producing tissues (the stroma). These rare types of cancerous growths account for less than 4 percent of adult testicle tumors and up to 20 percent of childhood testicular tumors. The two main types are LEYDIG'S CELL TUMORS and SERTOLI'S CELL TUMORS.

Leydig's Cell Tumors
Leydig's cell tumors develop from normal Leydig's cells (also called interstitial cells) of the testicle that normally produce ANDROGENS (male sex HORMONES, such as TESTOSTERONE). Leydig's cell tumors may develop in adults (75 percent of cases) or children (25 percent of cases). Although these tumors typically produce androgens, they also can produce female sex hormones (estrogens).

Most Leydig's cell tumors do not spread beyond the testicle and can be cured by surgical removal; however, a few spread to other parts of the body. After Leydig's cell tumors spread, the patient has a poor prognosis because the tumors do not respond well to chemotherapy or radiation therapy.

Sertoli's Cell Tumors
Sertoli's cell tumors develop from normal Sertoli's cells, which support and nourish sperm-producing GERM CELLS. Like the Leydig's cell tumors, they are usually benign; however, if they spread, they tend to be resistant to chemotherapy and radiation therapy.

subcapsular orchiectomy A surgical procedure in which the surgeon removes the testicle tissue from the capsule, which is then left in the scrotum. Although this procedure generally removes all of the viable testicular tissue, it does have the risk of leaving some TESTOSTERONE-producing cells behind after ORCHIECTOMY. It is preferable, however, for men who worry about the appearance of an empty scrotum.

See also TESTICULAR PROSTHESIS.

support groups Groups that give people affected by cancer an opportunity to meet and discuss ways to cope with the illness. People diagnosed with cancer and their families face many challenges that may lead to feelings of being overwhelmed, afraid, and alone. Cancer support groups can help people affected by cancer feel less alone and can improve their ability to deal with the uncertainties and challenges that cancer creates.

People who have been diagnosed with cancer sometimes find they need help coping with the emotional as well as the practical aspects of their disease. In fact, attention to the emotional burden of cancer is sometimes part of a patient's treatment plan. Cancer support groups are designed to provide a confidential atmosphere in which cancer patients or cancer survivors can discuss the challenges that accompany the illness with others who may have experienced the same challenges. Support groups have helped thousands of people cope with similar situations.

However, it is not only the cancer patient who may need a support group. Family and friends are affected when cancer touches someone they love, and they may need help in dealing with stresses such as family disruptions, financial worries, and changing roles within relationships. To help meet these needs, some support groups are designed for family members of people diagnosed with cancer; other groups encourage families and friends to participate along with the cancer patient or cancer survivor.

Several kinds of support groups are available to meet the individual needs of people at all stages of cancer treatment, from diagnosis through aftercare. Some are general cancer support groups; more specialized groups work with teens or young adults, family members, or people affected by a specific type of cancer.

Support groups may be led by a professional, such as a psychiatrist, psychologist, or social worker, or by cancer patients or survivors. In addition, support groups can vary in approach, size, and frequency with which they meet. Many groups are free; some require a fee (people can contact their health insurance company to find out whether their plan covers the cost).

Locating a Group

Many organizations offer support groups for people diagnosed with cancer and their family members or friends. Oncology health-care workers may have information about support groups, as may hospital social service departments. The local office of the American Cancer Society has lists of support groups. Additionally, many newspapers carry a special health supplement containing information about where to find this type of help. For a list of support groups, see Appendix I.

suppressor genes   Genes that are expressed in normal cells that help to suppress cancer. Through still poorly defined mechanisms, tumor suppressor genes are sometimes "turned off" in cells when they become damaged or deleted. When that happens, the affected cells are less able to elude malignant transformation, and they can more easily become tumor cells.

A wide range of suppressor genes are believed to cause some forms of PROSTATE CANCER. The largest pieces of DNA visible to the eye with the aid of a microscope are called chromosomes. Each cell has 22 pairs of chromosomes (autosomes) and one

pair of sex chromosomes (XX in females and XY in males). Scientists suspect these genes may be found on chromosomes 1, 8, 11, 16 and others.

Portions of one of the pairs of autosomes—chromosome 8—appear to be especially damaged in PROSTATE CANCER cells. Three different regions of chromosome 8 are deleted in most prostate tumors. Because these regions of chromosome 8 are missing in malignant but not normal prostate cells, scientists assume that these areas must harbor tumor suppressor genes.

sural nerve graft   A procedure in which the surgeon attempts to protect erection control during a radical PROSTATECTOMY. During the surgery, nerves are removed from the leg and ankle and grafted to replace nerve bundles that control erection that have been removed. If the procedure is successful, the new nerves take over the work of the removed nerves and restore sexual potency.

surgical castration   The removal of the testicles (ORCHIECTOMY) through a small incision in the scrotum, to reduce the production of TESTOSTERONE, which some reproductive cancers need in order to grow. Surgical castration is a type of HORMONAL THERAPY.

The surgery is permanent and the effects cannot be reversed. Most men who undergo surgical castration experience a loss of sexual desire and HOT FLASHES. Although surgical castration cannot cure cancer, it usually shrinks the tumor and slows the advance of disease.

surgical margins   See MARGINS.

surveillance   Another term for WATCHFUL WAITING, the practice of adjuvant RADIATION THERAPY, surgery, or CHEMOTHERAPY in favor of closely watching for evidence of relapse. People who choose surveillance agree to a thorough checkup schedule that may include blood testing for TUMOR MARKERS, chest X-rays, and computed tomography (CT) scans.

Surveillance, Epidemiology, and End Results (SEER)   A program of the NATIONAL CANCER INSTITUTE (NCI) that is the most authoritative source of information about cancer incidence and survival in the United States. The NCI's Surveillance, Epidemiology, and End Results (SEER) cancer registry program has been expanded to cover more of the racial, ethnic, and socioeconomic diversity of the United States, allowing for better description and tracking of trends in health disparities. Methodological studies are seeking better ways to measure socioeconomic factors and determine their relationship to cancer incidence, survival, and mortality rates.

Additionally, the NCI supports a growing body of research to examine the environmental, sociocultural, behavioral, and genetic causes of cancer in different populations and apply these discoveries through interventions in clinical and community settings. These interventions involve factors such as tobacco control, dietary modification, and adherence to screening practices.

survival Survival of male reproductive cancer (or any type of cancer) as described in medical literature can mean different things depending on the type of survival. When "survival" is discussed, it could mean anything from disease-free survival, disease-specific survival, event-free survival, progression-free survival, relative survival, or total survival.

Disease-Free Survival

Disease-free survival is the length of time after treatment that a man experiences a complete remission in which cancer is not detectable in his body, or the percentage of men who experience complete remission for a certain time. For example, if a type of male reproductive cancer treatment results in an 80 percent disease-free survival over five years, eight of every 10 men experience complete remission for five years after treatment.

Disease-Specific Survival

Disease-specific survival describes the proportion of men who have one type of male reproductive cancer who do not die of that cancer after a specific time. These men may still be alive or may have died of some other cause. For example, 70 percent disease-specific survival for a certain type of male reproductive cancer means that 30 percent of the

men who have that cancer die of the cancer and 70 percent either are alive or die of some other cause.

Event-Free Survival

Event-free survival is usually used only in clinical trials to describe the length of time after treatment that a man remains free of certain negative events determined by the type of clinical study. Negative events may include severe treatment side effects, recurrence or progression of cancer, or death due to treatment side effects or due to cancer.

Progression-Free Survival

Progression-free survival describes the length of time during and after treatment that a tumor does not grow, including the amount of time men have partially or completely responded, as well as the amount of time the disease has not progressed.

Relative Survival

Relative survival is the anticipated amount of time a person who has a particular disease will live, compared with people the same age who do not have that disease. Relative survival gives an idea of how much a particular disease is expected to shorten his life. Relative survival is often expressed as the percentage of people who have the disease who survive five years, divided by the percentage of the general population who will be alive at the end of five years. For example, if the five-year relative survival for early TESTICULAR CANCER is 98 percent, the proportion of men who have testicular cancer who are alive five years after diagnosis is 98 percent of the proportion of the general population who are alive five years later. In other words, five years after diagnosis, the population of men who have testicular cancer has 2 percent fewer survivors than the general population does, or the chance of a man's being alive five years after a testicular cancer diagnosis is 2 percent lower than it is for all men.

Relative survival is usually calculated for specific stages of cancer, which take into account the size of the tumor, whether or not it can be surgically removed, and spread to lymph nodes, bone, or other organs at the time of diagnosis. This is important, since survival is higher when male reproductive cancer is diagnosed early than when it is diagnosed after it has spread.

Relative survival considers only deaths due to the cancer, and not deaths due to accidents, heart disease, other cancers, or other causes.

Total Survival

This is the expected amount of time a person will live before dying of any cause. Total survival reflects the risk of dying of a specific cancer, plus the risk of dying of any other cause, such as an accident or heart disorder. Cancer experts calculate total survival as a way of figuring out how many years of life are lost as a result of having cancer. This has a major impact on choosing treatment. For example, a 90-year-old man who has a small prostate cancer is much more likely to die of another cause than of prostate cancer, so surgery to remove the prostate cancer may not be necessary. However, a 45-year-old who has a cancerous prostate has a higher risk of dying of metastatic prostate cancer if the mass is not completely removed.

See also SURVIVAL RATES.

survival rates   Survival rates for most types of male reproductive cancers are very good, especially for those patients who have very early stages of cancer. Almost all men diagnosed with early-stage TESTICULAR CANCER and PROSTATE CANCER survive with proper treatment, as do many men who have early-stage PENILE CANCER.

Prostate Cancer

Prostate cancer strikes about one in every 11 Caucasian men and one in every nine African-American men; the diagnosis usually is made at age 70 or older. However, the survival rate (especially in early cases) is excellent; mortality rates for prostate cancer are much lower than incidence rates, because survival of men with this cancer is generally quite high.

In fact, many older men have "silent" prostate cancer that produces few (if any) symptoms and does not affect life expectancy at all. Because most prostate cancers are tiny, are localized, and do not cause symptoms, another 9 million American men may have prostate cancer without knowing it.

Before they spread, up to 90 percent of these cancers can be cured with local treatment, such as radical prostatectomy (surgical removal of the prostate gland) or radiation therapy. Microscopic traces of prostate cancer can be identified in about 30 percent of men at age 60, and 50 percent to 70 percent at age 80. For every 10 years after age 40, the incidence of prostate cancer doubles.

Survival is lowest for older men; almost 80 percent of all deaths occur among men 70 years of age and older. However, in most older men, the prostate cancer does not grow, and many die of other causes and are not identified as having prostate cancer before they die.

Testicular Cancer

About 7,400 men in the United States are diagnosed with testicular cancer each year. Although testicular cancer accounts for only 1 percent of all cancers in men, it is the most common form of cancer in young men between the ages of 15 and 35. Survival rates are very high for most men who have early testicular cancer: More than 95 percent of men who have stage I or stage II testicular cancer are successfully treated. Stage III testicular cancer has about a 75 percent recovery rate.

Penile Cancer

Cancer of the tissues in the penis is rare in the United States: about 1,400 new cases of penile cancer are diagnosed each year, and an estimated 200 men die. Penile cancer strikes about one American man in every 100,000, accounting for just about 0.2 percent of cancers in men and 0.1 percent of cancer deaths in men in the United States.

sympathetic nervous system   The part of the autonomic nervous system that is involved in preparing the body to react to situations of stress or emergency. The nerves that allow normal ejaculation are part of the sympathetic nervous system. If these nerves are cut during a RETROPERITONEAL LYMPH NODE DISSECTION, normal ejaculation becomes impossible.

syncytiotrophoblastic cells   Giant cells with multiple nuclei that, together with cytotrophoblasts, form a highly malignant type of GERM CELL CANCER called CHORIOCARCINOMA. Syncytiotrophoblastic giant cells (STGs) also may be found alone, in which case they do not constitute choriocarcinoma. STGs produce HUMAN CHORIONIC GONADOTROPIN (hCG).

tadalafil (Cialis) A new anti-impotence drug approved in November 2003 that allows men to achieve an erection up to 36 hours after ingestion. The third anti-impotence pill to be approved since 1998, it will compete against the well-known sildenafil (Viagra), and VARDENAFIL (Levitra), a medication that was approved in August 2003. Cialis works by relaxing blood vessels in the penis, allowing the increased blood flow necessary for an erection.

Cialis, which is manufactured by Eli Lilly, sells for about the same price as Viagra ($10 a pill), but it lasts much longer than Viagra's four hours. Prior to approval in the United States, Cialis was available in 50 countries—including France, where its long-lasting effects won it the nickname "Le weekend" pill. Sexual therapists, urologists, and patients cite the 36-hour time frame as a potential advantage over similar products. It takes effect in about 30 minutes, especially on an empty stomach. Of the 40,000 records of sexual attempts chronicled during research studies, only a handful of men had sex more than once during the 36-hour period on one dose.

Side Effects

Like Viagra and Levitra, Cialis does have several side effects and restrictions. The drug should not be used in combination with nitroglycerin tablets or medicines used to treat high blood pressure; such combinations could cause a sudden, unsafe drop in blood pressure. It is also not recommended for men who have suffered a stroke or heart attack in the previous six months. Drinking alcohol to a level of intoxication while taking Cialis may increase a man's chances of getting dizzy or lowering blood pressure. In addition, Cialis does not protect a man or his partner from sexually transmitted diseases, including HIV.

The most common side effects with Cialis were headache and upset stomach. Backache and muscle ache were also reported, sometimes with delayed onset. Most men were not bothered by the side effects enough to stop taking Cialis. Although a rare occurrence, men who experience an erection for more than four hours (priapism) should seek immediate medical attention.

tazarotene-induced gene 1 (*TIG1*) A possible tumor suppressor gene that when present at low levels may allow some cases of PROSTATE CANCER to grow. British scientists compared genes expressed in malignant prostate cancer cells with those expressed in normal cells of the same tissue to identify ONCOGENES and tumor suppressor genes. *TIG1* was found in normal prostate tissue and in all 51 tissue samples of BENIGN PROSTATIC HYPERPLASIA, but in only four of 51 malignant prostate tissue samples. After inserting *TIG1* into a highly malignant prostate cancer cell line, the scientists showed that both the invasiveness and the ability of the cells to produce tumors were reduced. The scientists conclude that *TIG1* may be a tumor suppressor gene whose diminished expression may be involved in the malignant progression of prostate cancer.

tea A beverage drunk for 5,000 years in China and India and long regarded in those cultures as an aid to good health. Researchers now are studying tea for possible use in the prevention and treatment of cancer. Investigators are especially interested in the ANTIOXIDANTS (called catechins) found in tea that may selectively inhibit the growth of cancer. NATIONAL CANCER INSTITUTE (NCI) researchers who have investigated the therapeutic use of green tea conclude that drinking green tea has limited antitumor benefit for PROSTATE CANCER patients.

All varieties of tea are made from the leaves of a single evergreen plant (*Camellia sinensis*). All tea leaves are picked, rolled, dried, and heated; black tea is produced by an additional process of allowing the leaves to ferment and oxidize. Possibly because it is less processed, green tea contains higher levels of antioxidants than black tea. Although tea is drunk in different ways and varies in its chemical makeup, one study showed steeping either green or black tea for about five minutes released more than 80 percent of its catechins. Instant iced tea, on the other hand, contains negligible amounts of catechins.

In animal studies, catechins scavenged oxidants before cell damage occurred, reduced the number and size of tumors, and inhibited the growth of cancer cells. However, results of human studies have proved more contradictory, perhaps because of such factors as variations in diet, environment, and population. Some studies comparing tea drinkers to non–tea drinkers support the claim that drinking tea prevents cancer; others do not.

The human body constantly produces unstable molecules called oxidants (also known as free radicals). To become stable, oxidants steal electrons from other molecules and, in the process, damage cell proteins and genetic material. This damage may leave the cell vulnerable to cancer. Antioxidants are substances that allow the human body to scavenge and seize oxidants. As other antioxidants do, the catechins found in tea selectively interfere with specific enzyme activities that lead to cancer. They may also target and repair DNA aberrations caused by oxidants.

teratocarcinoma   A MIXED GERM CELL TUMOR made up of EMBRYONAL CELL CARCINOMA and TERATOMA.

teratoma   A benign tumor composed of a number of different normal types of tissue, growing in abnormal places. Although it is technically benign, it can act as a malignant tumor and spread throughout the body; eventually, it can become malignant. Because a teratoma is made up of normal cells, CHEMOTHERAPY does not affect it.

testicular cancer   A disease in which cells become malignant in one or both testicles. About 7,400 men in the United States are diagnosed with testicular cancer each year. Although testicular cancer accounts for only 1 percent of all cancers in men, it is the most common form of cancer in young men between the ages of 15 and 35. Although any man can have testicular cancer, it is more common in Caucasians than in African Americans.

More than 95 percent of men who have stage I or stage II testicular cancer are successfully treated. Stage III testicular cancer has about a 75 percent recovery rate.

Types of Testicular Cancer

About 95 percent of all testicular tumors are GERM CELL TUMORS. Germ cell tumors in men are classified as either SEMINOMAS or NONSEMINOMAS. The types grow and spread differently; treatment and prognosis also vary according to type.

About half of all testicular cancers are seminomas. Almost all men recover from this type of cancer if it is treated early.

Nonseminomas are a group of cancers that include CHORIOCARCINOMA, EMBRYONAL CELL CARCINOMA, TERATOMA, and YOLK SAC TUMORS. These cancers often develop earlier in life than seminomas and usually affect men in their 20s.

A testicular cancer may have a combination of both types.

Secondary Testicular Cancer

Secondary testicular tumors begin in another organ and then spread to the testicle. Lymphoma is the most common secondary testicular cancer. Among men older than 50 years of age, TESTICULAR LYMPHOMA is more common than primary testicular tumors. The disease prognosis depends on the type and stage of lymphoma. The usual treatment is surgical removal, followed by radiation therapy and/or chemotherapy.

Secondary testicular tumors also can affect children who have acute leukemia; in these cases, the leukemia cells can sometimes form a tumor in the testicle.

Cancers of the prostate, lung, skin (melanoma), kidney, and other organs also can spread to the testicles. The prognosis for these cancers is usually poor because these cancers generally spread quickly to other organs as well. Treatment depends on the specific type of cancer.

Risk Factors

Although the causes of testicular cancer are not known, studies show that several factors increase a man's risk of development of testicular cancer.

Undescended testicle (cryptorchidism) Normally, the testicles descend into the scrotum before birth. Men who have had a testicle that did not move down into the scrotum are at greater risk for the disease, even if surgery is performed to place the testicle into the scrotum. (However, most men who have testicular cancer do not have a history of undescended testicles.)

Abnormal testicular development Men whose testicles did not develop normally are at increased risk.

Klinefelter syndrome The sex chromosome disorder KLINEFELTER SYNDROME is characterized by low levels of male hormones, sterility, breast enlargement, and small testes. It has been linked to a greater risk of development of testicular cancer.

Personal history Men who have previously had testicular cancer are at increased risk of having cancer in the other testicle.

Age Testicular cancer affects younger men, particularly those between ages 15 and 35; it is uncommon in children and in men older than age 40.

Symptoms

The following symptoms can be caused by cancer or by other conditions:

- Painless lump or swelling in either testicle
- Enlargement of a testicle or change in the way it feels
- Heavy feeling in the scrotum
- Dull ache in the lower abdomen, lower back, or groin
- Sudden appearance of fluid buildup in the scrotum
- Pain or discomfort in a testicle or scrotum

Occasionally, men who have germ cell cancer notice breast tenderness or enlarged breasts, because certain types of germ cell tumors secrete high levels of a HORMONE called HUMAN CHORIONIC GONADOTROPIN (hCG), which stimulates breast development. Because blood tests can measure hCG levels, these tests are important in diagnosis, staging, and follow-up of some testicular cancers.

Some men who have testicular cancer have no symptoms; instead, their cancer is found during medical testing for other conditions. Sometimes, imaging tests or biopsies to find the cause of infertility can uncover a small testicular cancer.

Self-Exams

Because the earlier testicular cancer is found the better the chance for cure, experts recommend that men of all ages, starting in the midteenage years, examine their testicles regularly. The best time to do this is during or after a bath or shower, when the skin of the scrotum is relaxed.

To perform a testicular self-exam:

1. Stand in front of a mirror, looking for any swelling on the skin of the scrotum.
2. Hold the penis out of the way and examine each testicle separately.
3. Place the index and middle fingers under the testicle while placing the thumbs on the top and roll the testicle gently between the fingers.
4. Look and feel for any hard lumps or smooth round masses, or any change in the size, shape, or consistency of the testes. Each normal testis has an epididymis, which feels like a small bump on the upper or middle outer side of the testis. Normal testicles also contain blood vessels, supporting tissues, and tubes that conduct sperm.
5. It is normal for one testicle to be a little larger than the other. Sometimes, a testicle can be enlarged because fluid has collected around it. This is called a hydrocele. Veins in the testicle can dilate and cause enlargement and lumpiness around the testicle; this is called a varicocele. A doctor may need to examine these conditions to make sure cancer is not present.

Diagnosis

Men find most testicular cancers themselves, although a doctor usually examines the testicles during routine physical exams. When testicular cancer is found early, the treatment can often be less aggressive and may cause fewer side effects.

Blood tests Certain blood tests are sometimes helpful in diagnosing testicular tumors. Many testicular cancers secrete high levels of certain proteins such as ALPHA-FETOPROTEIN (AFP) and human chorionic gonadotropin (hCG). Tumors also may boost the levels of enzymes such as LACTATE DEHYDROGENASE (LDH). These proteins are important because their presence in the blood suggests that a testicular tumor is present. However, they can also be found in conditions other than cancer.

Nonseminomas often raise AFP and hCG levels; seminomas sometimes raise hCG levels but never AFP levels. A high LDH level often indicates widespread disease.

However, SERTOLI'S CELL TUMORS or LEYDIG'S CELL TUMORS do not produce these substances. Because these protein levels are not usually high if the tumor is small, blood tests can also estimate the size of the cancer and evaluate the response to therapy to ensure a tumor has not recurred.

Imaging tests Ultrasound of the scrotum can reveal the presence and size of a mass in the testicle or rule out other conditions, such as swelling due to infection. An ultrasound can help doctors determine whether a mass is solid or fluid filled, to distinguish some types of benign and malignant tumors from one another. If the mass is solid, it is probably cancer.

Surgical biopsy If a tumor is suspected, the doctor will suggest surgery to remove the testicle. In nearly all cases of suspected cancer, the entire affected testicle is removed through an incision in the groin. This procedure is called inguinal ORCHIECTOMY. The surgeon tries to remove the entire tumor together with the testicle and spermatic cord. The spermatic cord contains blood and lymph vessels that may provide a pathway that allows testicular cancer to spread to the rest of the body. To minimize the risk that cancer cells will spread, these vessels are tied off early in the operation. This is best done by performing the operation through an incision in the groin (inguinal) area.

In rare cases (for example, when a man has only one testicle or when cancer is not certain), the surgeon performs an inguinal BIOPSY before removing the testicle; in this case, only a sample of tissue from the testicle is removed through an incision in the groin. During this operation, the surgeon makes an incision in the groin, withdraws the testicle from the scrotum, and examines it without cutting the spermatic cord. If the mass is not cancerous, the testicle can often be returned to the scrotum. The testicle is removed only if the pathologist finds cancer cells. (The surgeon does not cut through the scrotum to remove tissue, because if there is cancer, this could potentially increase the risk of recurrence in the scrotum.)

Staging

If testicular cancer is found, more tests are needed to classify the cancer according to its stage (whether or not it has spread from the testicle to other parts of the body). A chest X-ray can determine whether cancer has spread to the lungs or lymph nodes. Computed tomography (CT) scans are helpful in staging the cancer to determine whether it has spread into the liver or other organs. CT scans can show the lymph nodes and distant organs where the cancer may have spread. MAGNETIC RESONANCE IMAGING (MRI) scans are particularly helpful in examining the brain and spinal cord. Positron emission tomography (PET) scans are very useful for detecting cancer that has spread beyond the testes and for checking enlarged lymph nodes to reveal whether they contain scar tissue or active tumor.

The following are the stages of testicular cancer:

Stage I: Testicular cancer is only found in the testicle.
Stage II: Testicular cancer has spread to the lymph nodes in the abdomen.
Stage III: Testicular cancer has spread beyond the lymph nodes to other areas, such as the lungs or liver.

Treatment

Most testicular cancer can be cured with surgery, radiation therapy, or chemotherapy. Because seminomas and nonseminomas grow in different ways, the two types may need different treatments. Treatment also depends on the stage of the cancer, the patient's age and general health, and other factors.

Men who have testicular cancer should discuss their concerns about sexual function and fertility with a doctor. If both testicles are removed, the man becomes infertile. However, male hormones can be administered to ensure that sexual function remains essentially normal. Testosterone can be replaced by intramuscular injection usually given every two weeks, by patches, applied to the skin daily, or by testosterone gel rubbed into the skin daily.

If a specific treatment might cause infertility, sperm can be frozen for future use. This procedure can allow some men to produce children after loss of fertility.

Surgery Surgery to remove the testicle through an incision in the groin is called a radical inguinal orchiectomy; as long as a man has one remaining healthy testicle, he can still have a normal erection and produce sperm. This means that an operation to remove one testicle does not make a man impotent and seldom interferes with fertility. An artificial testicle can be placed into the scrotum, providing the weight and feel of a normal testicle, if a man wishes.

Some of the lymph nodes located deep in the abdomen also may be removed. This type of surgery does not change a man's ability to have an erection or an orgasm, but it can cause sterility because it interferes with ejaculation. If this is a concern, the doctor may be able to remove the lymph nodes by using a special nerve-sparing surgical technique that may protect the ability to ejaculate normally.

Surgery may be combined with radiation therapy or chemotherapy or both.

Radiation therapy RADIATION THERAPY for testicular cancer is external and is usually aimed at lymph nodes in the abdomen. Seminomas are highly sensitive to radiation; however, because nonseminomas are less sensitive to radiation, men who have this type of cancer usually do not have radiation treatment. Radiation therapy interferes with sperm production, but most patients regain fertility within a few months after treatment ends. In the event that fertility might not be recovered, before treatment, many men store sperm at a special facility or bank, where it can be preserved for later use.

Chemotherapy CHEMOTHERAPY may be the first treatment if the cancer has spread outside the testicle. Some anticancer drugs interfere with sperm production, permanently in some patients and temporarily in others. Chemotherapy has made the biggest difference in reducing deaths of testicular cancer.

Bone marrow transplant In a BONE MARROW TRANSPLANT procedure, BONE MARROW is removed from the patient, treated with drugs to kill the cancer cells, and then frozen. The patient then is given chemotherapy, with or without radiation, to destroy the remaining cancer cells (the chemotherapy also destroys the remaining bone marrow). The frozen marrow is then thawed and injected back into the patient. This relatively new treatment for testicular cancer has shown some promising initial results, but it is not routinely recommended by doctors since traditional chemotherapy is typically very successful.

Follow-up Care

Men who have had testicular cancer have a higher risk of developing cancer in the remaining testicle, as well as of certain types of leukemia and other cancers. For this reason, regular follow-up is extremely important; it usually involves frequent exams and regular blood tests to measure tumor marker levels. X-rays and CT scans are usually performed at regular intervals.

testicular lymphoma A type of cancer that originates elsewhere in the body and spreads to the testicles. It is the most common secondary testicular cancer and is more common than primary testicular tumors among men older than 50 years of age. The prognosis in this type of malignancy depends on the type and stage of lymphoma. The usual treatment is surgical removal of the testicles, followed by radiation and/or CHEMOTHERAPY.

testicular prosthesis An artificial saline solution–filled testicle implanted into the scrotum after a cancerous testicle is removed. A testicular prostheses can create or restore the more normal cosmetic appearance of a testicle-containing scrotum.

Several studies have described the negative psychological effects that can result from the loss or absence of a testicle and have indicated that the cosmetic aspect of saline solution–filled testicular implants can provide emotional benefits. However, a testicular implant is used strictly for cosmetic appearances only and in no way functions as a natural testicle does. Before choosing to receive a testicular implant, patients should discuss their long-term expectations and the potential risks and complications of the procedure.

Types of Prostheses

There are two types of testicular prosthesis. A saline solution–filled type produced by the Mentor Corporation is the only prosthesis commercially available. The saline solution implant is about the same weight, shape, and texture of a normal testicle and is manufactured in four sizes: extra-small, small, medium, and large. The implant is made of a molded silicone elastomer shell about 0.035 inch thick that is not visible on X-ray.

A solid silicone elastomer produced by the Silimed Corporation is experimental and has not yet been approved by the U.S. Food and Drug Administration (FDA) for commercial use in patients.

The Process

The implant includes a self-sealing injection site at one end that allows the doctor to fill the device with a sterile saline solution immediately before surgery. On the opposite end of the implant is a silicone tab that the doctor can use to suture the implant into a secure position.

A testicular prosthesis is usually implanted under local anesthesia in an outpatient setting, the patient can return to work shortly afterward. With local anesthesia, patients are awake, but the lower part of the body is numb throughout the procedure.

Typically, testicular implant procedures are relatively simple and take 20 to 40 minutes. There are several different accepted surgical approaches that can be used to insert an implant. Once the implant has been filled and sutured into place, the doctor can add more saline solution for better cosmetic appearance.

Patients should be aware that implantation of a testicular prosthesis may not be a one-time procedure: Any surgical complications may require further procedures.

Contraindications

Implantation of the device should be carefully considered if the patient has a current infection, the scrotum is too small or damaged from prior surgery or radiation, the patient has uncontrolled diabetes or poor circulation, or the patient wants to avoid future surgery to remove it.

Risks

The known or potential risks of saline solution–filled testicular implants or the implant surgery include rupture or leakage of the implant, calcium deposits, pain, shifting, extrusion, fluid collection, infection, hardening, and hematoma.

Rupture and leakage Testicular implants, as for other medical implant devices, do not last a lifetime. There is a slight chance of the body's having an adverse reaction to the implant, and the implant may rupture or leak or both, necessitating removal. The long-term rates of deflation and resurgery are currently not known; however, a five-year study is currently being done to assess these possible problems. In terms of information from the clinical studies of the saline solution–filled testicular implant, about one in 30 patients needs surgery again within the first year either to remove or to adjust the implant. Infection or extrusion (the implant shifts and presses out through the skin) may also require additional surgery.

Discomfort or pain An uncomfortable feeling around the surgical site is usually temporary. The duration of this discomfort or pain should be discussed with the doctor or surgeon.

Migration or shifting In studies of the implant, the device moved from its original position about 2 percent of the time.

Extrusion In about 2 percent of cases, the implant shifts and presses out through the skin (extrusion). In addition, skin damage, shedding of dead skin, or wound separation may be caused by tight pull of skin over the implant, trauma to the skin during the surgery, or insufficient tissue to cover the implant.

Fluid collection In a natural process, occasionally excess fluid accumulates around the implant after surgery.

Hardening As a result of the body's natural reaction to an implanted device, scar tissue forms around the implant and contracts, causing discomfort. The implant may be difficult to remove if the degree of scar tissue is significant.

Hematoma A collection of blood (usually a clot) may be found in tissue after a blood vessel breaks. Large hematomas cause enlarged, tender, and discolored tissue that may, if untreated, lead to extrusion of the implant.

Infection Swelling, tenderness, pain, and fever may occur immediately after surgery or at any time after the implant is inserted. If an infection does not clear up promptly with proper treatment, the surgeon may have to remove the implant.

After the Procedure

Patients may experience some discomfort during the first one or two days after surgery; a small amount of bright red blood is to be expected. Most patients are instructed to keep surgical bandages on the scrotum for at least a few days. Most patients feel tired, and the scrotum is swollen, tender, and sensitive for some time. Swelling and black-and-blue bruises are normal. However, the ability to urinate should not be affected.

Although recovery times differ, patients should be able to resume most daily activities within a week to 10 days. Patients can usually begin to shower two days after the surgery. The dressing should be kept dry until then. However, patients should wait at least a month before resuming strenuous activities. The doctor can provide more specific details about recovery, including the amount of time to wait before resuming sex.

testicular self-examination Monthly self-exams of the testicles are an effective way of detecting TESTICULAR CANCER at an early, very curable stage. The self-exam is best performed after a warm bath or shower, since heat relaxes the scrotum, making it easier to see anything abnormal.

Standing in front of a mirror, the patient should check for any swelling on the scrotal skin, examining each testicle with both hands. The index and middle fingers should be placed under the testicle with the thumbs placed on top, rolling the testicle gently between the thumbs and fingers. There should be no pain during the exam. However, it is normal for one testicle to seem *slightly* larger than the other.

Next, the patient should find the EPIDIDYMIS (the soft, tubelike structure behind the testicle that collects and carries sperm). Cancerous lumps usually are found on the sides of the testicle but can also appear on the front. Lumps on the epididymis are not cancerous, and free-floating lumps in the scrotum that are not attached in any way to a testicle are not testicular cancer.

Any man who finds a lump on the testicle should see a doctor (preferably a urologist) immediately. The abnormality may be only an infection, but if it is testicular cancer, it spreads if it is not stopped by treatment. Other signs of testicular cancer should be kept in mind:

- Any enlargement of a testicle
- A significant loss of size in one of the testicles
- A feeling of heaviness in the scrotum
- A dull ache in the lower abdomen or in the groin
- A sudden collection of fluid in the scrotum
- Pain or discomfort in a testicle or in the scrotum
- Enlargement or tenderness of the breasts

The following symptoms are *not* normally signs of testicular cancer:

- A pimple, ingrown hair, or rash on the scrotal skin
- A free-floating lump in the scrotum, seemingly not attached to anything
- A lump on the epididymis or tubes from the testicle that feels like a third testicle
- Pain or burning during urination
- Blood in the urine or semen

testosterone The male sex HORMONE produced mainly by the testicles; a small amount is made by the adrenal glands. Testosterone is responsible for many physical and behavioral characteristics in a man, such as voice change and hair growth. PROSTATE CANCER is stimulated by the male hormones testosterone and dihydrotestosterone (a chemical that the body makes from testosterone); this is why there is a link between prostate cancer and high levels of testosterone. Men who have had their testicles removed at an early age (CASTRATION) rarely have this malignancy.

three-dimensional conformal therapy   A type of EXTERNAL BEAM RADIATION THERAPY that uses computers that aim focused beams of radiation from different directions into prostate cancer cells without damaging nearby healthy tissue. This procedure allows doctors to administer more radiation to kill cancer cells without increasing side effects.

thrombocytopenia   A drop in the number of platelets (blood cells responsible for clotting) that is often a side effect of RADIATION THERAPY or CHEMO-THERAPY. Certain types of cancer also may directly destroy platelets in the blood. Severe cases of thrombocytopenia can have grave consequences when minor injuries cause severe blood loss.

The condition can be treated with transfusions of platelets, intravenous gamma globulin, removal of the spleen, and medications to boost the platelet count. When radiation therapy or chemotherapy is stopped, the platelet count should return to normal.

TIG1   See TAZAROTENE-INDUCED GENE 1.

tomatoes and prostate cancer   Recent studies suggest that a diet that regularly includes tomato-based foods may help protect men from PROSTATE CANCER.

See also LYCOPENE.

transferrin   A chemical made by the liver and stored in the bones that appears to stimulate the growth of prostate cancer cells. As PROSTATE CANCER develops, it secretes chemicals that make blood vessels grow into the cancer and carry nutrients to nourish the malignant cells.

transrectal ultrasound of the prostate (TRUS/P)
An internal ultrasound test that uses sound wave echoes to create an image of the prostate. The test can be used to inspect the prostate visually for abnormal conditions such as gland enlargement, nodules, penetration of a tumor through the capsule of the gland, or invasion of seminal vesicles.

By gently inserting the ultrasound probe into the rectum, a doctor can identify potential cancer sites or remove tissue samples from suspicious areas of the prostate. This test is also extremely useful for guiding needle biopsies of the prostate gland and guiding probes or needles in cryosurgery.

transurethral hyperthermia   An investigative procedure that uses heat, usually provided by microwaves, to shrink the prostate.

transurethral incision of the prostate (TUIP)   A procedure that widens the urethra by making some small incisions in the bladder neck, at the site where the urethra joins the bladder, and in the prostate gland itself.

transurethral laser incision of the prostate (TULIP)   The use of a laser to remove tissue from an enlarged prostate. Rather than using a scalpel or an electrocautery device to remove the prostatic tissue, the surgeon uses a laser to vaporize it.

Because the prostatic tissue is vaporized, it cannot be sent to the hospital's pathology department for a biopsy. Therefore, patients who are selected for the laser procedure must be evaluated carefully for their risk of PROSTATE CANCER before a laser procedure is recommended.

Those who undergo the laser procedure must enter the hospital and undergo anesthesia, but because the laser involves no cutting, there is no bleeding. Thus, there are fewer postoperative complications of the laser treatment, and patients have a shorter recovery time and typically are discharged from the hospital within one to two days.

Patients who undergo laser treatment for BENIGN PROSTATIC HYPERPLASIA (BPH) can expect to experience more swelling at the operative site than those who undergo a TRANSURETHRAL RESECTION OF THE PROSTATE (TURP), in which excess prostate tissue is removed by shaving. This swelling inhibits the patient's ability to urinate immediately after the operation. Therefore, patients who undergo the laser treatment should expect to use a catheter for at least one week, whereas those who undergo TURP can expect to have the catheter removed on the second or third day after the operation.

transurethral prostatectomy   See TRANSURETHRAL RESECTION OF THE PROSTATE.

transurethral resection of the prostate (TURP)

A surgical procedure (also called a transurethral prostatectomy) in which obstructing prostate tissue is removed via the penis. A transurethral resection of the prostate (TURP) is the most common type of surgery for an enlarged prostate, or BENIGN PROSTATIC HYPERPLASIA (BPH): nine of 10 men who undergo prostate surgery have this procedure. BPH requires treatment only for symptoms that are severe enough to disrupt a man's life or threaten his health. During an annual prostate examination, if the doctor finds significant symptoms and an enlarged prostate gland, the patient and his doctor may decide to try a program of WATCHFUL WAITING. During this time, the physician examines the patient periodically (usually once a year) and may prescribe medication to lessen symptoms. If urination problems become difficult, a prostatectomy may be suggested.

In this type of surgery, no external incision is needed, because the surgeon reaches the prostate by inserting a resectoscope through the urethra, allowing removal of all of the prostate tissue that is bulging into the urethra and blocking the flow of urine. The prostate tissue is removed through the scope and sent to the pathologist for examination.

Recovery

Recovery can require two to eight weeks. During the first weeks after the operation, the patient may experience some of the same symptoms that he had before surgery. Sometime during the first postoperative month the scab inside the prostatic urethra may loosen and cause bleeding. The bleeding usually subsides if the patient increases fluid intake and decreases physical activity. However, if bleeding persists and blood clots are passed, the patient should consult a doctor.

By six to eight weeks after the operation, urination should be easier and less frequent, although nighttime urination may still occur. Generally, the longer the patient had the problem before it was treated, the longer the recovery time. Overall, patients should eat a balanced diet and try to prevent constipation. Straining to have a bowel movement can cause bleeding from the prostate. Patients should not resume sexual activity until the surgeon approves it.

Risks

There is a small chance that a TURP may cause conditions that require additional treatment, including uncontrolled urine leakage (very small risk), constriction of the urethra, or the necessity for a second operation at a later date. There is also a small risk of impotence after surgery. However, patients in good health who were capable of having an erection before the operation whose nerves were not affected by the procedure have a good chance of resuming normal sexual activity.

If There Are Cancer Cells

If the pathologist finds cancer cells in the tissue, the cells are graded and the percentage of cells with cancer is assessed. Normally if less than 5 percent of the tissue contains cancer and the Gleason score is low (below 6), the prostate cancer is considered to be insignificant. In this case, patient follow-up requires only an annual digital rectal exam (DRE) and prostate-specific antigen (PSA) level tests. However, if more than 5 percent of the tissue is malignant or the Gleason score is high, the cancer is considered to be potentially aggressive and may warrant further treatment.

Because not all of the prostate tissue is removed during a TURP, a man still needs annual prostate cancer screening. Prostate cancer is still a possibility, since surgical procedures such as TURP do not remove all of the prostate. A TURP does not make prostate cancer spread faster or more easily, but it can affect the risks of future treatment for prostate cancer. Patients who have had a TURP have more problems with interstitial seed radiation therapy, and there is a much higher risk of urinary incontinence. However, a radical PROSTATECTOMY (removal of the prostate) and external beam radiation treatment can be performed after TURP without increased risks.

See also TRANSURETHRAL INCISION OF THE PROSTATE (TUIP).

tumor marker   A substance that can be detected in the blood or urine that suggests the presence of cancer. Between 70 and 80 percent of TESTICULAR CANCER patients have elevated marker levels. Treatment of the cancer results in a drop in the level of the markers.

Examples of tumor markers in male reproductive cancers are ALPHA-FETOPROTEIN (AFP), HUMAN CHORIONIC GONADOTROPIN (hCG), PLACENTAL ALKALINE PHOSPHATASE (PLAP), and LACTATE DEHYDROGENASE (LDH).

Alpha-Fetoprotein (AFP)

Alpha-fetoprotein is found at high levels in the blood of some men who have testicular cancer. As the tumor grows, the blood level rises; AFP level falls as the cancer shrinks or after it has been surgically removed. This means that a blood test can sometimes measure the success of treatment and the spread of the disease. (However, high levels of AFP are also found in other diseases, such as liver disorders.)

Human Chorionic Gonadotropin (hCG)

The level of the hormone hCG rises significantly during pregnancy and in the presence of certain types of tumors, including GERM CELL TUMORS, and is therefore used as a marker for testicular cancer.

Placental Alkaline Phosphatase

The tumor marker PLAP is sometimes used to check for germ cell tumors (particularly SEMINOMA). However, it is not used very often and is more often used in examination of a specimen than in blood testing.

Lactate Dehydrogenase (LDH)

The enzyme LDH is normally found in blood produced by many tissues. At higher-than-normal levels, it is considered to be a marker for such possible malignancies as testicular cancer. However, cancer can recur without an increase in LDH level.

Tumor–Node–Metastasis staging system The most common method to determine the stage of cancer by assessing whether—or how far—cancer has spread. Several other methods are available to determine the spread of cancer, including the less common Jewett-Whitmore system developed by the AMERICAN UROLOGICAL ASSOCIATION.

The TNM classification system, which was developed by the AMERICAN JOINT COMMITTEE FOR CANCER, is considered so effective that it is used to stage all types of cancer.

Category T

In assessing prostate cancer, for example, in the TNM system, the *T* stands for "tumor," which is classified on the basis of its size, its location on one or both sides of the prostate, and its spread beyond the gland into other parts of the body. The doctor classifies the tumor numerically, ranging from the least dangerous (T1) through the most dangerous (T4). The classifications are furthered divided into (a), (b), and (c) categories. A classification ranging from T1, T1a, T1b, T1c, T2, T2a, T2b, to T2c is considered *local cancer:* cancer that has not spread beyond the prostate. T3, T3a, or T3b indicates cancer that has spread just slightly beyond the prostate, but not into other organs or throughout the body. T4 (there are no initialed subcategories) is the most advanced type of prostate cancer, which has spread to other organs or throughout the body.

Category N

The *N* in the TNM system is an assessment of whether the tumor has spread to the lymp nodes in the pelvis. In this classification N0 indicates no contamination of the lymph nodes; N1 indicates cancer spread into the lymph nodes.

Category M

M, the last part of the TNM staging system, is used to assess whether the tumor has spread (metastasized) beyond the lymph nodes in the pelvis. There are four categories in M: M0 (has not spread), M1a (spread into lymph nodes beyond the pelvis), M1b (spread to the bones), to M1c (spread to other parts of the body besides bones and lymph nodes).

TURP See TRANSURETHRAL RESECTION OF THE PROSTATE.

ultrasound (ultrasonography) A noninvasive scan that utilizes high-frequency sound waves to help a doctor visualize tissues deep within the body. Transrectal ultrasound is increasingly used in the diagnosis and treatment of PROSTATE CANCER. Ultrasounds are also used in conjunction with biopsy to help physicians visualize the tissues from which they extract samples.

undescended testicle See CRYPTORCHIDISM.

urethral cancer A rare type of cancer in which malignant cells are found in the urethra (the tube that empties urine from the bladder). It has often spread to nearby soft tissue before it is diagnosed. Although it can occur at any age, it appears most often in patients in their 60s. In men, 80 percent of cases are squamous cell carcinomas, most of which occur in the urethra at the base of the penis.

Symptoms

There may be no symptoms of early cancer of the urethra. If symptoms do appear, they may include the following:

- Lump or growth on the urethra
- Diminished urine stream
- Straining to void
- Frequent urination and increased nighttime urination
- Hardening of tissue in the perineum or penis
- Itching
- Incontinence
- Pain during or after sexual activity
- Painful urination
- Urinary tract infections

- Urethral discharge and swelling
- Swollen lymph nodes in the groin

Types of Urethral Cancer

Different types of urethral cancer develop in different types of cells in different areas of the urethra. In men, transitional cells line the upper portion and squamous cells line the urethra at the base of and within the penis.

Squamous cell carcinoma Squamous cell carcinoma develops in flat, scaly surface cells and is the most common type of urethral cancer.

Transitional cell carcinoma Transitional cell carcinoma appears in the surface cells of the urethra.

Adenocarcinoma Adenocarcinoma develops in glands located near the urethra.

Melanoma Melanoma is a urethral cancer that is extremely rare; it develops in the pigment-producing skin cells.

Sarcoma Another extremely rare type of cancer, sarcoma develops in blood vessels, smooth muscle, and connective tissue.

Risk Factors

The cause of urethral cancer is unknown; there are a number of known risk factors, including the following:

- *Bladder cancer:* The primary risk factor for urethral cancer is a history of bladder cancer.
- *Human papillomavirus (HPV):* Infection with HUMAN PAPILLOMAVIRUS (HPV) or other sexually transmitted diseases is also a risk factor. HPV is a group of more than 70 viruses that are transmitted sexually and cause genital warts. Two types of HPV are associated with warts that appear on the urethra. Having unprotected

sexual intercourse with multiple partners increases the risk for HPV infection.

- *Age:* People older than age 60 are at higher risk.
- *Chronic irritation:* Irritation of the urethra as a result of sexual intercourse or chronic urinary tract infection (UTI) increases risk.
- *Smoking:* Smoking increases the risk of bladder cancer, which is a risk factor for urethral cancer.

Diagnosis

If there are urethral cancer symptoms, a doctor examines the patient to feel for lumps in the urethra. In men, a thin lighted tube called a cystoscope may be inserted into the penis so the doctor can see inside the urethra. If cells or other signs that are not normal are present, the doctor may perform a biopsy, removing a piece of tissue to check for cancer cells.

Staging

If malignant cells are found, imaging tests are performed to find out whether cancer cells have spread to other parts of the body. These tests include X-ray, ultrasound, computed tomography (CT) scan, and magnetic resonance imaging (MRI). MRI is the preferred method to evaluate urethral cancer.

In cancer of the urethra, patients are grouped into stages, which depend on where the tumor is located and whether it has spread. The following stage groupings are used for cancer of the urethra:

- *Anterior urethral cancer:* The anterior urethra is the part of the urethra that is closest to the outside of the body. Urethral cancer that is superficial and located near the urethral opening often can be treated successfully.
- *Posterior urethral cancer:* The posterior urethra is the part of the urethra that connects to the bladder. Because this area is closer to the bladder, cancers that start here are more likely to grow through the inner lining of the urethra and affect nearby tissues. Cancer that develops here is usually invasive and rarely curable. In men, the condition may spread to the tissues of the penis and perineum, the prostate gland, the ligament that surrounds the urethra, the regional lymph nodes, and the penile and scrotal skin.

- *Recurrent urethral cancer:* The cancer has recurred after it has been treated, either in the same location or in another part of the body.

Treatment

There are treatments for all patients who have cancer of the urethra; treatment selection depends on the stage and location of the disease and the patient's age and overall health. Surgery, radiation therapy, and/or chemotherapy may be used.

Surgery Surgery is the most common treatment of cancer of the urethra. A doctor may remove the cancer by using one of the following operations:

- *Electrofulguration:* In this method, electric current is used to burn away the tumor and the area around it.
- *Laser therapy:* This method uses a narrow beam of intense light to kill cancer cells.
- *Cystourethrectomy:* The bladder and the urethra are removed.
- *Partial penectomy:* This type of surgery removes the part of the penis containing the urethra that has cancer.
- *Total penectomy:* Sometimes the entire penis is removed, necessitating plastic surgery to create a new penis.
- *Cystoprostatectomy:* The bladder and prostate are removed along with the penis. Lymph nodes in the pelvis may also be removed.

If the urethra is removed, the doctor fashions a new means for the urine to pass from the body; if the bladder is removed, a new mechanism to store and pass urine must be devised. Sometimes part of the small intestine can be used to make a tube through which urine can pass out of the body through an opening (stoma) on the outside of the body. (This is sometimes called an OSTOMY or UROSTOMY.)

Urethral cancer and invasive bladder cancer Because people who have bladder cancer sometimes also have cancer of the urethra, the urethra may be removed when the bladder is. If the urethra is not removed during surgery for bladder cancer, the doctor may follow the patient's condition closely in order to begin treatment if cancer of the urethra develops.

Radiation therapy RADIATION THERAPY may combined with surgery in advanced urethral cancer or may be the primary treatment of early urethral cancer that has not spread. Radiation can be applied by using external sources or by surgically implanting radioactive seeds or pellets (BRACHYTHERAPY) to destroy cancer cells. External radiation and brachytherapy are sometimes used together. External beam radiation usually entails treatment five days a week for about six weeks. Brachytherapy involves surgical implantation of the seeds, which become inactive over time and remain in place.

Chemotherapy A number of different drugs can be used in combination to destroy urethral cancer that has spread. Commonly used drugs include cisplatin (Platinol), vincristine (Oncovin), and methotrexate (Trexall).

Prognosis

The chance of recovery depends on the stage of the cancer and the patient's general state of health. The five-year survival rate for noninvasive urethral cancer treated by surgery or radiation therapy is about 60 percent. Recurrence rate for invasive urethral cancer treated with surgery, CHEMOTHERAPY, and radiation therapy combined is higher than 50 percent. Early diagnosis and treatment offer the best chance for cure.

urinary incontinence The loss of urine control or the inability to hold urine until the person can reach a toilet. It can range from the slight loss of urine to severe, frequent wetting and may be triggered by a condition such as BENIGN PROSTATIC HYPERPLASIA (BPH) or prostate cancer. It also is a problem for many men after the removal of the prostate (PROSTATECTOMY), and the older the man, the higher the risk of incontinence after prostatectomy.

Urine is formed in the kidneys and then flows down the ureters into the bladder, where it is stored until it is eliminated. Urination is controlled by the urinary sphincter (rings of muscles at the base of the bladder and in the wall of the urethra). The sphincter normally controls the flow and leakage of urine by tightening and closing around the neck of the bladder and urethra. When the bladder is full, the sphincter relaxes and allows urine to leave the bladder. At the same time, the bladder muscles contract and squeeze urine out of the bladder. When a man finishes urinating, the sphincter contracts and the bladder relaxes.

The PROSTATE GLAND lies directly below the bladder and completely encircles the urethra at the point where it leaves the bladder. When the prostate gland is removed in a radical prostatectomy or when it receives radiation therapy, damage can occur to the urinary sphincter, and can trigger temporary or permanent incontinence. However, when the operation is performed by an experienced surgeon who preserves the urinary sphincter and carefully rebuilds the urinary tract, there is a low risk of total incontinence.

A recent study at a medical center with extensive experience in performing radical prostatectomy reported that 93 percent of patients had complete continence 18 months after surgery. Studies from other health centers report patients had a consistently high rate of continence (between 85 percent and 100 percent) two months to 18 months after radical prostatectomy.

Types of Incontinence

There are several of incontinence: stress incontinence, urge incontinence, overflow incontinence, and functional incontinence.

Stress incontinence Stress incontinence is the most common type; in it urine leaks occur when pressure rises in the abdomen, as when a patient laughs, coughs, or bends. Leaking of urine during exercise, coughing, sneezing, laughing, lifting heavy objects, or other body movements that put pressure on the bladder is the most common type of incontinence and can almost always be cured.

Urge incontinence Urge incontinence is the inability to hold urine long enough to reach a toilet. It may be a sign of enlarged prostate, although it can also occur in otherwise healthy older men. It is often found in people who have conditions such as diabetes, stroke, dementia, Parkinson's disease, and multiple sclerosis, and it can also be a warning sign of early bladder cancer.

Mixed incontinence Mixed incontinence is a combination of stress and urge incontinence.

Overflow incontinence Overflow incontinence is leakage of small amounts of urine from a bladder that is always full.

Functional incontinence Functional incontinence is difficulty reaching a toilet in time because of physical conditions such as arthritis and is not related to male reproductive cancer.

Symptoms

There are a number of symptoms of urinary incontinence:

- Leaking of urine that prevents activities, causes embarrassment, and begins or continues after surgery
- Inability to urinate or retention of urine
- More frequent urination than usual without a proven bladder infection
- Need to rush to the bathroom
- Pain related to filling of the bladder
- Pain related to urination without a proven bladder infection
- Frequent bladder infections
- Progressive weakness of the urinary stream with or without a feeling of incomplete bladder emptying

Treatment

Treatment of incontinence depends on its type, cause, and severity, in general, the problem can be treated and often cured. When treatment is not completely successful, management plans can help reduce complications, anxiety, and stress.

First, a man who is experiencing incontinence problems should see a doctor for a complete medical examination, a detailed personal and family history of health and related problems, a physical examination that focuses on the urinary and nervous systems and reproductive organs, and urine samples. In many cases, patients are then referred to a UROLOGIST.

Treatment may include behavioral techniques such as pelvic muscle exercises, biofeedback, and bladder training; medication; or surgery if the incontinence is related to a structural problem such as an enlarged prostate.

Incontinence also may be managed by inserting a catheter into the urethra and collecting the urine in a container. An alternative to the catheter for men is an external collecting device that fits over the penis and connects to a drainage bag.

In addition, special absorbent underwear can be worn easily under clothing.

urologic oncologist A UROLOGIST who has received specialized training experience in treating urologic cancers, including PROSTATE CANCER, TESTICULAR CANCER, PENILE CANCER, bladder cancer, and kidney cancer. These subspecialists usually work in medical centers and perform research in addition to patient care.

urologist A doctor who specializes in diseases of the urinary tract. Urology is the study of diseases and disorders of the kidneys, urinary tract, prostate gland, and the male sex organs. Problems that urologists treat include urinary incontinence; kidney and bladder stones; kidney, bladder, prostate, and testicular cancer; prostate disorders; and sexual dysfunction. Urologists provide both medical and surgical treatment options.

Although urology is classified as a surgical subspecialty, because of the wide variety of clinical problems encountered, a knowledge of internal medicine, pediatrics, gynecology, and other specialties is required by the urologist. In recognition of the wide scope of urology, the American Urological Association has identified eight subspecialty areas, including urologic oncology. Urologic oncologists treat cancers of the male and female urinary tract and the male reproductive organs, including prostate, bladder, penile, and testicular cancers of men.

Urologists often work closely with other specialists, such as nephrologists, endocrinologists, and oncologists; they may work in a clinic that offers various services and procedures to patients.

To be certified by the American Board of Urology, the urologist must have met a standard in urology by fulfilling specified educational and examination requirements, including four years of medical school and five years in a residency program in urology. Completion of the qualifying licensing examinations is required to practice medicine; licensure by a regional licensing authority is also required. Once certified, the urologic surgeon who wishes to maintain certified status on expiration of the original certificate must complete a recertification process every 10 years for certificates issued on or after January 1, 1985.

Us TOO International   The world's largest independent charitable network of education and support groups for men who have PROSTATE CANCER and their families. Us TOO International and hundreds of local affiliated support group chapters offer education, publications, fellowship, peer counseling, treatment option information, and discussion of medical alternatives. The group's goals include education, advocacy, patient and family support, and public awareness of prostate cancer and prostate disease. For contact information, see Appendix I.

vaccine A potential form of BIOLOGICAL THERAPY that would encourage a cancer patient's immune system to recognize and destroy cancer cells. In order to understand how a cancer vaccine would theoretically work, it is important to comprehend how the immune system functions, constantly scanning the body looking for foreign invaders. Because cancer cells originate in the body, they are usually not detected by the immune system.

In cancer vaccine technology, tumor cells would be removed, marked as "foreign" by adding a special gene, and then injected beneath the skin along with an immunostimulant (such as interleukin-2). This stimulates the immune system to react as if it has been newly infected with cancer, so that it will destroy this "new" antigen. Scientists hope such a vaccine would help the body recognize cancer, rejecting tumors and preventing cancer recurrence.

Unlike vaccines against infectious diseases, cancer vaccines are designed to be injected after disease is diagnosed, rather than before it develops. Cancer vaccines given when a tumor is small may be able to eradicate the cancer.

Although the first cancer vaccines targeted melanoma, scientists are also testing vaccines for many other types of cancer, including PROSTATE CANCER. In one study of vaccines against prostate cancer that had spread to the bone, patients were given 13 shots of the vaccine for four months; 41 percent who had a low dosage and 70 percent who had a high dosage were alive two years later. The vaccine, known as GVAX, is also being tested for lung, pancreas, and colon cancers.

In a slightly different approach, Californian and German scientists have successfully used an oral vaccine to stop cancerous tumor growth in animals by choking off the tumor's blood supply.

Researchers first targeted a protein produced in new blood vessels (vascular endothelial growth factor [VEGF] receptor 2), one of several substances that trigger new blood vessel growth (a process called angiogenesis). New blood vessel growth is critical to allow cancerous tumors to grow and spread. When researchers administered genetically engineered bacteria that contained a gene to express the VEGF receptor 2 protein, the bacteria triggered the animals' immune system to fight off the mild infection from the bacteria—and, in the process, killed the protein that spurs new blood vessel growth to the tumors. The vaccine was effective against melanoma, colon cancer, and lung cancer in the animals. The immune response triggered by the vaccine destroys the blood vessels that nourish the tumor. Researchers estimate that studies in humans may not begin until at least 2010.

vacuum pump A mechanical, nonsurgical method of producing an engorged, erect penis that is rigid enough for sex. The external vacuum device consists of a clear plastic cylinder, a vacuum pump, and a tension ring. The cylinder is placed over the penis and the vacuum pump draws blood into the penis. The tension ring is placed around the base of the penis, traps blood inside the penis, and maintains the erection. With this noninvasive technique, an erection may be obtained within a few minutes.

Side Effects

At first, some men may develop reddish pinpoint dots or bruising on the penis caused by the negative pressure of the vacuum pump. Some men find use of the vacuum device awkward. The penis is cooler to the touch because fresh blood is not circulating through the penis.

Although the tension ring must be removed within 30 minutes, after several minutes the process may be repeated. Although an erection may be achieved, ejaculation may be difficult.

vardenafil (Levitra)   A prescription medicine used to treat erectile dysfunction, approved in August 2003. Levitra belongs to a class of drugs called PDE-5 inhibitors, one of three (the other two are VIAGRA and Cialis) approved since 1999, which increase blood flow to the penis, helping men to achieve and keep an erection long enough to enable sexual activity. Once a man has completed sexual activity, blood flow to his penis should decrease, and his erection should go away. Levitra can improve erectile function even in men who have other negative health factors, such as diabetes or prostate surgery.

Who Should Not Take Levitra

Patients should not take Levitra if they take any form of nitrate medication, such as nitroglycerin, isosorbide mononitrate, and isosorbide dinitrate (used to relieve chest pain that can occur as a result of heart disease). Taking Levitra in combination with nitrates may cause serious side effects. Patients also should avoid Levitra if they are taking alpha-blockers sometimes prescribed for prostate problems or high blood pressure; the combination could lower blood pressure to an unsafe level.

Side Effects

The most common side effects of Levitra are headaches, flushing, and stuffy nose. It may cause an erection that will not go away (priapism), though this is rare. Patients who get an erection that lasts more than four hours should get medical help right away, because without treatment, priapism can cause lasting damage, including the inability to have erections. Rarely, Levitra may cause vision changes, such as seeing a blue tinge to objects or having difficulty telling the difference between the colors blue and green.

vasectomy and cancer   About one of every six American men older than age 35 has had a vasectomy, and some studies have suggested there may

be a relationship between vasectomy and cancer (especially PROSTATE CANCER or TESTICULAR CANCER). However, scientists who have carefully reviewed all the data believe that there is no consistent link between vasectomy and prostate cancer. Nor could experts find a convincing biological explanation for a link between vasectomy and an increased risk of prostate cancer.

As a result, in 1993 a National Institutes of Health (NIH) panel stated that providers should continue offering and performing vasectomy and recommended that further research be conducted to clarify any possible risk.

Although most studies find no connection, a few reported a link between vasectomy and prostate cancer. It is possible that other factors, including chance, may be responsible for the increased prostate cancer risk seen in these studies. Scientists expect that additional research will clarify this issue.

Several studies that are examining a possible connection between vasectomy and prostate cancer are currently under way. The largest of these studies is the National Cancer Institute's (NCI) Prostate, Lung, Colorectal, and Ovarian (PLCO) Cancer Screening Trial, which began in 1992 and will end in 2015. The PLCO Trial is evaluating screening procedures for prostate cancer and will prospectively examine potential risk factors, including vasectomy, associated with prostate cancer.

Testicular cancer is much less common than prostate cancer, accounting for only 1 percent of cancers in American men. A few studies have suggested a link between vasectomy and an increased risk of testicular cancer, but experts suspect this increase may be due to factors other than vasectomy. It is also possible that the vasectomy procedure increases the rate at which an existing, but undetected, testicular cancer progresses. At this time, experts believe there is either no association or only a weak link between vasectomy and testicular cancer.

vesicant   An intravenous CHEMOTHERAPY drug capable of damaging tissue and causing pain and swelling if it leaks into the skin. Many chemotherapy drugs cause local tissue damage if they leak out of the vein. They include the following:

- Anthracyclines: daunorubicin, doxorubicin (Adriamycin), epirubicin, idarubicin
- Antibiotics: bleomycin, mitomycin, actinomycin
- Mustards: mustine
- Vinca alkaloids: vincristine, vinblastine, vindesine
- Others: etoposide, tenoposide, amsacrine, mitoxantrone

Viagra (sildenafil)   Medication used to treat impotence and help improve a man's ability to have an erection in response to stimulation. It is a common treatment for the impotence that often results after treatment for PROSTATE CANCER. Unlike local medications that act directly on the penis, this pill circulates throughout the entire body.

The drug was originally designed to improve blood flow in the heart's blood vessels. However, research subjects soon began to report that the drug triggered a remarkable improvement in their ability to achieve and maintain an erection. Further studies were completed, and on March 27, 1998, the medication was approved by the U.S. Food and Drug Administration (FDA) for the treatment of impotence.

Within 30 to 60 minutes, the drug is absorbed in the bloodstream, where it inhibits an enzyme found primarily in the penis. Blocking this enzyme allows the smooth muscle in the penis to remain relaxed, boosting blood flow into the penis and generating an erection. Sildenafil (Viagra) is unique in that it simply enhances a natural-occurring process; therefore, erection occurs only as the result of sexual stimulation. In one study, 83 percent of patients reported a better erection after taking Viagra compared to 12 percent who took a dummy pill.

However, if Viagra is taken with a high-fat meal, its effectiveness can be much lower. If the patient is not sexually stimulated after taking Viagra, the medication is simply eliminated from the body in a few hours.

Viagra effectively treats ERECTILE DYSFUNCTION (impotence) years after prostate cancer patients receive treatment, according to the first study to look at the effectiveness of the medication in a large number of patients over an extended period. The new study was presented in October 2003 at the annual meeting of the American Society for Therapeutic Radiology and Oncology. The drug successfully treated impotence in 75 percent of patients four years after external beam radiation therapy or BRACHYTHERAPY (internal radiation) for prostate cancer. Among patients who reported success with the drug after the initial trial, 96 percent continued to use and find the medication effective. However, Viagra was less effective for men who had received stronger external radiation doses.

Side Effects

There are relatively few side effects of Viagra, and those that do occur are usually short-lived. However, some patients have reported congestion, diarrhea, facial flushing, headaches, or mild, temporary visual changes in perception of blue-green colors, or increased sensitivity to light. Viagra also may cause a drop in blood pressure and should not be used by men who have a history of coronary problems or by anyone who is using nitroglycerin or other blood pressure medications. Because there is also a potential for heart risk during sexual activity for patients who have preexisting heart disease, Viagra should not be used by men for whom sexual activity is inadvisable because of underlying heart problems.

Viagra and Prostate Cancer

Despite its popularity, there had been some initial concern that Viagra had certain chemical effects that could help prostate cancers grow. However, in a 2003 Chinese study of mice with human prostate cancer cells injected into their prostate gland, scientists found no evidence that Viagra caused the growth or spread of prostate cancer.

vitamin E   A vitamin that has been linked to a lower risk of PROSTATE CANCER. Vitamin E helps to mop up excess FREE RADICALS in the body—harmful substances that have been linked to the development of several kinds of cancer. However, men who have a history of bleeding problems or who use blood thinners should discuss vitamin E use with their doctor.

watchful waiting The decision not to treat PROSTATE CANCER when it is first diagnosed. The patient receives no immediate medical or surgical treatment, and the doctor monitors regular PROSTATE-SPECIFIC ANTIGEN (PSA) level testing and DIGITAL RECTAL EXAM (DRE). The PSA values are watched at small intervals to determine whether the level is rising or dropping (PSA velocity).

This strategy generally is reserved for men who have a low Gleason score and for elderly men who are too weak to tolerate radiation therapy or surgery or who also have other severe medical conditions that limit life expectancy. Men younger than age 72, healthy men, and those who have a higher Gleason score are more likely to live long enough to have symptoms of prostate cancer and are better suited to more active treatment.

A trial is currently comparing watchful waiting with radical PROSTATECTOMY to see which is more effective: the 15-year U.S. Prostate Cancer Intervention Versus Observation Trial (PIVOT). A European study (RIVOT) is comparing watchful waiting with RADIATION THERAPY for localized prostate cancer.

Many experts endorse watchful waiting for some patients because rarely does low-grade, low-stage disease advance within five years, and the risk of cancer progression of these cancers is low even within 10 years (between 10 and 25 percent). Moreover, the risk of complications of active treatment (including INCONTINENCE and ERECTILE DYSFUNCTION) is significant (especially in younger men).

There are some negative aspects of watchful waiting, however. Sixty percent of men whose prostate cancer does not spread who survive more than 10 years die of prostate cancer. Younger patients whose disease was initially confined and who undergo watchful waiting have a higher risk of development of a fatal incurable prostate cancer.

weight Under certain conditions, heavier men have a lower risk of developing PROSTATE CANCER than men who weigh less, according to a recent study of 2,896 men who had prostate cancer. Men who had a higher body mass index also had a lower risk of prostate cancer than men who had a lower body mass index, but only if they were younger than age 60 or had a family history of prostate cancer. Such an association was not seen in men who had sporadic prostate cancers.

Whitmore-Jewett staging A system of staging the extent of PROSTATE CANCER composed of alphabetical classifications A through D, followed by numerical prefixes 1 through 3 (A1, A2, B1, B2, B3, and so on, to D1, D2, D3). In this system, A is the earliest type of cancer and D is the most severe. This system has been largely replaced by the more common TUMOR–NODE–METASTASIS STAGING SYSTEM, although a few physicians still use this method. The Whitmore-Jewett staging system was developed by the AMERICAN UROLOGICAL ASSOCIATION.

wine and cancer There are many biologically active plant-based chemicals in wine. Some scientists believe that specific compounds called polyphenols found in red wine (such as catechins and RESVERATROL) may have antioxidant or anticancer properties.

Polyphenols are ANTIOXIDANT compounds found in the skin and seeds of grapes, which are dissolved by alcohol produced by the fermentation process. Red wine contains more polyphenols than white wine because when white wine is made, the skins are removed after the grapes are crushed. The phenols in red wine include catechin, gallic acid, and epicatechin.

Polyphenols have been found to have antioxidant properties: That is, they can protect cells from damage caused by molecules called FREE RADICALS. These free radicals can damage important parts of cells, including proteins, membranes, and DNA, and that damage may lead to cancer. Research on the antioxidants found in red wine has shown that they may help inhibit the development of certain cancers.

Resveratrol is a type of polyphenol that is produced as part of a plant's defense system in response to an invading fungus, stress, injury, infection, or ultraviolet irradiation. Red wine contains high levels of the antioxidant resveratrol, as do grapes, raspberries, peanuts, and other plants. Resveratrol has been shown to reduce tumor incidence in animals by affecting one or more stages of cancer development and has been shown to inhibit growth of many types of cancer cells in culture. It also appears to reduce inflammation and activation of a protein produced by the body's immune system when it is under attack. This protein affects cancer cell growth and metastasis.

However, experts believe it is still too early to draw conclusions about the association between red wine consumption and cancer in humans. Although consumption of large amounts of alcoholic beverages may increase the risk of some cancers, there is growing evidence that the health benefits of red wine consumption are related to its nonalcoholic components.

yohimbine The active ingredient of the West African yohimbe plant that has been promoted as an aphrodisiac and that is sometimes used by some men to treat impotence that results from treatment for PROSTATE CANCER. Yohimbine contains an alkaloid that produces blood vessel engorgement in the pelvic area, stimulating the lower center of the spinal cord. However, self-medication is strongly discouraged because of its side effects, including weakness, paralysis, gastrointestinal problems, and psychosis.

yolk sac carcinoma A malignant tumor that produces ALPHA-FETOPROTEIN and is thought to be derived from primitive endodermal cells. As a pure tumor, the yolk sac tumor, so called for its resemblance to a yolk sac, is the most common testicular tumor among infants and children up to age three. A pure yolk sac tumor is extremely rare in adults, but it is seen as a component in a MIXED GERM CELL TUMOR in about 30 percent of cases. It is also known as an endodermal sinus tumor or infantile EMBRYONAL CELL CARCINOMA.

See also TESTICULAR CANCER.

APPENDIXES

APPENDIX I
HELPFUL ORGANIZATIONS

ADVOCACY

National Patient Advocate Foundation
753 Thimble Shoals Boulevard
Suite A
Newport News, VA 23606
(757) 873-0438
(800) 532-5274 (toll-free)
http://www.npaf.org

A national health care reform network that supports legislation to enable cancer survivors to obtain insurance funding for medical care and participation in clinical trials. Services include referrals, information, advocacy, benefits, and health insurance assistance.

National Prostate Cancer Coalition (NPCC)
1158 15th Street NW
Washington, DC 20005
(202) 463-9455
(888) 245-9455 (toll-free)
http://www.pcacoalition.org

National Prostate Cancer Coalition, a grassroots awareness and advocacy group, offers services that include advocacy, public education, referrals, and education information.

AIRLINE TRANSPORTATION (FREE)

Air Care Alliance
1515 E. 71st Street
Suite 312
Tulsa, OK 74136
(918) 745-0384
(888) 260-9707 (toll-free)
http://www.aircareall.org/

The Air Care Alliance is a nationwide league of humanitarian flying organizations dedicated to community service. Member group activities involve health care, patient transport, and related kinds of public-benefit flying.

AirLifeLine
50 Fullerton Court
Suite 200
Sacramento, CA 95825
(916) 641-7800
(877) AIRLIFE (toll-free)
http://www.airlifeline.org

The organization provides transportation to and from medical destinations for patients in financial need within 1,000 air miles of any departure point in the United States.

Corporate Angel Network
Westchester County Airport, Bldg. 1
White Plains, NY 10604
(914) 328-1313
(866) 328-1313 (toll-free)
http://www.corpangelneetwork.org

Corporate Angel Network finds free air transportation on corporate planes for cancer patients who need medical attention. Patients must be ambulatory.

National Patient Air Transport Hotline
P.O. Box 1940
Manassas, VA 22110-0804
(800) 296-1217 (toll-free)
http://www.npath.org

National Patient Air Transport Hotline is a clearinghouse for patients who cannot afford travel for medical care.

ALTERNATIVE HEALTH

Office of Cancer Complementary and Alternative Medicine
National Cancer Institute, NIH
Executive Boulevard North
Suite 102
Bethesda, MD 20892
(800) 4CANCER (toll-free)
http://www.cancer.gov/cam

The Office of Cancer Complementary and Alternative Medicine (OCCAM) was established in 1998 to enhance the activities of the National Cancer Institute in the arena of complementary and alternative medicine. The OCCAM's goal is to increase the amount of high-quality cancer research and information about the use of complementary and alternative modalities.

BLACK ISSUES

See RACIAL ISSUES IN CANCER.

BONE MARROW TRANSPLANT

Blood & Marrow Transplant Information Network
2900 Skokie Valley Road
Suite B
Highland Park, IL 60035
(847) 433-3313
(888) 597-7674 (toll-free)
http://www.marrow.org

A nonprofit organization, the network provides publications and support services to bone marrow, peripheral blood stem cell, and cord blood transplant patients and survivors. Services include publishing a quarterly newsletter (*Blood & Marrow Transplant Newsletter*), a resource directory, a "patient-to-survivor" telephone link, and a 157-page book describing physical and emotional aspects of marrow and stem cell transplantation. A second book, *Mira's Month* ($5), helps prepare young children for their parent's transplant. Addi-

tional resources include a directory of transplant centers and an attorney list for assistance in resolving insurance problems.

Bone Marrow Foundation, The
70 East 55th Street
20th Floor
New York, NY 10022
(212) 838-3029
(800) 365-1336 (toll-free)
http://www.bonemarrow.org

The foundation gives eligible transplant candidates financial assistance limited to helping defray the cost of ancillary services needed to ensure proper care during the transplant procedure, as well as in pre- and posttransplant treatment phases.

Bone Marrow Transplant Family Support Network
P.O. Box 845
Avon, CT 06001
(800) 826-9376 (toll-free)

The national telephone support network for patients and their families offers referrals, bone marrow transplant information, counseling, children's services, and health insurance information. The network answers callers' questions and connects newly diagnosed patients with recovered bone marrow transplant (BMT) patients of the same age who have the same diagnosis or are in the same stage of disease.

National Bone Marrow Transplant Link
20411 W. 12 Mile Road
Suite 108
Southfield, MI 48076
(800) LINK-BMT (or (800) 546-5268, toll-free)
http://www.comnet.org

National Bone Marrow Transplant Link is a national clearinghouse for a variety of bone marrow transplant issues. Services include patient advocacy, referrals, research funding, and an excellent resource guide on bone marrow transplant (BMT).

National Marrow Donor Program
3001 Broadway Street NE
Suite 500
Minneapolis, MN 55413-1753
(800) MARROW2 (or [800] 627-7692, toll-free)

(888) 999-6743 (Office of Patient Advocacy)
http://www.marrow-donor.org

The National Marrow Donor Program maintains a registry of bone marrow donors, provides information on how to become a donor, and organizes donor recruitment drives.

BRACHYTHERAPY

American Brachytherapy Society
11250 Roger Bacon Drive
Suite 8
Reston, VA 20190-5202
(703) 234-4078
http://www.americanbrachytherapy.org

The society is a nonprofit organization consisting of physicists, physicians, and other health care providers interested in brachytherapy that conducts research into the use of brachytherapy in malignant and benign conditions. The group supplies information, promotes the highest standards of practice, and encourages continuing education for radiation oncologists and other cancer experts.

CANCER

AMC Cancer Research Center-Cancer Information and Counseling Line
1600 Pierce Street
Denver, CO 80214
(303) 233-6501
(800) 525-3777 (toll-free)
(800) 321-1557 (toll-free)
http://www.amc.org

A nonprofit research institute dedicated to the prevention of cancer, the organization has services that include providing up-to-date facts about all aspects of cancer as well as personal assistance from counselors trained and experienced in dealing with the fear, confusion, conflicts, and other problems often associated with the disease. All staff are paid professionals with degrees in counseling or related health areas. The group also offers members of the general public access to the latest information on cancer prevention, detection, diagnosis, treatment, and rehabilitation, including the Physi-

cians' Data Query (PDQ), a database of research studies and treatment protocols from the nation's cancer centers. The service mails out thousands of free brochures and other literature every year and helps put callers in touch with cancer-related resources in their community. In addition, the service funds research.

American Cancer Society (ACS)
1599 Clifton Road NE
Atlanta, GA 30329-4251
(800) 227-2345 (toll-free)
http://www.cancer.org

The society is a nationwide community-based organization dedicated to eliminating cancer as a major health problem through research, education, and service. Chartered divisions exist in every state plus Washington, D.C., and Puerto Rico. Services include a variety of programs such as Reach to Recovery, Cansurmount, I Can Cope, Road to Recovery, Man to Man, International Association of Laryngectomees, Look Good . . . Feel Better, and Resources, Information, and Guidance (RIG). The society operates Hope Lodges for temporary housing in selected areas.

American Joint Committee on Cancer
633 N. Saint Clair
Chicago, IL 60611
(312) 202-5290
E-mail: sburkhardt@facs.org

The organization was established in 1959 to publish systems of classification of cancer, including staging and end results reporting, for doctors' use in selecting most effective treatment, determining prognosis, and continuing their evaluation of cancer control measures. Included are six founding organizations, four sponsoring organizations, and seven liaison organizations.

Association of Cancer Online Resources
173 Duane Street
Suite 3A
New York , NY 10013
(212) 226-5525
http://www.acor.org

The association gives patients and families access to numerous cancer-specific mailing lists.

Cancer Care
275 Seventh Avenue
New York, NY 10001
(212) 712-8080
(800) 813-HOPE (or [800] 813-4673, toll-free)
http://www.cancercare.org

The national nonprofit agency offers a range of free support services to cancer patients and their families, including professional individual and group counseling, bereavement counseling, online support and counseling, educational programs, workshops, teleconferences, financial assistance, and referrals. Services are offered at all stages of the disease to patients and families. Supplementary financial assistance is awarded for home care, transportation, and pain medication. Funds are limited to cancer treatment in New York, New Jersey, and Connecticut. Cancer Care has offices in New Jersey, Connecticut, and Long Island and offers African-American and Hispanic Outreach programs.

Cancer Hope Network
Two North Road
Chester, NJ 07930
(877) 467-3638 (or [877] HOPENET, toll-free)
http://www.cancerhopenetwork.org

Cancer Hope Network is a nonprofit organization that provides free and confidential one-on-one support to cancer patients and their families. Services include volunteer training programs and a toll-free information number. It matches cancer patients and/or family members with trained volunteers who have recovered from a similar cancer experience.

Cancer Information and Counseling Line
1600 Pierce Street
Denver, CO 80214
(800) 525-3777 (toll-free)
http://www.amc.org

A toll-free telephone service, the line is part of the psychosocial program of the American Medical Center (AMC) Cancer Research Center. Professional counselors provide up-to-date medical information, emotional support through short-term counseling, and resource referrals to callers nationwide between the hours of 8:30 a.m. and 5:00 p.m.

MST. Individuals may also submit questions about cancer and request resources via e-mail.

Cancer Information Service
Building 31, Room 10A16
9000 Rockville Pike
Bethesda MD 20892
(301) 402-5874
(800) 4 CANCER (9:00 A.M. to 4:30 P.M. local time, Monday through Friday, toll-free)
(800) 332-8615 (toll-free)
http://www.icic.nci.nih.gov

The Nationwide network was founded by the National Cancer Institute (NCI). Calls are routed to local Cancer Information Service (CIS) offices, where trained cancer information specialists answer virtually any question on cancer. More than 100 free pamphlets are offered. The CIS Outreach Coordinator is available to groups to help them set up their own education programs.

Cancer Net
Building 31, Room 10A03
31 Center Drive, MSC 2580
Bethesda, MD 20892-2580
(301) 435-3848
http://cancernet.nci.nih.gov

The Web site offers a wide range of cancer information from the National Cancer Institute, including details of treatment options, clinical trials, reduction of cancer risk, and coping with cancer. Resources on support groups, financial assistance, and educational materials are also offered.

Cancer Research Institute
681 Fifth Avenue
New York, NY 10022-4209
(212) 688-7515
http://www.cancerresearch.org

A nonprofit organization, the institute funds research projects and scientists across the country. Publications include *The Cancer Research Institute Help Book* and information about clinical trials of immunological treatments.

Cancer Survivors Network
American Cancer Society (ACS)
1599 Clifton Road NE

Atlanta, GA 30329-4251
(877) 333-4673
http://www.cancer.org

The network is a telephone and Internet-based service for cancer survivors, their families, caregivers, and friends. Survivors may access prerecorded discussions via phone or join live chat sessions and find virtual support groups, prerecorded talk shows, and personal stories online. Cancer Survivors Network is supported by the American Cancer Society.

Cancervive
11636 Chayote Street
Suite 500
Los Angeles, CA 90049
(310) 203-9232
(800) 4-TO-CURE (toll-free)
http://www.cancervive.org

Cancervive helps cancer survivors to face and overcome the challenges of "life after cancer." Services include support groups, educational materials, insurance information and assistance, and advocacy for cancer survivors.

Exceptional Cancer Patient, Inc. (EcaP)
522 Jackson Park Drive
Meadville, PA 16335
(814) 337-8192
http://www.ecap-online.org

EcaP offers programs and services to cancer patients, people who have terminal illness, and health professionals. Services are based in Connecticut only; referrals are national.

Information and Referral Network
http://www.ir-net.com/index.html

The network is an online "one-stop" shopping center for human services, information, referrals, and other community services.

International Cancer Alliance for Research and Education
4853 Cordell Avenue
Suite 206
Bethesda, MD 20814
(800) ICA-RE61 (toll-free)
(301) 654-7933
http://www.icare.org/frontpage.htm

This nonprofit organization provides high-quality cancer information to patients and their doctors and has developed several unique patient-centered programs through an extensive process of collection, evaluation, and dissemination of information that puts the cancer patient in contact with top physicians and scientists around the world. This organization is operated by a network of scientists, clinicians, caring staff, and lay volunteers, many of whom are patients.

International Union against Cancer
3 rue du Conseil General
1205 Geneva
Switzerland
http://www.uicc.org

International Union against Cancer (IUAC) is devoted to advancing scientific and medical knowledge in research, diagnosis, treatment, and prevention of cancer and promoting all other aspects of the campaign against cancer throughout the world. Particular emphasis is placed on professional and public education. IUAC is an independent non-government association of more than 290 member organizations in about 85 countries. Members are voluntary cancer leagues and societies, cancer research and/or treatment centers, and, in some countries, ministries of health.

CAREGIVERS

National Family Caregivers Association (NFCA)
10400 Connecticut Avenue
Suite 500
Kensington, MD 20895-3944
(301) 942-6430
(800) 896-3650 (toll-free)
http://www.nfcacares.org

National Family Caregivers Association provides educational and emotional support for family caregivers and services including advocacy; individual, family, group, peer, and bereavement counseling; and information.

Well Spouse Foundation
P.O. Box 30093
Elkins Park, PA 19027

(800) 838-0879 (toll-free)
http://www.wellspouse.org

A membership organization, the foundation provides emotional support and information for the "well spouse" or the caregiver of the chronically ill. Services include publication of a newsletter, local support groups, round robin letter writing, an annual weekend conference, and bereavement counseling.

CHEMOTHERAPY

CHEMOcare
231 N. Avenue
Westfield, NJ 07090
(800) 552-4366 (toll-free)
(908) 233-1103
http://www.chemocare.com

This program and Web site sponsored by the Scott Hamilton Cancer Alliance for Research Education and Survivorship (CARES) initiative is designed to provide the latest information about chemotherapy to patients and their families. The site contains information about having chemotherapy, managing side effects, and living well during treatment.

Chemotherapy Foundation
183 Madison Avenue
Suite 302
New York NY 10016
(212) 213-9292
http://www.neoplastics.mssm.edu/
   sympbrochure.html

The public foundation was established in 1968 dedicated to the control, cure, and prevention of cancer through innovative medical therapies including chemotherapy, chemoimmunotherapy, chemohormonal therapy, chemoprevention, and biotechnologies. The foundation is also dedicated to the education of physicians, patients, and the public through educational literature and currently sponsors selected basic and clinical research initiatives at six major New York City medical centers.

CLINICAL TRIALS

Cancer Liaison Program (CLP)
Food and Drug Administration (FDA Room 9-
   49CFH-12)

5600 Fishers Lane
Rockville, MD 20857
(888) INFO-FDA (toll-free)
http://www.fda.gov/oashi/cancer/cancer.html

A division of the FDA, the Cancer Liaison Program works directly with cancer patients and advocacy programs to provide information on the FDA drug approval process, cancer clinical trials, and access to investigational therapies when admission to an existing clinical trial is not possible.

Coalition of National Cancer Cooperative Groups, Inc.
1818 Market Street
Suite 1100
Philadelphia, PA 19103
(877) 520-4457
http://www.ca-coalition.org

The Coalition of National Cancer Cooperative Groups, Inc., is the nation's premier network of cancer clinical trials specialists. Services include a variety of programs and information for physicians, patient advocate groups, and patients designed to improve the clinical trials process.

DEATH AND DYING

See also HOSPICE.

Partnership for Caring
1620 I Street NW
Suite 202
Washington, DC 20006
(202) 296-8071
(800) 989-9455 (toll-free)
http://www.partnershipforcaring.org

Partnership for Caring is an advocacy and research organization protecting the rights of dying patients that provides information to help people prepare for end-of-life decisions. Services include referrals; guest speakers; counseling; legal assistance; patient advocacy; pain management; volunteer services; hospice care; and distribution of advance directives, including living wills, durable power of attorney, and explanatory guidelines appropriate to state of residence. The group also furnishes various publications, videos, and audios that deal with advance care planning and end-of-life issues.

Widowed Persons Service
NY Service Program
  for Older People, Inc. (SPOP)
188 West 88th Street
New York, NY 10024
(212) 787-7120 ext 139
(212)721-6279
http://www.spop.org

SPOP's Widowed Persons Service, cosponsored by the American Association of Retired Persons, serves widows, men, and women of all ages, offering peer support and information to the newly widowed.

FINANCIAL AID

Bone Marrow Foundation, The
70 East 55th Street, 20th Floor
New York, NY 10022
(212) 838-3029
(800) 365-1336
http://www.bonemarrow.org

The foundation gives eligible transplant candidates financial assistance to help defray the cost of ancillary services needed to ensure proper care during the transplant procedure, as well as in pre- and posttransplant treatment phases.

Cancer Fund of America
2901 Breezewood Lane
Knoxville, TN 37921-1009
(865) 938-5281
http://www.cfoa.org

Cancer Fund of America is dedicated to providing direct aid in the form of goods to financially indigent patients.

Ensure Health Connection
P.O. Box 29139
Shawnee, KS 66201
(800) 986-8501 (toll-free)
http://www.ensure.com

The connection provides coupons and valuable information to people who need the nutritional supplement Ensure. Ensure donates their product to food banks, where a person in need may be able to receive a free supply.

Hill-Burton Free Hospital Care
5600 Fishers Lane
Rockville MD 20857
(800) 638-0742 (toll-free)
(301) 443-5656
http://www.hrsa.gov/osp/dfcr/
Email: dfcrcomm@hrsa.gov

Hill-Burton is a program run by the U.S. government that can arrange for certain medical facilities or hospitals to provide free or low-cost care.

Medicine Program, The
P.O. Box 520
Doniphan, AL 63935
(573) 996-7300
http://www.themedicineprogram.com

The program provides free prescription medicine to those who qualify; a processing fee is required for each medication requested.

Mission of Hope Cancer Fund
802 First Street
Jackson, MI 49023
(517) 782-4643
(888) 544-6423
http://www.cancerfund.org

A nonprofit organization, the fund was established by a cancer survivor to help cancer patients and their families who have specific financial needs relieve some of the extra financial burdens of cancer patients and their families while dealing with cancer treatment and recovery. Services include education, counseling, housing, and financial medication assistance.

National Association of Hospital Hospitality
4915 Auburn Avenue
Bethesda MD 20814
(800) 542-9730 (toll-free)
http://www.nahhh.org

A nonprofit corporation, the association serves facilities that provide lodging and other supportive services to patients and their families when confronted with medical emergencies. It also provides referrals.

National Patient Air Transport Hotline
P.O. Box 1940
Manassas, VA 22110-0804

(800) 296-1217 (toll-free)
http://www.npath.org

The hotline is a clearinghouse for patients who cannot afford travel for medical care.

Patient Advocate Foundation (PAF)

753 Thimble Shoals Boulevard
Suite B
Newport News, VA 23606
(757) 873-6668
(800) 532-5274 (toll-free)
http://www.patientadvocate.org

Patient Advocate Foundation helps cancer patients deal with insurance coverage, pay for managed care treatment, and understand managed care. Services include mediation, negotiation, and education on behalf of patients experiencing problems related to preauthorization, coding and billing, the insurance appeal process, debt crisis, job retention, access to pharmaceutical agents, access to chemotherapy, access to medical devices, access to surgical procedures, and expedited applications for Social Security, Medicare, Medicaid, and other agencies.

GENETICS INFORMATION

National Society of Genetic Counselors

233 Canterbury Drive
Wallingford, PA 19086-6617
(610) 872-7608
http://www.nsgc.org/

The National Society of Genetic Counselors promotes the genetic counseling profession as a recognized integral part of health care delivery, education, research, and public policy. Services include referrals, educational programs, and genetic screening.

GOVERNMENT AGENCIES

Cancer Liaison Program (CLP)

Food and Drug Administration (FDA Room 9-49CFH-12)
5600 Fishers Lane
Rockville, MD 20857
(888) INFO-FDA (toll-free)
http://www.fda.gov

As a division of the FDA, the Cancer Liaison Program works directly with cancer patients and advocacy programs to provide information about the FDA drug approval process, cancer clinical trials, and access to investigational therapies when admission to an existing clinical trial is not possible.

Centers for Disease Control and Prevention Division of Cancer Prevention and Control (DCPC)

4770 Buford Highway NE
MS K-64
Atlanta, GA 30341-3717
(770) 488-4751
(800) 311-3435 (toll-free)
http://www.cdc.gov/cancer

The Division of Cancer Prevention and Control of the Centers for Disease Control serves as a leader for nationwide cancer prevention and control and as a partner with state health agencies and other key groups.

National Cancer Institute

Building 31, Room 10A03
31 Center Drive, MSC 2580
Bethesda, MD 20892-2580
(301) 435-3848
(800) 422-6237 (toll-free)
http://www.cancer.gov

National Cancer Institute is the federal government's principal agency for cancer research. Services include the Physician's Data Query (PDQ) comprehensive database, which contains peer-reviewed summaries and most current information on cancer treatment, screening, prevention, genetics, and supportive care; a registry of cancer clinical trials being conducted worldwide; and directories of physicians, professionals who provide genetic services, and organizations that provide care to people with cancer.

National Center for Complementary and Alternative Medicine

NCCAM Clearinghouse
P.O. Box 7923
Gaithersburg, MD 20893-7923
(301) 519-3153

(866) 464-3615 (TTY)
(888) 644-6226 (toll-free)
http://www.nccam.nih.gov

The National Center for Complementary and Alternative Medicine supports rigorous research on complementary and alternative medicine (CAM), trains researchers in CAM, and disseminates information to the public and professionals on which CAM modalities are effective, which are not, and why. Services include a toll-free telephone line, information packages, fact sheets, a newsletter, referrals, meetings and workshops, and treatment information.

Social Security Administration (SSA)
Office of Public Inquiries
6401 Security Boulevard
Room 4-C-5 Annex
Baltimore, MD 21235
(800) 772-1213 (toll-free)
http://www.ssa.gov

The Social Security Administration is the U.S. government agency that runs the Social Security program. It also provides information about retirement and disability benefits, Supplemental Security Income (SSI), and Medicare (the government program that pays for the medical care of the elderly). Services include a toll-free number, referrals, financial assistance, and information.

HOME CARE

See also HOSPICE.

Visiting Nurse Association of America (VNAA)
11 Beacon Street
Suite 910
Boston, MA 02108
(617) 523-4042
(800) 426-2547 (toll-free)

The Visiting Nurse Association of America (VNAA) provides information on all aspects of home health care, including general nursing; physical, occupational, and speech therapy; medical social service; home health aide and homemaker services; nutritional counseling; and hospice care. Callers are referred to a local VNAA service.

HOSPICE

Hospice Education Institute
3 Unity Square
P.O. Box 98
Machiasport, Maine 04655-0098
(207) 255-8800
http://www.hospiceworld.org

An independent, nonprofit organization that offers the public and health care professionals information about the many facets of caring for the dying and the bereaved. Services include a toll-free information and referral service (HospiceLink), regional seminars, professional education, advice, and assistance.

HospiceLink
Hospice Education Institute
190 Westbrook Road
Essex CT 06426
(800) 331-1620 (toll-free)
(203) 767-1620

A service offered by the Hospice Education Institute that maintains a computerized directory of all hospice and palliative care programs in the United States. The toll-free telephone number provides referrals to hospice and palliative care programs and general information about the principles and practices of good hospice and palliative care.

National Hospice and Palliative Care Organization, The
1700 Diagonal Road
Suite 625
Alexandria, VA 22314
(703) 837-1500
http://www.nhpco.org

The National Hospice and Palliative Care Organization provides information and referrals to nationwide hospice programs via a toll-free phone number. Services include referrals, patient advocacy, research, public engagement, and professional education.

National Hospice Foundation
1700 Diagonal Road
Suite 625
Alexandria, VA 22314

(703) 516-4928
http://www.nhpco.org

A charitable organization, the foundation was created in 1992 to broaden understanding of hospice through research and education, expanding America's vision for end-of-life care. In doing so, it engages and informs the public about the quality of that care that hospice provides.

Visiting Nurse Association of America (VNAA)
11 Beacon Street
Suite 910
Boston, MA 02108
(617) 523-4042
(800) 426-2547

The Visiting Nurse Association of America (VNAA) provides information on all aspects of home health care, including general nursing; physical, occupational, and speech therapy; medical social service; home health aide and homemaker services; nutritional counseling; and hospice care. Callers are referred to a local VNAA service. Services include educational information, referrals, and home care and hospice care.

HOUSING (TEMPORARY)

American Cancer Society (ACS)
1599 Clifton Road NE
Atlanta, GA 30329-4251
(800) 227-2345 (toll-free)
http://www.cancer.org

The American Cancer Society operates Hope Lodges for temporary housing in selected areas.

National Association of Hospital Hospitality Houses, Inc.
P.O. Box 18087
Asheville, NC 28814-0087
(828) 253-1188
(800) 542-9730 (toll-free)

A nonprofit corporation, the association serves facilities that provide lodging and other supportive services to patients and their families when confronted with medical emergencies. Services include referrals and housing and lodging facilities.

INFERTILITY

Fertile Hope
P.O. Box 624
New York, NY 10014
(888) 994-HOPE
http://www.fertilehope.org

Fertile Hope is a national nonprofit organization addressing the reproductive needs of cancer patients and survivors. Services include awareness, education, financial assistance, research, and support.

INTERNATIONAL HELP

Canadian Prostate Cancer Network (CPCN)
P.O. Box 1253
Lakefield, ON KOL 2HO
Canada
(705) 652-9200
http://www.cpcn.org

CPCN is a national organization of 125 support groups throughout Canada offering help to men with prostate cancer. The CPCN Web site features a map of Canada for easy location of support groups by province.

International Cancer Alliance for Research and Education (ICARE)
4853 Cordell Avenue
Suite 206
Bethesda, MD 20814
(800) ICA-RE61; (301) 654-7933
http://www.icare.org/frontpage.htm

A nonprofit organization, ICARE provides high-quality cancer information to patients and their doctors. It has developed several unique patient-centered programs through an extensive process of collection, evaluation, and dissemination of information, putting the cancer patient in contact with top physicians and scientists around the world. This organization is operated by a network of scientists, clinicians, caring staff, and lay volunteers, many of whom are patients.

International Union against Cancer (UICC)
3 rue du Conseil General
1205 Geneva

Switzerland
http://www.uicc.org

UICC is devoted exclusively to all aspects of the worldwide fight against cancer. Its objectives are to advance scientific and medical knowledge in research, diagnosis, treatment, and prevention of cancer and to promote all other aspects of the campaign against cancer throughout the world. Particular emphasis is placed on professional and public education. UICC is an independent nongovernment, association of more than 290 member organizations in about 85 countries. Members are voluntary cancer leagues and societies, cancer research and/or treatment centers, and, in some countries, ministries of health.

Planet CANCER
1804 E. 39th Street
Austin, TX 78722
(512)481-9010
http://www.planetcancer.org

Planet Cancer is an international network of young adults (between ages 18 and 35) who have cancer who support each other in online and face-to-face communities. Services include peer support; the Planet Cancer Forum, in which patients communicate directly with each other; advocacy; and Adventure Therapy, an outdoor expedition for young adults.

Us TOO International
930 North York Road
Suite 50
Hinsdale, IL 60521
(800) 808-7866; (630) 323-1002
http://www.ustoo.com

Us TOO is an international network of chapters that offer support and services to prostate cancer survivors. Services include support groups, referrals for clinical trials, information, and advocacy. Support groups are located throughout the United States and Canada; the organization's Web site lists clinical trials for men with prostate cancer. Some support groups also sponsor Side by Side, a group of women partners of prostate cancer patients. Us TOO also provides professional education.

KLINEFELTER SYNDROME

Klinefelter Syndrome and Associates
P.O. Box 119
Roseville, CA 95678-0119
(916) 773-2999
http://www.genetic.org/ks

A nonprofit organization and international support organization that provides information, encourages research, and fosters treatment and cures for symptoms of sex chromosome variations. The organization distributes a newsletter three times a year to more than 1400 Klinefelter syndrome males, families, physician, and support organizations. The group also produces brochures about Klinefelter syndrome and actively participates in research and educational projects on Klinefelter syndrome and other male sex chromosome variations.

LEGAL ISSUES

Cancer Legal Resource Center
919 S. Albany Street
Los Angeles, CA 90019-0015
(213) 736-1455
http://www.wlcdr.org/clrc.html

The center provides information for cancer patients about their legal rights and the legal issues they face while battling cancer. It also has access to a panel of volunteer attorneys and other professionals willing to assist people with cancer.

PAIN

American Chronic Pain Association (ACPA)
P.O. Box 850
Rocklin, CA 95677
(800) 533-3231
http://www.theacpa.org

A self-help organization, the ACPA offers educational material and peer support to help people combat chronic pain, as well as referrals to pain control facilities. It publishes a quarterly newsletter and a book on coping with pain for which a donation is requested and organizes support groups.

American Pain Society
4700 West Lake Avenue
Glenview, IL 60025
(847) 375-4715
http://www.ampainsoc.org

A multidisciplinary educational and scientific organization, the society is dedicated to serving people in pain. Members research and treat pain and act as advocates for patients who have pain. Services include the publication of *Pain Facilities Directory,* information on more than 500 specialized pain treatment centers across the country; counseling for pain; referrals; and education programs.

National Chronic Pain Outreach Association, Inc.
P.O. Box 274
Millboro, VA 24460
(540) 862-9437
http://www.chronicpain.org

A nonprofit organization, the association was formed to lessen the suffering of people who have chronic pain by educating pain sufferers, health care professionals, and the public about chronic pain and its management.

PROFESSIONAL GROUPS

The American Association for Cancer Education
9500 Euclid Avenue (R30)
Cleveland, OH 44195
(216) 444-9827
http://www.aaceonline.com/index.asp

A professional organization of educators in many disciplines working to improve cancer education, advance cancer prevention, expedite early cancer detection, promote individualized therapy, and develop rehabilitation programs for cancer patients, the American Association for Cancer Education has members of the faculties of schools of medicine, dentistry, osteopathy, education, pharmacy, nursing, public health, and social work. The association encourages projects for the training of paramedical personnel and educational programs for the general public, populations at risk, and cancer patients.

American College of Radiology
1891 Preston White Drive
Reston, VA 20191
(703) 648-8912
(703) 648-8900
(800) 227-5463 (toll-free)
http://www.acr.org

A medical professional organization, the college was designed to advance the science of radiology, improve radiologic service to the patient, study the economic aspects of the practice of radiology, and encourage improved and continuing education for radiologists and allied professional fields.

American Society of Clinical Oncology
1900 Duke Street
Suite 200
Alexandria, VA 22314
(703) 299-0150
http://www.asco.org

An organization that represents more than 10,000 cancer professionals worldwide, the society offers scientific and educational programs and other initiatives intended to foster the exchange of information about cancer. Services include ASCO OnLine for both professionals and people who have cancer; extensive information is offered on its patient page.

American Urological Association
1120 North Charles Street
Baltimore, MD 21201
(410) 727-1100
http://www.auanet.org

The world's preeminent urological organization, the association conducts a wide range of activities to ensure that more than 13,000 members have current knowledge of the latest research and best practices in the field of urology. Services include publications, an annual meeting, continuing medical education, and health policy advocacy.

Association of Community Cancer Centers
11600 Nebel Street
Suite 201
Rockville, MD 20852-2557
(301) 984-9496 ext. 200
http://www.accc-cancer.org

An association designed to help oncology professionals deal with program management, cuts in reimbursement, hospital consolidation and mergers, and legislation and regulations, ACCC counts as members medical and radiation oncologists, surgeons, cancer program administrators and medical directors, senior hospital executives, practice managers, oncology nurses, oncology social workers, and cancer program data managers. ACCC Institution/Group Practice members include more than 650 medical centers, hospitals, oncology practices, and cancer programs across the United States.

National Society of Genetic Counselors

233 Canterbury Drive
Wallingford, PA 19086-6617
(610) 872-7608
http://www.nsgc.org/

The National Society of Genetic Counselors promotes the genetic counseling profession as a recognized integral part of health care delivery, education, research, and public policy. Services include referrals, educational programs, and genetic screening.

PROSTATE CANCER

Alliance for Prostate Cancer Prevention (APCaP)

1010 Jorie Boulevard
Suite 124
Oak Brook, IL 60523
(630) 990-7100
http://www.apcap.org/contact.html

The group was designed to include public and private business leaders, legislators, health providers and administrators, researchers, and federal, state, and local health officials in a coordinated cohesive forum to enhance and promote prostate cancer awareness, education, research, and primary and secondary prevention programs.

American Foundation for Urologic Disease (AFUD)

1128 North Charles Street
Baltimore, MD 21201
(410) 468-1800
(800) 242-2383 (toll-free)
http://www.afud.org

A charitable organization established to raise funds for research, lay education and patient advocacy for the prevention, detection, management and cure of urologic disease.

American Prostate Society

P.O. Box 870
Hanover, MD 21076 USA
(800) 308-1106
http://www.ameripros.org

A nonprofit organization, the society provides timely free information and the latest treatments/cures for prostate cancer, prostatitis, prostate growth, and impotence. In addition to a Web site featuring FAQs and other information, the society provides a free newsletter on request and e-mailed answers to e-mailed questions.

CaP CURE (Association for the Cure of Cancer of the Prostate)

1250 Fourth Street
Suite 360
Santa Monica, CA 90401
(310) 458-2873
(800) 757-2873 (or [800] 757-CURE)
http://www.capcure.org

CaP CURE is dedicated to finding a cure for prostate cancer through support of research, education, and prevention. Services include advocacy; identification and support of prostate cancer research, referrals, and information on clinical trials.

Man to Man

American Cancer Society
1599 Clifton Road NE
Atlanta, GA 30329
(800) 227-2345 (toll-free)
(404) 320-3333
http://www.cancer.org

The program is a support group that offers an educational presentation by a health care professional, support, and one-on-one visitation and telephone services by specially trained prostate cancer survivors.

Men's Cancer Resource Group

1001 South MacDill Avenue
Tampa, FL 33629
(813) 273-3652 3
(800) 309-6467 (24-hour hotline, toll-free)

Organized by prostate cancer survivors and concerned professionals, the Men's Cancer Research Group offers a support network as well as an education clearinghouse for current information on research and treatment. The group offers support group meetings and community outreach in the Tampa Bay area.

National Prostate Cancer Coalition (NPCC)

1158 15th Street NW
Washington, DC 20005
(202) 463-9455
(888) 245- 9455 (toll-free)
http://www.pcacoalition.org

The National Prostate Cancer Coalition, a grassroots awareness and advocacy group, is interested in outreach and advocacy to benefit men who have prostate cancer. Services include advocacy, public education, referrals, and information.

Patient Advocates for Advanced Cancer Treatments (PAACT)

1143 Parmelee NW
P.O. Box 141695
Grand Rapids, MI 49514
(616) 453-1477
http://www.paactusa.org

A nonprofit prostate cancer advocacy organization, the PAACT informs prostate cancer patients of the most advanced methods of detection, diagnostic procedures, evaluations, and treatments. The legal action committee can help patients with insurance problems. Services include referrals, a public library, information, the quarterly *Cancer Communication* newsletter, counseling, sex therapy, advocacy, volunteer services, medical assistance, alternative therapies, support group information, elderly services, and health insurance information.

Us Too International

930 North York Road
Suite 50
Hinsdale, IL 60521

(800) 808-7866 (toll-free)
(630) 323-1002
http://www.ustoo.com

An international network of support groups, the group has a Web site that lists clinical trials for men who have prostate cancer. Some support groups also sponsor Side by Side, a group of women partners of prostate cancer patients.

RACIAL ISSUES IN CANCER

Intercultural Cancer Council

PMB-C
1720 Dryden
Houston, TX 77030
(713) 798-4617

The council promotes policies, programs, partnerships, and research to eliminate the unequal burden of cancer among racial and ethnic minorities and medically underserved populations in the United States and its associated territories. The Intercultural Cancer Council works in partnership with both federal and private agencies and institutions.

Native American Cancer Research

3022 South Nova Road
Pine, CO 80470
(303) 838-9359
http://members.aol.com/natamcan/aboutnac.htm

The goals of Native American Cancer Research (NACR) are to reduce Native American cancer incidence and mortality rates and to increase the cancer survival rate among Native Americans through primary prevention, secondary prevention, risk reduction, screening (early detection), education, training, research, diagnosis, control, treatment, support, quality of life, and/or studies.

Native CIRCLE: The American Indian/Alaska Native Cancer Information Resource Center and Learning Exchange

Charlton 6, Room 282
200 First Road SW
Rochester, MN 55905
(877) 372-1617
http://www.mayo.edu/nativecircle/native.html

The American Indian/Alaska Native Cancer Information Resource Center and Learning Exchange (Native C.I.R.C.L.E.) exists to stimulate, develop, maintain, and disseminate culturally appropriate cancer information materials for Native American/Alaska Native educators, health-care leaders, and students.

RADIATION THERAPY

American College of Radiology
1891 Preston White Drive
Reston, VA 20191
(703) 648-8912
(703) 648-8900
(800) 227-5463 (toll-free)
http://www.acr.org

A medical professional organization, the college was designed to advance the science of radiology, improve radiologic service to the patient, study the economic aspects of the practice of radiology, and encourage improved and continuing education for radiologists and allied professionals.

RESEARCH

American Institute for Cancer Research (AICR)
1759 R Street NW
Washington, DC 20009
(202) 328-7744
(800) 843-8114 (toll-free)
http://www.aicr.org

A national cancer organization, the AICR focuses exclusively on the relationship between nutrition and cancer. Services include a wide array of education materials for consumers to help them lower their cancer risk through diet. A nutrition toll-free hot line allows consumers to speak personally with a registered dictitian.

Cancer Research Foundation of America
1600 Duke Street
Suite 110
Alexandria, VA 22314
(703) 836-4412
(800) 227-2732 (or [800] 227-CRFA)
http://www.preventcancer.org

Cancer Research Foundation of America is a nonprofit organization dedicated to cancer prevention through research and education. Services include funding peer-reviewed research grants and fellowship, and developing educational programs that focus on prevention and early detection, including free newsletters, brochures, videos, public service announcements and CD-roms.

Cancer Research Institute
681 Fifth Avenue
New York, NY 10022-4209
(212) 688-7515
http://www.cancerresearch.org

Since 1953, the nonprofit institute has supported cancer immunology research, which is based on the premise that the body's immune system can be mobilized against cancer. The institute has supported more than 2,750 scientists and clinicians at leading universities and research centers worldwide.

SPERM BANKS

American Association of Tissue Banks (AATB)
1350 Beverly Road
Suite 220-A
McLean, VA 22101
(703) 827-9582
http://www.aatb.org

A scientific, nonprofit organization founded in 1976, the association sets guidelines for sperm banking systems to ensure the safety and availability of high-quality transplantable human tissue. The reproductive tissues most commonly provided by members of the AATB are human sperm and embryos.

SUPPORT GROUPS (GENERAL)

Cancer Care Connection (CCC)
3 Innovation Way
Suite 210
Newark, DE 19711
(302) 266-8050
(866) 266-7008 (toll-free)
http://www.cancercareconnection.org

A nonprofit agency, the CCC provides information, referrals, and compassionate listening to people affected by cancer through a free phone service. Cancer Care Connection also provides referrals to physician locator services and to clinical trial principal investigators. Services are offered in Delaware, southern Pennsylvania, southern New Jersey, and northern Maryland.

The Center for Attitudinal Healing

33 Buchanan Drive
Sausalito, CA 94965
(415) 331-6161
http://www.healingcenter.org

The Center for Attitudinal Healing is an agency that provides nonsectarian spiritual and emotional support.

Comfort Connection

269 East Main Street
Newark, DE 19711
(302) 455-1501

The Comfort Connection is committed to improving overall well-being and making life more peaceful through services aimed at supporting the mind, body, and soul, which include massage therapy, relaxation for stress management (including muscle relaxation, guided imagery, meditation, and problem-solving tactics), counseling, nutrition support, cosmetic services, and volunteer services.

Group Room Radio Talk Show, The

Vital Options TeleSupport Cancer Network
15821 Ventura Boulevard
Suite 645
Encino, CA 91436
(818) 788-5225
(800) GRP-ROOM (toll-free)
http://www.vitaloptions.org

A weekly syndicated call-in cancer talk show, the program links patients, survivors, and health care professionals.

Make Today Count

1235 E. Cherokee
Springfield, MO 65804
(800) 432-2273 (toll-free)

Make Today Count is an organization that draws together people who have life-threatening illnesses for mutual support. Services include cancer counseling and general counseling.

National Association of Hospital Hospitality Houses, Inc.

P.O. Box 18087
Asheville, NC 28814-0087
(828) 253-1188
(800) 542-9730 (toll-free)

A nonprofit corporation, the association serves facilities that provide lodging and other supportive services to patients and their families when confronted with medical emergencies. Services include referrals, housing and lodging facilities and volunteer services.

R. A. Bloch Cancer Foundation

4435 Main Street
Kansas City, MO 64111
(816) 932-8453
(800) 433-0464 (toll-free)
http://www.blochcancer.org

The foundation provides a toll-free hotline that matches newly diagnosed patients with people who have survived the same cancer. It also offers free information lists of multidisciplinary second-opinion centers. Services include Cancer Hotline, provision of home volunteers with similar diagnoses, support groups, educational and special interest presentations, and a list of medical multidisciplinary second opinion boards.

The Wellness Community

35 East 7th Street
Suite 412
Cincinnati, OH 45202
(513) 421-7111
(888) 793-WELL (toll-free)
http://www.wellness-community.org

The Wellness Community provides free psychosocial support to people who are fighting to recover from cancer. There are 20 Wellness Community facilities nationwide. Services include counseling, support groups, networking groups, information, nutritional information, volunteer services, and survivor concerns.

SURVIVORS

National Coalition for Cancer Survivorship
1010 Wayne Avenue
Suite 770
Silver Spring, MD 20910
(301) 650-9127
(877) NCCS-YES (toll-free)
http://www.canceradvocacy.org

The National Coalition for Cancer Survivorship (NCCS) is a survivor-led organization that works on behalf of all cancer survivors. NCCS's mission is to ensure high-quality cancer care for all Americans. Services include referrals, information, and advocacy.

Well Spouse Foundation
P.O. Box 30093
Elkins Park, PA 19027
(800) 838-0879 (toll-free)
http://www.wellspouse.org

A membership organization, the foundation provides emotional support and information to the well spouse or the caregiver of the chronically ill. Services include a newsletter, local support groups, round robin letter writing, an annual weekend conference, and bereavement counseling.

TEENS/YOUNG ADULTS

Planet CANCER
1804 E. 39th Street
Austin, TX 78722
(512) 481-9010
http://www.planetcancer.org

Planet CANCER is an international network of young adults (between ages 18 and 35) who have cancer who support each other in online and face-to-face communities. Services include peer support; Planet Cancer Forum, in which patients communicate directly with each other; advocacy; Adventure Therapy, an outdoor expedition for young adults.

The Ulman Cancer Fund for Young Adults
PMB # 505
4725 Dorsey Hall Drive
Suite A
Ellicott City, MD 21042

(410) 964-0202
(888) 393-FUND (toll-free)
http://www.ulmanfund.org

The Ulman Cancer Fund for Young Adults was founded to provide support programs, education, and resources, free of charge, to benefit young adults affected by cancer and their families and friends and to promote awareness and prevention. Services include support groups, a guidebook (*"No Way, It Can't Be": A Young Adult Faces Cancer*), a nationwide skin protection campaign, and scholarship program.

TESTICULAR CANCER

Klinefelter Syndrome and Associates
P.O. Box 119
Roseville, CA 95678-0119
(916) 773-2999
http://www.genetic.org/ks/

The nonprofit organization distributes a newsletter three times a year and actively participates in research and educational projects related to Klinefelter syndrome and other male sex chromosome variations.

Lance Armstrong Foundation (LAF)
P.O. Box 161150
Austin, TX 78716-1150
(512) 236-8820
http://www.laf.org

A nonprofit group, the foundation was created in 1997 by the champion cyclist and cancer patient Lance Armstrong. The LAF promotes the best physical, psychological, and social recovery and care of cancer survivors and their loved ones, focusing on survivorship education and resources, community programs, national advocacy, and research.

Testicular Cancer Resource Center
http://tcrc.acor.org

A charitable organization, the center is devoted to helping people understand testicular and extragonadal germ cell tumors by providing accurate and timely information about these tumors and their treatment. Services include information for patients, caregivers, family, friends, and physicians.

APPENDIX II
CANCER CENTERS

ALABAMA

University of Alabama at Birmingham Comprehensive Cancer Center*
1824 Sixth Avenue South
Birmingham, AL 35294
(205) 975-8222
(800) 822-0933 or (800) UAB-0933
http://www.ccc.uab.edu/

ARIZONA

Arizona Cancer Center*
The University of Arizona
P.O. Box 245024
1515 North Campbell Avenue
Tucson, AZ 85724
(520) 626-2900 (new patient registration line)
(800) 622-2673 or (800) 622-COPE
http://www.azcc.arizona.edu/

CALIFORNIA

USC/Norris Comprehensive Cancer Center and Hospital*
1441 Eastlake Avenue
Los Angeles, CA 90033
(323) 865-3000
(800) 872-2273 or (800) USC-CARE
E-mail: cainfo@ccnt.hsc.usc.edu (for general information)
http://www.ccnt.hsc.usc.edu/

Jonsson Comprehensive Cancer Center at UCLA*
UCLA Box 951781
8-684 Factor Building
Los Angeles, CA 90095

(310) 825-5268
E-mail: jcccinfo@mednet.ucla.edu
http://www.cancer.mednet.ucla.edu/

City of Hope*
Cancer Center and Beckman Research Institute
1500 East Duarte Road
Duarte, CA 91010
(626) 359-8111
(800) 826-4673 or (800) 826-HOPE
E-mail: becomingapatient@coh.org
http://www.cityofhope.org/

Chao Family Comprehensive Cancer Center*
University of California at Irvine
Building 23
Route 81
101 The City Drive
Orange, CA 92868
(714) 456-8200
http://www.ucihs.uci.edu/cancer/

University of California, San Diego Cancer Center*
9500 Gilman Drive
La Jolla, CA 92093
(858) 534-7600
http://www.cancer.ucsd.edu

University of California, San Francisco Comprehensive Cancer Center*
Box 0128, UCSF
2340 Sutter Street
San Francisco, CA 94143
(415) 476-2201 (general information)
(800) 888-8664 (cancer referral line)
E-mail: cceditor@cc.ucsf.edu
http://www.cc.ucsf.edu/

---

*Comprehensive cancer centers
**Clinical cancer centers

Salk Institute
10010 North Torrey Pines Road
La Jolla, CA 92037
(858) 453-4100 (ext.1386) (Cancer Center)

The Burnham Institute
10010 North Torrey Pines Road
La Jolla, CA 92037
(858) 646-3400 (Cancer Center)

UC Davis Cancer Center**
University of California, Davis
4501 X Street
Suite 3003
Sacramento, CA 95817
(916) 734-5800

COLORADO

University of Colorado Cancer Center*
Box F-704
1665 North Ursula Street
Aurora, CO 80010
(720) 848-0300
(800) 473-2288 (cancer referral line)
http://www.uch.uchsc.edu/uccc/

CONNECTICUT

Yale Cancer Center*
Yale University School of Medicine
P.O. Box 208028
333 Cedar Street
New Haven, CT 06520
(203) 785-4095 (administrative offices)
http://www.info.med.yale.edu/ycc/

DISTRICT OF COLUMBIA

Lombardi Cancer Center*
Georgetown University Medical Center
3800 Reservoir Road, NW
Washington, DC 20007
(202) 784-4000
http://www.lombardi.georgetown.edu/

FLORIDA

**H. Lee Moffitt Cancer Center & Research
  Institute at The University of South Florida***
12902 Magnolia Drive
Tampa, FL 33612
(813) 972-4673 or (813) 972-HOPE
http://www.moffitt.usf.edu/

HAWAII

Cancer Research Center of Hawaii**
1236 Lauhala Street
Honolulu, HI 96813
(808) 586-3010
http://www.hawaii.edu/crch/

ILLINOIS

**The Robert H. Lurie Comprehensive Cancer
  Center***
Northwestern University
Olson Pavilion 8250
710 North Fairbanks Court
Chicago, IL 60611
(312) 908-5250
E-mail: s-markman@northwestern.edu
http://www.lurie.nwu.edu/

**University of Chicago Cancer Research
  Center***
Mail Code 9015
5758 South Maryland Avenue
Chicago, IL 60637
(773) 702-9200
(888) 824-0200 (new patients)
E-mail: aholub@mcis.bsd.uchicago.edu
http://www.-uccrc.uchicago.edu/

INDIANA

Indiana University Cancer Center**
535 Barnhill Drive
Indianapolis, IN 46202
(317) 278-4822
(888) 600-4822
http://www.iucc.iu.edu

Purdue University Cancer Center
Hansen Life Sciences Research Building
South University Street
West Lafayette, IN 47907
(765) 494-9129 (Cancer Center)

IOWA

**The Holden Comprehensive Cancer Center
  at The University of Iowa***
5970-Z JPP
200 Hawkins Drive
Iowa City, IA 52242
(800) 777-8442 (patient referral)
(800) 237-1225 (general information)

E-mail: Cancer-Center@uiowa.edu
http://www.uihealthcare.com/
   DeptsClinicalServices/CancerCenter

MAINE

The Jackson Laboratory
600 Main Street
Bar Harbor, ME 04609
(207) 288-6041 (Cancer Center)

MARYLAND

The Johns Hopkins Oncology Center*
Weinberg Building
401 North Broadway
Baltimore, MD 21231
(410) 502-1033 (information)
http://www.hopkinskimmelcancercenter.org

**The Sidney Kimmel Comprehensive Cancer
   Center***
at Johns Hopkins
Room l57
North Wolfe Street
Baltimore, MD 21287
(410) 955-8822

MASSACHUSETTS

Dana-Farber Cancer Institute*
44 Binney Street
Boston, MA 02115
(617) 632-3000 (ask for patient information)
http://www.dana-farber.org/

Center for Cancer Research
Massachusetts Institute of Technology
Room E17-110
77 Massachusetts Avenue
Cambridge, MA 02139
(617) 253-8511(Cancer Center)

MICHIGAN

**Barbara Ann Karmanos
   Cancer Institute***
Operating the Meyer L. Prentis Comprehensive
   Cancer Center of Metropolitan Detroit
Wertz Clinical Center
4100 John R Street
Detroit, MI 48201
(800) 527-6266
(800) KARMANOS

E-mail: info@karmanos.org
http://www.karmanos.org/

**University of Michigan Comprehensive
   Cancer Center***
1500 East Medical Center Drive
Ann Arbor, MI 48109
(800) 865-1125
E-mail: wwwcancer@umich.edu
http://www.cancer.med.umich.edu/

MINNESOTA

Mayo Clinic Cancer Center*
200 First Street SW
Rochester, MN 55905
(507) 284-2111 (appointment information desk)
http://www.mayo.edu/cancercenter/

University of Minnesota Cancer Center*
Box 806 Mayo
420 Delaware Street SE
Minneapolis, MN 55455
(612) 624-8484
http://www.cancer.umn.edu/

MISSOURI

Siteman Cancer Center**
Barnes-Jewish Hospital and
Washington University School of Medicine
Box 8100
660 South Euclid
St. Louis, MO 63110
(314) 747-7222
(800) 600-3606
E-mail: info@ccadmin.wustl.edu
http://www.siteman.wustl.edu/

NEBRASKA

UNMC Eppley Cancer Center**
University of Nebraska Medical Center
986805 Nebraska Medical Center
Omaha, NE 68198
(402) 559-4238
http://www.unmc.edu/cancercenter/

NEW HAMPSHIRE

Norris Cotton Cancer Center*
Dartmouth-Hitchcock Medical Center
One Medical Center Drive

Lebanon, NH 03756
(603) 650-6300 (administration)
(800) 639-6918 (cancer help line)
E-mail: cancerhelp@dartmouth.edu
http://www.dartmouth.edu/dms/nccc

NEW JERSEY

The Cancer Institute of New Jersey**
Robert Wood Johnson Medical School
195 Little Albany Street
New Brunswick, NJ 08901
(732) 235-2465 or (732) 235-CINJ
http://www.cinj.umdnj.edu

NEW YORK

Memorial Sloan-Kettering Cancer Center*
1275 York Avenue
New York, NY 10021
(800) 525-2225
http://www.mskcc.org/

Roswell Park Cancer Institute*
Elm and Carlton Streets
Buffalo, NY 14263
(800) 767-9355 or (800) ROSWELL
http://www.roswellpark.org/

Kaplan Comprehensive Cancer Center*
New York University School of Medicine
550 First Avenue
New York, NY 10016
(212) 263-6485
http://www.nyucancerinstitute.org/

Herbert Irving Comprehensive Cancer Center*
Columbia Presbyterian Center, New York–Presbyterian Hospital
PH 18, Room 200
622 West 168th Street
New York, NY 10032
(212) 305-9327 (office of administration)
http://www.ccc.columbia.edu/

Albert Einstein Comprehensive Cancer Center*
Albert Einstein College of Medicine
1300 Morris Park Avenue
Bronx, NY 10461
(718) 430-2302

E-mail: aeccc@aecom.yu.edu
http://www.aecom.yu.edu/cancer

NORTH CAROLINA

Duke Comprehensive Cancer Center*
Duke University Medical Center
Box 3843
301 MSRB
Durham, NC 27710
(919) 684-3377
http://www.cancer.duke.edu

UNC Lineberger Comprehensive Cancer Center*
University of North Carolina at Chapel Hill
School of Medicine
Campus Box 7295
Chapel Hill, NC 27599
(919) 966-3036
E-mail: dgs@med.unc.edu
http://www.cancer.med.unc.edu/

Comprehensive Cancer Center of Wake Forest University*
Wake Forest University Baptist
Medical Center
Medical Center Boulevard
Winston-Salem, NC 27157
(336) 716-4464
http://www.bgsm.edu/cancer/

OHIO

The Ohio State University Comprehensive Cancer Center*
The Arthur G. James Cancer Hospital and
Richard J. Solove Research Institute
Suite 519
300 West 10th Avenue
Columbus, OH 43210
(800) 293-5066 (The James Line)
E-mail: cancerinfo@jamesline.com
http://www.jamesline.com

Ireland Cancer Center*
University Hospitals of Cleveland
11100 Euclid Avenue
Cleveland, OH 44106
(216) 844-5432
(800) 641-2422

E-mail: info@irelandcancercenter.org
http://www.irelandcancercenter.org

OREGON

The Oregon Cancer Center**
The Oregon Health Sciences University
CR145
3181 Southwest Sam Jackson Park Road
Portland, OR 97201
(503) 494-1617
http://www.ohsu.edu/oci/

PENNSYLVANIA

Fox Chase Cancer Center*
7701 Burholme Avenue
Philadelphia, PA 19111
(215) 728-2570 (to schedule an appointment)
(888) 369-2427
(888) FOX CHASE
E-mail: info@fccc.edu
http://www.fccc.edu/

University of Pennsylvania Cancer Center*
Penn Tower
3400 Spruce Street
15th Floor
Philadelphia, PA 19104
(215) 662-4000 (main)
(800) 789-7366 or (800) 789-PENN (referral/to
  schedule an appointment)
http://www.oncolink.upenn.edu/

The Wistar Institute
3601 Spruce Street
Philadelphia, PA 19104
(215) 898-3926 (Cancer Center)

University of Pittsburgh Cancer Institute*
Iroquois Building
3600 Forbes Avenue
Suite 206
Pittsburgh, PA 15213
(800) 237-4724 or (800) 237-4PCI
E-mail: PCI-INFO@msx.upmc.edu
http://www.upci.upmc.edu/

Kimmel Cancer Center**
Thomas Jefferson University
Bluemle Life Sciences Building

233 South 10th Street
Philadelphia, PA 19107
(215) 503-4500
(800) 533-3669 or (800) JEFF-NOW (Jefferson
  Cancer Network)
(800) 654-5984 (TDD)
http://www.kcc.tju.edu/

TENNESSEE

St. Jude Children's Research Hospital**
332 North Lauderdale Street
Memphis, TN 38105
(901) 495-3300
http://www.2.stjude.org

The Vanderbilt-Ingram Cancer Center*
Vanderbilt University
649 The Preston Building
Nashville, TN 37232
(615) 936-1782
(615) 936-5847
(800) 811-8480 (clinical trial or treatment option
  information)
(888) 488-4089 (all other calls)
http://www.vicc.org/

TEXAS

The University of Texas M.D. Anderson Cancer Center*
1515 Holcombe Boulevard
Houston, TX 77030
(713) 792-6161
(800) 392-1611
http://www.mdanderson.org/

San Antonio Cancer Institute*
8122 Datapoint Drive
San Antonio, TX 78229
(210) 616-5590
http://www.ccc.saci.org/

UTAH

Huntsman Cancer Institute**
University of Utah
2000 Circle of Hope
Salt Lake City, UT 84112
(801) 585-0303
(877) 585-0303
http://www.hci.utah.edu/

VERMONT

Vermont Cancer Center*
University of Vermont
Medical Alumni Building
Burlington, VT 05401
(802) 656-4414
E-mail: vcc@uvm.edu
http://www.vermontcancer.org

VIRGINIA

Massey Cancer Center**
P.O. Box 980037
Virginia Commonwealth University
401 College Street
Richmond, VA 23298
(804) 828-0450
http://www.vcu.edu/mcc/

The Cancer Center at The University of Virginia**
Box 800334
University of Virginia Health System
Charlottesville, VA 22908
(804) 924-9333
(800) 223-9173
http://www.med.virginia.edu/medcntr/cancer/
home.html

WASHINGTON

Fred Hutchinson Cancer Research Center*
P.O. Box 19024
LA-205
1100 Fairview Avenue North
Seattle, WA 98109
(206) 288-1024
(800) 804-8824 (appointments and medical
referral—Seattle Cancer Care Alliance)
E-mail: hutchdoc@seattlecca.org (patient information)
http://www.fhcrc.org/

WISCONSIN

University of Wisconsin Comprehensive Cancer Center*
600 Highland Avenue, K5/601
Madison, WI 53792
(608) 263-8600
(608) 262-5223 (Cancer Connect)
(800) 622-8922 (Cancer Connect)
E-mail: uwccc@uwcc.wisc.edu/
http://www.cancer.wisc.edu

APPENDIX III
DRUGS USED TO TREAT MEN'S REPRODUCTIVE CANCER

acridine carboxamide A substance in the family of drugs called topoisomerase inhibitors that is being studied as a potential chemotherapy agent.

actinomycin D See DACTINOMYCIN.

Actiq See FENTANYL CITRATE.

Adriamycin See DOXORUBICIN.

Adrucil See 5-FU.

AE-941 A substance made from shark cartilage being studied for its ability to prevent the growth of new blood vessels to solid tumors. It belongs to the family of drugs called angiogenesis inhibitors.

aldesleukin See INTERLEUKIN-2.

alemtuzumab (Campath 1H) A monoclonal antibody used to treat cancer. Monoclonal antibodies are laboratory-made substances designed to find cancer cells and bind to them.

alendronate sodium A drug that affects bone metabolism that is being studied as a possible treatment for bone pain caused by cancer. Alendronate sodium belongs to the family of drugs called bisphosphonates.

allopurinol sodium (Zyloprim) An orally administered drug used before chemotherapy to reduce some toxic side effects.

ALVAC-CEA vaccine A cancer vaccine that contains a canary pox virus (ALVAC) combined with the human carcinoembryonic antigen (*CEA*) gene.

amethopterin See METHOTREXATE.

amifostine (Ethyol) A drug used to control some of the side effects of chemotherapy (especially platinum therapy) and radiation therapy. It works by neutralizing the platinum in noncancerous tissue and protects kidneys from platinum damage. It also seems to protect the nervous system and possibly the bone marrow. Side effects include nausea, vomiting, and low blood pressure; less common side effects include chills, sneezing, sleepiness, and facial flushing. Very rarely, a drop in calcium level in the blood may occur.

aminoglutethimide (Cytadren, Elipten) An oral chemotherapy agent in the family of drugs called nonsteroidal aromatase inhibitors used to treat prostate cancer as well as breast and adrenal cancers. Aminoglutethimide is used to decrease the production of sex hormones (estrogen or testosterone) and suppress the growth of tumors that need sex hormones for growth. Because of its function, it may also be called a "medical adrenalectomy." Since this medication blocks vital steroid hormones, patients must also take corticosteroid replacement therapy (usually hydrocortisone) with this drug.

Common side effects include skin rash, low-grade fever, and malaise. Less common side effects include drowsiness and lethargy, blurred vision, mild nausea and vomiting, dizziness when standing quickly, and mild appetite loss. Rarely, this drug may cause rhythmic eye movements, lowering of blood pressure, and uncoordinated gait.

androgens (Testex, Halotestin, Teslac) Androgens include testosterone propionate, obfluoxymesterone, and obtestolactone, which belong to the general group of hormone drugs. Androgens seem to change the hormonal levels within cells, removing the stimulus to divide and thereby interfering with the division of cancer cells. Side effects include fluid retention; less commonly, androgens may cause nausea or an increase in blood calcium level. Rarely, it may cause painful erections.

Anzemet See DOLASETRON.

Apo-Prednisone See PREDNISONE.

arginine butyrate A substance that is being studied as a treatment for cancer.

asparaginase (Elspar) An enzyme used in the treatment of cancer that belongs to the family of drugs called antineoplastics, which interfere with the growth of cancer cells. Side effects include mild nausea and vomiting, appetite loss, fatigue or drowsiness, depression, allergic reactions, and altered liver function test results. Less common side effects include mild anemia and increase in the blood sugar level. Rarely, the drug may lower white blood or platelet count, causing a risk of bleeding or infection.

bacille Calmette-Guérin (BCG) A type of bacteria used in cancer treatment to stimulate the immune system.

BEP A common combination of chemotherapeutic drugs (bleomycin, etoposide, and Platinol [cisplatin]) used to treat germ cell tumors.

bevacizumab A monoclonal antibody that may prevent the growth of blood vessels from surrounding tissue to a solid tumor.

Biafine cream A topical preparation used to reduce the risk of, and treat skin reactions to, radiation therapy.

bicalutamide (Casodex) An oral antiandrogen used as a type of chemotherapy drug in combination with luteinizing hormone–releasing hormone (LHRH) analog to treat advanced prostate cancer. This drug works by stopping the growth of cancer cells that depend on male hormones.

More common side effects include swelling or tenderness of breasts; less common side effects include hot flashes and constipation. Rarely, nausea and diarrhea or headache may occur.

Blenoxane See BLEOMYCIN.

bleomycin (Blenoxane) A commonly used injectable chemotherapy drug in the family of drugs called antitumor antibiotics derived from *Streptomyces verticillus*. It is used to treat penile and testicular cancer, as well as cancers of the head and neck, vulva, cervix, skin, kidney, lung, and esophagus, and lymphomas, soft tissue sarcomas, Kaposi's sarcoma, and melanoma. Bleomycin interferes with cell division, thereby killing the cell. It is given as an intravenous infusion over 20 to 30 minutes or as a continuous infusion. It also can be administered as an injection.

Side effects include fever and chills, appetite loss and nausea, hair loss, mouth sores, and skin changes. Less commonly, there may be pain at the injection or tumor site and irritation of lungs or in the vein where the drug was given. Rarely, it may cause an allergic reaction or lung fibrosis.

broxuridine A drug that makes cancer cells more sensitive to radiation and is also used as a diagnostic agent to determine how fast cancer cells grow.

buserelin An anticancer drug that belongs to the family of drugs called gonadotropin-releasing hormones. In prostate cancer therapy, buserelin blocks the production of testosterone in the testicles.

Campath 1H See ALEMTUZUMAB.

Camptosar See IRINOTECAN.

camptothecin-11 See IRINOTECAN.

CAP A combination of the chemotherapy drugs cisplatin, Adriamycin (doxorubicin), and Cytoxan (Cyclophosphamide) sometimes used to treat prostate cancer as well as non–small cell lung cancer and cancers of the kidney and bladder.

carbogen An inhalant of oxygen and carbon dioxide that increases the sensitivity of tumor cells to the effects of radiation therapy.

carboplatin (Paraplatin) A platinum-based anticancer drug similar to cisplatin but somewhat less toxic; however, it is not as effective as cisplatin in treatment of testicular cancer. This intravenous drug belongs to the family of drugs called alkylating agents, which disrupt cancer cell growth, destroying the malignant cells.

Common side effects include decreased platelet and white blood cell counts (causing risk of bleeding and infection), brittle hair, altered kidney function at high dosages, and fetal abnormalities. Less common side effects include nausea and vomiting, appetite loss, diarrhea or constipation, taste changes, or pins and needles sensations. Rarely, it may cause confusion, visual changes, rash, tinnitus, severe allergic reaction, or dizziness.

carboxypeptidase G2 A bacterial enzyme used to neutralize the toxic effects of the chemotherapy drug methotrexate.

Casodex See BICALUTAMIDE.

celecoxib A nonsteroidal anti-inflammatory drug that reduces pain; it is currently being studied as a possible cancer prevention treatment.

CF A combination of chemotherapy drugs that includes cisplatin and fluorouracil (5-FU) that may be used to treat gestational trophoblastic tumor.

CFL A combination of the chemotherapy drugs cisplatin, fluorouracil (5-FU), and leucovorin calcium that is sometimes used to treat gestational trophoblastic tumor.

chlorambucil (Leukeran) A chemotherapy agent in the family of drugs called alkylating agents that is sometimes used to treat testicular cancer as well as cancers of the breast and ovary. Chlorambucil disrupts the growth of cancer cells, destroying them.

Common side effects include decreased platelet and white blood cell counts (increasing the risk of bleeding or infection). Less common effects include appetite and weight loss; rarely, it may cause nausea and vomiting, liver damage, confusion or seizures, and visual problems.

CISCA A combination of the chemotherapy drugs cisplatin, Cytoxan (Cyclophosphamide), and Adriamycin (Doxouracil) sometimes used to treat prostate cancer.

***cis*-diamminedichloroplatinum** See CISPLATIN.

cisplatin (Platinol) A very commonly used intravenous chemotherapy agent that belongs to the family of drugs called platinum compounds and is sometimes used to treat testicular, penile, or prostate cancer, as well as cancers of the head and neck, bladder, ovary, breast, lung, esophagus, and cervix. Cisplatin disrupts the growth of cancer cells, destroying them.

More common side effects include nausea and vomiting, taste changes, pins and needles sensations, and kidney damage. Less common side effects include fatigue, appetite loss, hair thinning, diarrhea, and decreased platelet and white blood counts (causing risk of bleeding or infection). Rarely, cisplatin may cause chest pain and heart attack, severe allergic reaction, hearing loss, or walking problems.

clodronate A drug used as treatment for abnormally high levels of calcium in the blood (hypercalcemia) and for cancer that has spread to the bone (bone metastasis). It may decrease pain, the risk of fractures, and the development of new bone metastases.

combretastatin A4 phosphate   A chemotherapy drug that reduces the blood supply to tumors.

Compazine   See PROCHLORPERAZINE.

Cosmegen   See DACTINOMYCIN.

COX-2 inhibitors   The abbreviated term for *cyclooxygenase-2 inhibitors,* a family of nonsteroidal anti-inflammatory drugs used to relieve pain and inflammation. COX-2 inhibitors are being studied as chemotherapy drugs.

CVEB   A combination of the chemotherapy drugs cisplatin, vinblastine, etoposide, and bleomycin sometimes used to treat prostate cancer.

cyclobutane dicarboxylate platinum   See CARBO-PLATIN.

cyclooxygenase-2 inhibitors   See COX-2 INHIBITORS.

cyclophosphamide (Cytoxan)   One of the most commonly used chemotherapy drugs, sometimes used to treat testicular cancer, among other types. Administered intravenously or orally, it belongs to the family of alkylating agents, which disrupt the growth of cancer cells, killing them.

Common side effects include hair loss, nausea and vomiting, appetite loss, mouth sores, diarrhea, and decreased white blood cell count, causing an increased risk of infection. Less common side effects include a drop in platelet count (increasing risk of bleeding), blood in urine, acne, fatigue, and fetal changes. Rarely, cyclophosphamide may cause heart changes at high dosages or lung fibrosis; it very rarely can induce certain types of cancer.

cyclosporine   A drug used to help reduce the risk of rejection of organ and bone marrow transplants by the body that is also used in clinical trials to make cancer cells more sensitive to chemotherapy drugs.

cyproterone acetate   A synthetic hormone being studied for treatment of hot flashes in men who have prostate cancer who have had both testicles removed by surgery.

Cytadren   See AMINOGLUTETHIMIDE.

Cytovene   See GALLIUM NITRATE.

Cytoxan   See CYCLOPHOSPHAMIDE.

DACT   See DACTINOMYCIN.

dactinomycin (actinomycin D [Cosmegen])   An intravenous antibiotic chemotherapy drug sometimes used to treat testicular cancer, among other types of cancer. It disrupts the growth of cancer cells, killing them.

More common side effects include decreased platelets and white blood cell counts (causing increased risk of bleeding or infection), hair loss, nausea and vomiting, appetite loss, mouth sores, diarrhea, rash, and radiation recall. Less common side effects include fatigue, fever, depression, muscle or bone aches, and fetal changes. Rarely, there may be liver or kidney damage, or second malignancies that occur later.

DDP   Diamminedichloroplatinum.   See CISPLATIN.

Decadron (dexamethasone [Hexadrol])   See DEXAMETHASONE.

Demerol   See MEPERIDINE.

2'-deoxycytidine   A drug that protects healthy tissues from the toxic effects of anticancer drugs.

Deltasone   See PREDNISONE.

DES   See DIETHYLSTILBESTROL.

dexamethasone (Decadron)   An antinausea drug and synthetic adrenocorticoid prescribed to ease nausea and vomiting in chemotherapy patients. Because it can irritate the stomach in pill form, it must be taken with food.

More common side effects include weight gain, sodium or fluid retention, depression, increased blood sugar level and appetite, sleep problems, increased risk of infection, bruising, mood changes, or delayed wound healing. Less common side effects include thirst, increased urination, fungal infections, bone fractures, sweating, diarrhea, nausea, headache, increased heart rate, or calcium loss. Rarely, dexamethasone may cause cataracts, personality changes, blurry vision, or stomach ulcer.

dexrazoxane (Zinecard)   A drug used to protect the heart from the toxic effects of anthracycline drugs. It is one of the family of drugs called chemoprotective agents. Side effects may include decreases in white blood cell and platelet counts; less commonly, there may be pain at the injection site or changes in kidney or liver blood test results.

diethylstilbestrol (DES, stilbestrol [Stilphostrol])   An estrogen used to treat advanced prostate cancer, it stops the growth of cancer cells that depend on male hormones to grow and divide. Side effects include breast swelling or tenderness, voice changes, and decreased sexual desire. Less common side effects include temporary nausea and vomiting, uterine bleeding, or loss of bladder control. Rarely, DES may cause blood clots in legs or lungs or an increased calcium level.

Dilaudid   See HYDROMORPHONE.

dipyridamole   A drug that prevents blood cell clumping and enhances the effectiveness of fluorouracil and other chemotherapeutic agents.

DMC   A combination of the chemotherapy drugs dactinomycin (Cosmegen), methotrexate, and Cytoxan (Cyclophosphamide) sometimes used to treat gestational trophoblastic tumor.

dolasetron (Anzemet)   An antiemetic drug that prevents or reduces nausea and vomiting that typically occur during chemotherapy. It can be given intravenously or orally and works by blocking the serotonin pathway through which chemotherapy stimulates the vomiting center in the brain.

Occasionally this drug may cause a headache; rarely, it may cause fever, fatigue, bone pain, muscle aches, constipation, heartburn, appetite loss, pancreatic inflammation, electrical changes in the heart, flushing, abnormal dreams, sleep problems, confusion and anxiety, anaphylaxis, or itching.

doxercalciferol   A substance being studied as a possible preventive treatment for recurrent prostate cancer. It belongs to the family of drugs called vitamin D analogs.

docetaxel (Taxotere)   A type of taxane that when used alone or together with estramustine is helpful in the treatment of prostate cancer. Docetaxel works by disrupting the growth of cancer cells. Side effects include nausea and vomiting, rash, appetite loss, diarrhea, hair thinning or loss, and decreased platelet and white cell counts. Steroids are usually given at the time of its administration to minimize side effects.

dolasetron (Anzemet)   An antiemetic drug that prevents or reduces nausea and vomiting that typically occur during chemotherapy.

doxorubicin (Adriamycin)   An anthracycline antibiotic used in combination with other drugs to treat prostate cancer. Doxorubicin disrupts the growth of cancer cells, destroying them. Side effects include loss of appetite, nausea and vomiting, hair loss, and decreased white blood cell and platelet counts. Less common side effects include mouth or lip sores, radiation recall, and irregular heartbeat. Rarely, it may cause heart damage, leading to congestive heart failure.

dronabinol (Marinol)   A synthetic pill form of delta-9-tetrahydrocannabinol (THC), an active ingredient in marijuana that is used to treat nausea and vomiting associated with cancer chemotherapy. For some patients this member of the cannabinoid class prevents nausea and vomiting when other antinausea drugs are ineffective. It can also be used to boost appetite through a mechanism that is not fully understood. Side effects include disorientation, drowsiness, muddled thinking, mood changes, dry mouth, decreased coordination, and change in the ability to perceive surroundings. Less common side effects include increased heart rate and decreased blood pressure.

edrecolomab   A type of monoclonal antibody (a laboratory-produced substance that can locate and bind to cancer cells) used in cancer therapy.

Efudex   See 5-FU.

eniluracil (5-ethynyluracil)   A chemotherapy drug that increases the effectiveness of fluorouracil.

Epogen   See EPOETIN ALFA.

Eprex   See EPOGEN.

erythropoietin (EPO epoetin alfa, [Epogen, Procrit, Eprex])   A colony-stimulating factor that stimulates the production of red blood cells and is sometimes used to treat certain chemotherapy patients. This injected drug is made by recombinant DNA technology; it is similar to hormones the body makes in the bone marrow to produce blood cells. Less common side effects include fever, fatigue, headache, and hives.

Estracyte   See ESTRAMUSTINE.

estramustine (Estracyt, Estracyte, Emcyt)   A combination of the hormone estradiol (an estrogen) and nitrogen mustard (an anticancer drug) used in the palliative therapy of prostate cancer. This oral drug is an alkylating chemotherapy agent, which affects cells with estrogen receptors, killing them.

More common side effects include itchy, dry skin; night sweats; and breast enlargement and nipple tenderness. Less common side effects include nausea and vomiting, itching and pain in the perineal area, rash and peeling fingertip skin, oral numbness, thinning hair, and pain in the eyes. Rarely it may cause blood clots in legs, lungs, heart, or brain.

etanidazole (Nitrolmidazole)   A radiosensitizing drug that increases the effectiveness of radiation therapy. Cancer cells are injured more extensively by radiation when they have adequate oxygen; this drug mimics oxygen, increasing the damaging effect of radiation. It also makes cell self-repair more difficult.

More common side effects include decreased sensations in hands and feet or pins and needles feelings. Less common side effects include nausea and vomiting; rarely, it may cause a rash or muscle aches.

5-ethynyluracil (eniluracil)   An anticancer drug that increases the effectiveness of fluorouracil.

etidronate (Didronel)   An oral and intravenous drug in the family of drugs called bisphosphonates that is used as treatment for cancer that has spread to the bone. Given intravenously, it prevents bone from breaking down. Etidronate should not be given with milk, which interferes with its absorption. Rarely, it may cause diarrhea, nausea and vomiting, abdominal pain, or rash.

Ethyol   See AMIFOSTINE.

etoposide (Toposar, Etopophos, VePesid)   An important chemotherapy drug derived from podophyllotoxin that belongs to the family of drugs called mitotic inhibitors and is sometimes used to treat testicular cancer, among other types. It can be given either intravenously or orally.

More common side effects include decreased platelet and white blood cell counts (causing increased risk of bleeding and infection), mild nausea and vomiting, appetite loss, taste changes, and hair loss. Less common side effects include constipation or diarrhea, stomach pain, and radiation recall. Rarely, etoposide may cause a drop in blood pressure, breathing problems during infusion, rash or itching, heart changes, numbness, fever and chills, or allergic reactions.

Eulexin   See FLUTAMIDE.

fentanyl citrate   A narcotic pain medication in the form of a raspberry-flavored lollipop, prescribed for cancer patients whose extreme pain is not controlled by oral narcotics. Pain relief occurs while the patient sucks on (but does not chew) the lollipop and for several hours afterward. The patient should remove the lollipop if the pain is relieved or if a side effect occurs.

To discard unused portions of this lollipop, wrap it in toilet tissue with the stick removed and flush it down the toilet; it can severely harm children who mistake it for candy. This drug binds to opioid receptors in the brain and central nervous system, altering the perception of pain as well as the emotional response. Relief begins within about five minutes.

Patients must already be taking opioid drugs in order to use this drug, because it is very strong and can be dangerous if other opioid pain relievers have not been taken for at least a week. This short-acting drug is intended to give relief between doses of long-acting opioid pain relievers. The smallest effective dose should be used to prevent dependence or tolerance.

More common side effects include sleepiness, dizziness, headache, fever, fatigue, and constipation. Less common side effects include breathing problems, cough, sore throat, walking problems, anxiety and confusion, depression, sleeping problems, muscle aches, itching, rash, sweating, nausea and vomiting, appetite loss, or heartburn. Rarely, fentanyl citrate may cause bowel rupture as a result of severe constipation, or vision changes.

filgrastim (granulocyte colony-stimulating factor [Neupogen]) A protein cytokine that belongs to the synthetic drug class of biologic response modifiers, produced by recombinant (DNA) techniques. It is used to boost neutrophil (white blood cell) count after chemotherapy. Filgrastim is very similar to a substance made by the body's own immune system, which stimulates bone marrow to produce neutrophils dedicated to fighting infection. This drug may cause bone pain.

finasteride (Proscar) An oral drug used to treat benign prostatic hyperplasia (BPH); it is also being studied as a possible chemotherapy agent for prostate cancer.

FL A combination of the chemotherapy drugs flutamide and leuprolide (Lupron) sometimes used to treat prostate cancer.

flecainide A drug used to treat abnormal heart rhythms that also may relieve nerve pain—the burning, stabbing, or stinging pain that may arise from damage to nerves caused by some types of cancer or cancer treatment.

Fluoroplex See 5-FU.

fluorouracil See 5-FU.

5-Fluracil See 5-FU.

flusol DA (20%) An investigational drug being studied as a possible radiosensitizer, used to boost the effectiveness of radiation therapy. Radiation can injure cancer cells more quickly if the cells have plenty of oxygen; flusol mimics oxygen, which makes cancer cells more vulnerable to radiation and slower to repair themselves when damaged. This is an investigational drug not yet approved by the U.S. Food and Drug Administration (FDA) for the treatment of cancer. Side effects may include facial flushing, chest pressure, chills, and fever that occur immediately after administration of the first dose.

flutamide (FLUT, Eulexin) An anticancer hormone drug in the family of drugs called antiandrogens that is sometimes used to treat advanced prostate cancer. It works by blocking the effects of male hormones on cancer cells, stopping their growth. It is sometimes combined with leuprolide (Lupron) for prostate cancer patients.

More common side effects include hot flashes and sweating. Less common side effects include decreased sexual interest and ability, breast swelling, and nausea and diarrhea.

5-FU (5-fluorouracil, fluorouracil [Adrucil]) A standard intravenous (IV) chemotherapy agent in the family of drugs called antimetabolites that is sometimes used to treat prostate cancer as well as cancers of the colon, breast, ovary, stomach, liver, and pancreas. This drug may also be administered by infusion over days or months; it prevents cells from making deoxyribonucleic acid (DNA) and ribonucleic acid (RNA) by interfering with the synthesis of nucleic acids, disrupting the growth of cancer cells. This is a very commonly used drug, often in combination with other chemotherapy agents.

More common side effects include decreased platelet and white blood cell counts (causing increased risk of bleeding and infection), nausea and vomiting, mouth sores, thinning hair, diarrhea, and increased sensitivity to sunlight. Less common side effects include appetite loss, headache, weakness, and muscle aches. Rarely, 5-FU may cause walking problems, eye irritation, and blurred vision.

Folex   See METHOTREXATE.

gallium nitrate (Ganite, Cytovene)   A drug that lowers blood calcium level, it is used as treatment for cancer that has spread to the bone, blocking bone breakdown. It is given intravenously as a 24-hour infusion.

Less common side effects include diarrhea, nausea, or constipation. Rarely, gallium nitrate may cause kidney damage or vomiting.

Ganite   See GALLIUM NITRATE.

gemtuzumab ozogamicin   A type of monoclonal antibody used in cancer detection and therapy. Monoclonal antibodies are laboratory-produced substances that can locate and bind to cancer cells.

genistein   An isoflavone found in soy products. Soy isoflavones are being studied to determine whether they help prevent cancer.

goserelin acetate (Zoladex)   A drug that blocks the production of male hormones that is used to treat advanced prostate cancer. It is administered monthly as a pellet injected under the skin of the abdomen, where it slowly releases the drug. Goserelin is a synthetic version of the body's lutenizing hormone–releasing hormone (LHRH), which blocks the release of testosterone. Cancers that are dependent on male hormones for growth are thus no longer stimulated.

More common side effects include drop in sexual desire and ability, hot flashes, and breast swelling. A less common side effect is breast tenderness. Rarely,

the drug may cause chills and fever, anxiety, constipation or diarrhea, weight gain, irregular heartbeat or high blood pressure, depression, chest pain, increased blood sugar level, urinary tract infection, kidney damage, headache, stroke, or heart attack.

G-CSF (granulocyte colony-stimulating factor, filgrastim [Neupogen])   Substance that stimulates the growth of a type of white blood cell (granulocyte) and serves as a growth factor for peripheral blood stem cells. Side effects may include flulike symptoms and bone pain; less common side effects include facial flushing, rash, or redness at site of injection. Rarely, G-CSF may cause breathing problems, weight gain, and foot swelling.

granisetron (Kytril)   An antinausea drug given intravenously or orally to chemotherapy patients to prevent or control nausea and vomiting. It belongs to a general class of drugs called serotonin antagonists and acts by blocking two pathways of serotonin to prevent nausea and vomiting. It binds to the serotonin receptors in the lining of the stomach, preventing the stimulation of the vomiting center in the brain.

Less common side effects include headache, constipation, or diarrhea. Rarely, it may cause fatigue.

halofuginone hydrobromide   A substance that is being studied for its ability to slow the growth of connective tissue and prevent the growth of new blood vessels to a solid tumor. It belongs to the family of drugs called quinazolinone alkaloids.

Halotestin   See ANDROGENS.

hematoporphyrin derivative   A drug used in photodynamic therapy that is absorbed by tumor cells. When exposed to light, it becomes active and kills the cancer cells.

Hexadrol   See DEXAMETHASONE.

hydrazine sulfate   A substance that has been studied as a treatment for cancer and as a treatment for cachexia (body wasting) associated with advanced stages of cancer.

hydromorphone (Dilaudid) A prescription narcotic painkiller that is stronger than heroin and is effective longer, for up to six hours. It can be given to cancer patients in severe pain as either an oral medication, a rectal suppository, or an intramuscular injection. It binds to opioid receptors in the brain, altering the perception of pain as well as the emotional response to it.

More common side effects include constipation, drowsiness, sedation, dizziness, nausea, or dry mouth. Less common side effects include mood changes, euphoria, mental clouding, decreased breathing rate, vomiting, delayed digestion, and decreased heart rate and blood pressure. Rarely, hydromorphone may cause seizures, urination problems, decreased sexual interest, and bowel rupture due to constipation.

Ifex See IFOSFAMIDE.

ifosfamide (Ifex) An anticancer drug related to the nitrogen mustards. It is active in a number of cancers, including germ cell cancers. Because this drug is very irritating to the bladder, it is combined with mesna to protect the bladder (sometimes called "mesna rescue"). It works by disrupting the growth of cancer cells, killing them.

More common side effects include nausea and vomiting, hair loss, bladder irritation, and kidney function problems. Less common side effects include decreased white blood cell count (causing increased risk of infection) and pain at the injection site. Rarely, ifosfamide may cause decreased platelet count (causing increased risk of bleeding), fatigue, confusion, or dizziness.

imiquimod A substance that improves the body's natural response to infection and disease that is being studied as a topical agent to prevent some types of cancer. It belongs to the family of drugs called biological response modifiers.

Indocin See INDOMETHACIN.

indomethacin (Indocin, Indocin SR, Indotech) A drug that belongs to the family of drugs called nonsteroidal anti-inflammatory drugs (NSAIDs), used to reduce tumor-induced suppression of the immune system and to increase the effectiveness of anticancer drugs. Indomethacin blocks the synthesis of prostaglandins, thereby preventing pain receptors from sending pain messages to the brain. This drug also reduces inflammation and fever. Side effects include headache, vomiting, tinnitus, tremor, and sleep problems. Less common side effects include dizziness, depression, fatigue, nausea, appetite loss, heartburn, and gastrointestinal bleeding.

Indotech See INDOMETHACIN.

interleukin-3 (IL-3) A type of biological response modifier (a substance that can improve the body's natural response to disease) that enhances the immune system's ability to fight tumor cells. These substances are normally produced by the body; they are also made in the laboratory for use in treating cancer and other diseases. Side effects include fever, headache, stiff neck, and facial flushing. Less common effects may include mild bone pain or foot swelling. Rarely, there may be a drop in blood pressure or a rash or bruises on skin.

interleukin-4 (IL-4) A type of biological response modifier (a substance that can improve the body's natural response to disease) that enhances the immune system's ability to fight tumor cells. These substances are normally produced by the body and are also made in the laboratory for use in treating cancer and other diseases.

interleukin-6 (IL-6) A type of biological response modifier (a substance that can improve the body's natural response to infection and disease). These substances are normally produced by the body, and can also be made in the laboratory. Side effects may include fever and chills, headache, and decreased red blood cell count with increased risk of anemia. Less commonly, there may be appetite loss or joint aches.

interleukin-11 (IL-11) A type of biological response modifier (a substance that can improve the body's natural response to disease) that stimulates immune response and may reduce toxicity to the gastrointestinal system that results from cancer therapy. These substances are normally produced by the body; they are also made in the laboratory for use in treating cancer. IL-11 is also called oprelvekin.

interleukin-12 (IL-12) A type of biological response modifier (a substance that can improve the body's natural response to disease) that enhances the ability of the immune system to kill tumor cells and may interfere with blood flow to the tumor. These substances are normally produced by the body and are made in the laboratory for use in treating cancer.

irinotecan (CPT-11, camptothecin-11 [Camptosar]) A topoisomerase inhibitor used to treat several types of cancer, including prostate cancer, by disrupting the growth of cancer cells. Side effects include nausea and vomiting, sweating, diarrhea, fatigue, anemia, and decreased white blood cell count.

Isophosphamide See IFOSFAMIDE.

ketoconazole (Nizoral) An antifungal drug used as a treatment for prostate cancer because it can block the production of male sex hormones. More common side effects include nausea; less common side effects include diarrhea and vomiting. Rarely, ketoconazole may cause stomach pain, rash or hives, constipation, breast enlargement, dizziness, nervousness, sleeping problems, fever, decreased sexual ability, headache, and increased sensitivity to sunlight.

Kytril See GRANISETRON.

Leukeran See CHLORAMBUCIL.

Leup See LEUPROLIDE.

leuprolide (Lupron) A chemotherapy drug that blocks the production of male hormones by the testicles. Leuprolide is a luteinizing hormone–releasing hormone (LHRH) that tells the brain to stop producing its own LHRH; subsequently, the testicles stop producing testosterone. Leuprolide reduces testosterone levels in about five to eight days. At first, when a man takes leuprolide there is an increase in luteinizing hormone and testosterone levels; this increase may affect men who have cancer that has spread to the bone by worsening bone pain temporarily. This response is called a flare reaction; medication can prevent the problem.

When leuprolide is combined with flutamide or bicalutamide (Casodex), it may be used instead of surgical removal of the testicles in the treatment of prostate cancer. However, the drug treatment is expensive and requires more visits to the doctor. Leuprolide can either be given daily as a self-administered injection under the skin or monthly as a long-acting pellet injected under the skin.

These drugs do have side effects, including hot flashes, erectile dysfunction, anemia, and osteoporosis. Erectile dysfunction occurs in about 80 percent of men who use leuprolide, together with decreased interest in sex. It also may cause weight gain and fatigue. Rarely, leuprolide may cause nausea and vomiting, loss of appetite, and swelling of hands, feet and breasts.

Levo-Dromoran See LEVORPHANOL.

levorphanol (Levo-Dromoran) A narcotic injectible and oral drug that is similar to morphine and used to control pain, binding to receptors in the brain to mute the perception of pain.

More common side effects include constipation, drowsiness, sedation, nausea, and dry mouth. Less common side effects include mood changes, euphoria, depression, mental clouding, slowed breathing, vomiting, low blood pressure, and lowered heart rate. Rarely, levorphanol may cause urination problems, facial flushing, itching, sweating, decreased sexual interest, and bowel rupture due to constipation.

LHRH agonist leuprolide Luteinizing hormone–releasing hormone.
See also LEUPROLIDE.

Lupron See LEUPROLIDE.

L-VAM A combination of the anticancer drugs Lupron (leuprolide), vinblastine, Adriamycin (doxorubicin), and mutamycin sometimes used to treat prostate cancer as well as cancers of the kidney and bladder.

Marinol   See DRONABINOL.

meperidine (Demerol)   A strong narcotic used to treat pain for a short period (between two and three hours). For this reason, it is not given for chronic pain, but for occasional episodes of pain after surgery.

More common side effects include constipation, sedation, nausea and vomiting, dizziness, and dry mouth. Less common side effects include mood changes, including euphoria or mental clouding and decreased breathing rate, blood pressure, and heart rate. Rarely, meperidine may cause urination problems, seizures, and lack of sexual interest. Patients should drink fluids every hour to prevent constipation.

mesna (Mesnex)   A drug that belongs to a class of medications known as cytoprotective agents, used in combination with other drugs to treat testicular cancer. Occasionally, mesna may cause nausea, vomiting or diarrhea.

Mesnex   See MESNA.

methotrexate (amethopterin [Mexate, Folex])   An important antimetabolite chemotherapy drug sometimes used to treat testicular cancer as well as cancers of the breast, cervix, head and neck, colon, and lung, and acute leukemia sarcoma, lymphoma, and mycosis fungoides. This drug can either be given intravenously or orally. It prevents cells from making DNA and RNA by interfering with the synthesis of nucleic acids, disrupting the growth of cancer cells.

More common side effects include nausea and vomiting at high dosages, mouth sores, diarrhea, increased sunburn risk, radiation recall, and appetite loss. Less common side effects include decreased platelet and white blood cell counts (causing increased risk of bleeding and infection), and kidney damage at high dosages. Rarely, methotrexate may cause liver toxicity, lung collapse at high dosages, hair loss, rash or itching, dizziness, and blurred vision. Drinking alcohol while taking this drug can increase the risk of liver damage.

2-methoxyestradiol   An angiogenesis inhibitor drug derived from estrogen that prevents the formation of new blood vessels that tumors need in order to grow.

metoclopramide (Reglan)   An antinausea drug that may be given to chemotherapy patients before treatment to prevent nausea and vomiting, either intravenously or orally. In low dosages, it increases stomach emptying to reduce the chance of nausea and vomiting caused by food in the stomach. At high dosages it blocks the messages to the part of the brain responsible for nausea and vomiting.

More common side effects include sedation, sleepiness, diarrhea, or dry mouth. Rarely, it may cause rash, hives, or a drop in blood pressure. Metoclopramide may cause extrapyramidal side effects, which include restlessness, tongue protrusion, and involuntary movements, which stop when the patient is given diphenhydramine.

Mexate   See METHOTREXATE.

mifepristone (RU486)   A French abortion drug that is currently being studied as a possible chemotherapy drug to treat prostate cancer as well as metastatic breast cancer, ovarian cancer, and some brain tumors.

MITH   See MITHRAMYCIN.

Mithracin   See MITHRAMYCIN.

mithramycin (MITH [Mithracin])   A chemotherapy drug sometimes used to treat testicular cancer and Paget's disease of the bone. It is also given as a means of lowering calcium level of patients who have hypercalcemia, which occurs in a number of cancers. More common side effects include nausea and vomiting, hair loss, appetite loss, mouth sores, and decreased platelet and white blood cell counts (causing increased risk of bleeding and infection).

mitoxantrone (DHAD [Novantrone])   An important antibiotic intravenous chemotherapy drug sometimes used to treat prostate cancer as well as leukemia, lymphoma, and breast cancer. It is also used in combination with steroids to ease symptoms of patients who have advanced prostate cancer. This drug was developed as an alternative to doxorubicin (Adriamycin), because it has a milder side effect profile. It disrupts the growth of cancer cells, killing them.

More common side effects include mild nausea and vomiting and a decreased white blood count. Less common side effects include hair loss; rarely, it may cause an allergic reaction, mouth sores, decreased platelet count, or heart damage with congestive heart failure.

monoclonal antibodies (MOABs)   Certain antibodies made in the laboratory that are produced by a single type of cell and are specific for a particular antigen. Researchers are examining ways to create MOABs specific to the antigens found on the surface of the cancer cell being treated. MOABs are made by injecting human cancer cells into mice so that the mouse immune system makes antibodies against these cancer cells. The mouse cells producing the antibodies are then removed and fused with laboratory-grown cells to create "hybrid" cells called hybridomas. Hybridomas can indefinitely produce large quantities of these pure antibodies, or MOABs.

MOABs may be used in cancer treatment in a number of ways: They may react with specific types of cancer to enhance a patient's immune response to the cancer, or they may be programmed to act against cell growth factors, thus interfering with the growth of cancer cells. MOABs may be linked to anticancer drugs, radioactive substances, or other toxins. When the antibodies latch onto cancer cells, they deliver these poisons directly to the tumor, helping to destroy it. MOABs may help destroy cancer cells in bone marrow that has been removed from a patient in preparation for a bone marrow transplant. MOABs carrying radioisotopes may also prove useful in diagnosing certain cancers, such as prostate cancer. Researchers are testing MOABs in clinical trials to treat prostate cancer and other types of cancer.

Side effects include fever and chills, sweating, fatigue, hives or itching, flu-like symptoms, or swollen lymph nodes two to four weeks after treatment. Less common side effects include nausea and vomiting or diarrhea. Rarely, MOABs may cause fluid accumulation in the lungs.

Neosar   See CYTOXAN.

Neupogen   See FILGRASTIM.

Nilandron   See NILUTAMIDE.

nilutamide (Nilandron)   An oral antiandrogen drug used after surgical removal of the testes to treat prostate cancer that has spread.

Nitrolmidazole   See ETANIDAZOLE.

Oncovin   See VINCRISTINE.

ondansetron (Zofran)   An antinausea drug especially helpful for patients who are taking cisplatin, dramatically reducing nausea and vomiting. This drug blocks the serotonin pathway by which chemotherapy stimulates the vomiting center in the brain. It is given immediately before intravenous chemotherapy or within an hour if chemotherapy is given by mouth. Occasionally it may cause diarrhea or constipation, or headache.

Orasone   See PREDNISONE.

oxycodone (Percodan, Percocet, Endodan, Oxy-Contin)   A prescription narcotic drug used to ease pain that is given either orally or by injection. It binds to opioid receptors in the brain, altering the perception of pain and the emotional response to it.   Oxycodone may cause constipation, drowsiness or sedation, nausea, dizziness, or dry mouth. Less common side effects include vomiting, mood changes of depression or euphoria, mental clouding, and decreased breathing and heart rates and blood pressure.

paclitaxel (Taxol)   A type of taxane (also called a mitotic inhibitor) that is derived from the yew tree, which kills cancer cells by depriving them of hormones they need to grow and divide. In prostate cancer paclitaxel is not very effective when used alone, but when combined with estramustine it can lower prostate-specific antigen (PSA) level in 60 percent of patients, by up to 80 percent.

Side effects include hair loss, nausea and vomiting, mild diarrhea, stomatitis, muscle and bone aches, numbness and tingling, fatigue, and decreased white blood count. The drug should not be used by patients who have a pacemaker or abnormal heart rhythm.

Paraplatin   See CARBOPLATIN.

Percodan   See OXYCODONE.

Platinol   See CISPLATIN.

platinum   See CISPLATIN.

plicamycin (mithramycin, Mithracin)   An antibiotic used to treat testicular cancer that works by disrupting the growth of cancer cells, destroying them. Side effects include nausea and vomiting, hair loss, appetite loss, mouth or lip sores, and decreased platelet or white blood cell count.

prednisone (Apo-Prednisone, Deltasone, Orasone)   A glucocorticoid steroid that decreases inflammation by interfering with the action of white blood cells. It is an important drug used in combination with other chemotherapy agents to treat many different kinds of cancer. Side effects include delayed wound healing, depression or mood changes, weight gain and increased appetite, increase in blood sugar level, skin bruises, increased risk of infection, fluid retention, and sleep disturbances. Less common side effects include weakness, bone fractures, fungal infections, sweating, diarrhea, nausea, headache, or increased heart rate. Rarely, personality changes, cataracts, blurred vision, and stomach ulcer may occur.

prochlorperazine (Compazine)   An antinausea drug commonly prescribed for chemotherapy patients to control severe nausea and vomiting, because it blocks messages to the part of the brain responsible for these side effects. It can be given intravenously or orally.

More common side effects include dry mouth, constipation, sedation, and sleepiness. Less common side effects include blurred vision, restlessness, involuntary muscle movements, tremor, increased appetite and weight gain, increased heart rate, and decreased blood pressure. Rarely, prochlorperazine may cause jaundice, rash or hives, and increased sensitivity to sunlight.

Procrit   See EPOGEN.

Proscar   See FINASTERIDE.

Reglan   See METOCLOPRAMIDE.

stilbestrol   See DIETHYLSTILBESTROL.

Stilphostrol   See DIETHYLSTILBESTROL.

suramin   A drug currently used to treat certain infections that is being studied as a possible chemotherapy drug against prostate cancer as well as cancers of the lung, ovary, and bladder. Many studies are currently assessing its usefulness in combination with other chemotherapy drugs.

Teslac   See ANDROGENS.

Testex   See ANDROGENS.

Toposar   See ETOPOSIDE.

VB   A combination of the chemotherapy drugs vinblastine and bleomycin sometimes used to treat prostate cancer as well as cancers of the kidney or bladder.

VBP   A combination of the chemotherapy drugs vinblastine, bleomycin, and prednisone sometimes used to treat prostate cancer or cancers of the kidney, bladder, or prostate.

Velban   See VINBLASTINE.

VelP   A chemotherapy protocol that uses vinblastine, ifosfamide, and cisplatin to treat testicular cancer.

VePesid See ETOPOSIDE.

vinblastine (Velban) An alkaloid-based anti-cancer drug obtained from the periwinkle plant to treat testicular cancer, among others. Vinblastine disrupts cell division, killing the cell. This drug may cause decrease white blood and platelet counts, increasing the risk of infection or bleeding. It also may cause hair loss. Less common side effects include constipation and numbness in hands or feet. Rarely, vinblastine may cause headache, depression, jaw pain, nausea and vomiting, mouth sores, problems in emptying the bladder, dizziness, vision changes, or increased heart rate.

VIP A chemotherapy protocol using etoposide, ifosfamide, and cisplatin to treat testicular cancer.

vincristine (Oncovin) An intravenous chemotherapy drug sometimes used to treat prostate or testicular cancer as well as cancers of the brain, breast, and cervix, and lymphoma, acute leukemia, Wilms' tumor, neuroblastoma, or rhabdomyosarcoma. Vincristine, derived from the periwinkle plant, disrupts and kills cancer cells.

Vincristine can cause constipation that may lead to a serious problem. Other common side effects include hair loss and numbness or tingling. Less common side effects include weakness, muscle aches, cramping, and stomach pain. Rarely, it can cause double vision, depression, taste changes, decreased platelet and white blood cell counts (causing increased risk of bleeding and infection), jaw pain, and headache.

vindesine (vinblastine amide sulfate [Eldisine]) An investigational intravenous drug being studied as a possible treatment for testicular cancer as well as lymphoma, melanoma, leukemia, and cancers of the lung, colon, and breast. It belongs to the group of drugs derived from a plant alkaloid (vinca) and works by disrupting cell division.

Common side effects include constipation, hair loss, pins and needles sensations, and decreased white blood cell count. Less common side effects include nausea and vomiting, muscle weakness, and stomach cramps. Rarely, vindesine may cause hoarseness, jaw pain, diarrhea, or decreased platelet count.

Zinecard See DEXRAZOXANE.

Zoladex See GOSERELIN ACETATE.

Zyloprim See ALLOPURINOL SODIUM.

APPENDIX IV
CLINICAL TRIALS IN MALE REPRODUCTIVE CANCERS

PENILE CANCER

The following clinical trials are listed as a service for anyone interested in more information about joining a particular trial studying treatments for men's reproductive cancers. For more information, see the Web site of the National Cancer Institute at www.cancer.gov/clinicaltrials.

PHASE II PILOT STUDY OF HUMAN PAPILLOMAVIRUS 16 (HPV16) E6 AND E7 PEPTIDE VACCINES IN PATIENTS WITH ADVANCED OR RECURRENT CARCINOMA OF THE CERVIX OR OTHER TUMORS CARRYING HPV16

This Phase II trial will study the effectiveness of human papillomavirus vaccine therapy in treating patients who have advanced or recurrent cancer of the penis, among other sites. Vaccines made from certain human papillomaviruses may be able to help the body to kill more tumor cells. Peripheral stem cells will be collected and treated in the laboratory to make the vaccine. Patients will receive vaccinations in weeks 1, 3, 7, and 11, and treatment may be repeated for as long as benefit is shown. Patients will receive a follow-up evaluation one month after the final vaccination.

TESTICULAR CANCER

DIAGNOSTIC STUDY OF FLUDEOXYGLUCOSE F 18 POSITRON EMISSION TOMOGRAPHY IN THE PREDICTION OF RELAPSE IN PATIENTS WITH HIGH-RISK STAGE I NON-SEMINOMATOUS OR MIXED SEMINOMA/NON-SEMINOMATOUS GERM CELL TUMOR OF THE TESTIS

This diagnostic trial will study the effectiveness of positron emission tomography (PET) using fludeoxyglucose F 18 in predicting relapse in patients who have stage I germ cell tumor of the testicle. Imaging procedures such as PET may improve the ability to detect the extent of cancer and allow doctors to plan more effective treatment for patients who have testicular cancer. Patients will receive an infusion of fludeoxyglucose F 18 followed by positron emission tomography one hour later. Some patients may receive chemotherapy and will be evaluated every six months; other patients may be treated on another clinical trial. These patients will be evaluated once a month for one year, every two months for a year, every three months for a year, and every four to six months thereafter.

DIAGNOSTIC STUDY TO CORRELATE HISTOPATHOLOGY, IMMUNOCHEMISTRY, AND QUANTITATIVE RADIOLOGY WITH OUTCOME IN PATIENTS WITH EARLY STAGE NONSEMINOMATOUS GERM CELL TUMOR OF THE TESTIS

This diagnostic trial is designed to detect the risk of recurrent disease in patients who have stage I testicular cancer and who have undergone orchiectomy within the previous 12 weeks. Diagnostic procedures may improve a doctor's ability to predict the recurrence of testicular cancer.

Some patients will undergo surgery to remove lymph nodes in the abdomen; all patients will undergo radiology and blood tests to predict the risk of recurrence. Some patients may receive chemotherapy or radiation therapy. Patients will receive periodic follow-up evaluations.

GENETIC AND ETIOLOGIC MULTIDISCIPLINARY STUDY OF FAMILIAL TESTICULAR CANCER

This study will identify new families with familial testicular cancer to determine genetic susceptibility.

Studying members of families with testicular cancer may help to identify genetic susceptibility.

DNA samples will be collected from all participants. Participants will also complete questionnaires, undergo a physical examination and imaging studies, and have blood samples drawn for testing. However, patients will not receive the results of genetic testing, and the results will not influence treatment. Participants will be evaluated once a year for five years.

PHASE I STUDY OF PACLITAXEL AND IFOSFAMIDE FOLLOWED BY CARBOPLATIN AND ETOPOSIDE WITH STEM CELL SUPPORT IN PATIENTS WITH ADVANCED GERM CELL TUMORS WITH UNFAVORABLE PROGNOSTIC FACTORS AND RESISTANCE TO CISPLATIN

This Phase I trial is studying the effectiveness of combination chemotherapy (paclitaxel, ifosfamide, carboplatin and etoposide plus peripheral stem cell transplantation) in patients who have cisplatin-resistant advanced germ cell tumors. Drugs used in chemotherapy use different ways to stop tumor cells from dividing so they stop growing or die. Peripheral stem cell transplantation may allow doctors to give higher doses of chemotherapy drugs and kill more tumor cells.

Bone marrow will be collected and preserved before beginning chemotherapy. Patients will receive a 24-hour continuous infusion of paclitaxel followed by infusions of ifosfamide once a day for three days. Patients will then receive injections of filgrastim twice a day until day 13. On days 11 through 13, peripheral stem cells will be collected. Treatment may be repeated every two weeks for two courses. Two weeks later, patients will receive infusions of carboplatin and etoposide for three days followed by injections of filgrastim until blood counts return to normal. Peripheral stem cells or bone marrow will be reinfused on day 5. Treatment will be repeated every two weeks for three courses. After treatment has been completed, some patients may undergo surgery.

PHASE I STUDY OF RECOMBINANT FOWLPOX-CEA-TRICOM VACCINE WITH OR WITHOUT SARGRAMOSTIM (GM-CSF) OR RECOMBINANT FOWLPOX-GM-CSF IN PATIENTS WITH ADVANCED OR METASTATIC CEA-EXPRESSING ADENOCARCINOMAS

In this Phase I trial, scientists will study the effectiveness of vaccine therapy with or without sar-gramostim in treating patients who have advanced or metastatic cancer. Vaccines may make the body build an immune response to kill tumor cells. Colony-stimulating factors such as sargramostim may increase the number of immune cells found in bone marrow or peripheral blood. Combining vaccine therapy with sargramostim may make tumor cells more sensitive to the vaccine and may kill more tumor cells.

Patients will be assigned to one of three groups. Patients in group one will receive an injection of the vaccine every two weeks for four doses and then every two months for as long as benefit is shown. Patients in group two will receive injections of the vaccine as in group one and an injection of sargramostim once a day for four days beginning on the day of each vaccination. Patients in group three will receive injections of the vaccine as in group one and an injection of a sargramostim vaccine on the day of each vaccination as in group two. Patients will be evaluated once a month for four months.

PHASE II STUDY OF ARSENIC TRIOXIDE IN MEN WITH REFRACTORY TESTICULAR OR EXTRAGONADAL GERM CELL MALIGNANCIES

This Phase II trial will study the effectiveness of arsenic trioxide in treating men who have germ cell cancer that has not responded to previous treatment. Patients will receive a one- to two-hour infusion of arsenic trioxide once a day for five days. Treatment may be repeated every four weeks for up to three years. Patients will be evaluated every two months for three years.

PHASE II STUDY OF IMATINIB MESYLATE IN PATIENTS WITH PROGRESSIVE, REFRACTORY, OR RECURRENT PURE TESTICULAR SEMINOMA OR OVARIAN GERM CELL DYSGERMINOMA AFTER CISPLATIN-BASED CHEMOTHERAPY

This Phase II trial will study the effectiveness of imatinib mesylate in treating patients who have progressive, refractory, or recurrent testicular or ovarian cancer following cisplatin-based chemotherapy. Imatinib mesylate may stop the growth of tumor cells by blocking the enzymes necessary for tumor cell growth.

Patients will receive imatinib mesylate by mouth once a day for as long as benefit is shown. Some patients may undergo surgery. Patients will be evaluated every three months for a year and every six months for a year.

PHASE II STUDY OF PACLITAXEL, IFOSFAMIDE, AND CISPLATIN IN PATIENTS WITH METASTATIC NONSEMINOMATOUS GERM CELL TUMOR OF THE TESTIS IN FIRST RELAPSE FOLLOWING FIRST LINE TREATMENT WITH BLEOMYCIN, ETOPOSIDE, AND CISPLATIN

This phase II trial will study the effectiveness of combining paclitaxel, ifosfamide, and cisplatin in treating patients who have metastatic testicular cancer that has recurred following treatment.

Patients will receive a three-hour infusion of paclitaxel, in addition to infusions of ifosfamide and cisplatin daily for five days. Treatment may be repeated every three weeks for four courses.

PHASE II/III RANDOMIZED STUDY OF BLEOMYCIN/CISPLATIN/ETOPOSIDE (BEP) VERSUS BLEOMYCIN/CISPLATIN/ ETOPOSIDE/PACLITAXEL (T-BEP) IN MEN WITH INTERMEDIATE PROGNOSIS GERM CELL CANCER

This randomized Phase II/III trial will compare the effectiveness of two regimens of combination chemotherapy in treating men who have germ cell cancer. It is not yet known which regimen of combination chemotherapy may be more effective for germ cell cancer.

Patients will be randomly assigned to one of two groups. Group one will receive infusions of cisplatin and etoposide for five days plus infusions of bleomycin once a week for three weeks. Patients in group two will receive an infusion of paclitaxel on the first day of treatment plus chemotherapy as in group one. Patients in group two may also receive injections of G-CSF. Treatment in both groups may be repeated every three weeks for up to four courses. Quality of life will be assessed before treatment and one and two years following treatment. All patients will receive follow-up evaluations once a month during year 1, every two months during year 2, every three months during year 3, every 6 months during year 4, and once a year thereafter.

PHASE III RANDOMIZED STUDY OF BLEOMYCIN, ETOPOSIDE, AND CISPLATIN (BEP) WITH OR WITHOUT HIGH-DOSE CARBOPLATIN, ETOPOSIDE, AND CYCLOPHOSPHAMIDE PLUS AUTOLOGOUS BONE MARROW OR PERIPHERAL BLOOD STEM CELL TRANSPLANTATION IN MALE PATIENTS WITH PREVIOUSLY UNTREATED POOR- OR INTERMEDIATE-RISK GERM CELL TUMORS

This randomized Phase III trial is comparing the effectiveness of combination chemotherapy with or without bone marrow or peripheral stem cell transplantation in treating men with previously untreated germ cell tumors. It is not known whether combining chemotherapy with bone marrow or peripheral stem cell transplantation is more effective than combination chemotherapy alone in treating men with germ cell tumors.

Patients will be randomly assigned to one of two groups. Patients in group one will receive combination chemotherapy plus G-CSF for 10 days or until blood counts return to normal. Treatment may be repeated every three weeks for four courses. Patients in group two will receive two courses of chemotherapy as in group one. Bone marrow or peripheral stem cells will be collected before or after chemotherapy. Some patients will receive two additional courses of chemotherapy; other patients will receive high-dose chemotherapy followed by reinfusion of bone marrow or peripheral stem cells. Some patients from both groups may undergo radiation therapy and/or surgery.

PHASE III RANDOMIZED STUDY OF STANDARD CISPLATIN, ETOPOSIDE, AND IFOSFAMIDE (VIP) FOLLOWED BY SEQUENTIAL HIGH DOSE VIP AND STEM CELL RESCUE VERSUS BLEOMYCIN, ETOPOSIDE, AND CISPLATIN (BEP) IN CHEMOTHERAPY NAIVE MEN WITH POOR PROGNOSIS GERM CELL CANCER

This randomized Phase III trial is comparing the effectiveness of combination chemotherapy with or without peripheral stem cell transplantation in treating men who have previously untreated germ cell cancer. Patients in group one will receive four courses of chemotherapy consisting of etoposide, cisplatin, and bleomycin. Patients in group two will receive one course of chemotherapy consisting of etoposide, cisplatin, and ifosfamide followed by daily injections of filgrastim. Peripheral stem cells will then be collected. Patients will receive high-dose chemotherapy followed by reinfusion of stem cells, and daily injections of filgrastim until blood counts return to normal. Treatment may be repeated every three weeks for three courses. Quality of life will be assessed before chemotherapy, at six months, and at two years after treatment. Patients will receive follow-up evaluations once a month for a year, every two months for a year, every three months for a year, every six months for a year, and once a year thereafter.

RANDOMIZED STUDY OF CT SCAN FREQUENCY IN PATIENTS WITH STAGE I TESTICULAR TERATOMA AFTER ORCHIECTOMY

This randomized clinical trial will determine if there is a different result from two different schedules of CT scans in treating patients with stage I testicular cancer after undergoing orchiectomy. Imaging procedures such as CT scans help the doctor in detecting cancer or the recurrence of cancer. Increasing the number of times a CT scan is given may improve the ability to detect stage I testicular cancer.

Patients in group one will be given CT scans at three and 12 months after orchiectomy; patients in group two will be given scans at three, six, nine, 12, and 24 months after orchiectomy. Patients will be evaluated once a month for the first year after orchiectomy, every two months for the second year, every three months for the third year, and every four to six months thereafter.

PROSTATE CANCER

DIAGNOSTIC STUDY OF MAGNETIC RESONANCE IMAGING AND MAGNETIC RESONANCE SPECTROSCOPIC IMAGING FOR THE LOCALIZATION OF PROSTATE CANCER PRIOR TO RADICAL PROSTATECTOMY

This diagnostic trial will compare the effectiveness of combination magnetic resonance imaging (MRI)/ magnetic resonance spectroscopic imaging (MRSI) to that of MRI alone in determining the extent of prostate cancer in patients who are scheduled to undergo surgery to remove the prostate gland. Imaging procedures such as MRI and MRSI may improve the ability to detect the extent of prostate cancer. It is not yet known if MRI combined with MRSI is more effective than MRI alone in detecting the extent of prostate cancer.

At least six weeks after biopsy, patients will undergo various combinations of MRI and MRSI, followed by surgery to remove the prostate gland within six months.

DIAGNOSTIC STUDY OF SERUM AND URINE PROTEOMIC PROFILES AS PREDICTORS OF CLINICAL OUTCOME IN PATIENTS WITH LOCALIZED PROSTATE CANCER TREATED WITH RADIOTHERAPY

In this diagnostic trial, researchers will study blood and urine proteins to try to predict treatment outcome in patients undergoing radiation therapy for localized prostate cancer. They believe that proteins found in blood and urine samples may help predict outcome and allow doctors to plan more effective treatment.

Urine and blood samples will be collected from patients before or after radiation therapy, and samples will be studied in the laboratory. Results of the studies will not influence patient treatment.

GENETIC MAPPING OF INTERACTIVE SUSCEPTIBILITY LOCI IN PATIENTS AND SIBLINGS WITH BREAST, COLON, LUNG, OR PROSTATE CANCER

In this clinical trial, scientists will try to identify genes that may be associated with cancer in patients and siblings who have cancer of the breast, prostate, lung, or colon. Identification of genes that may be associated with developing certain types of cancer may someday provide important information about a person's risk of getting cancer.

A questionnaire will be completed about the incidence of cancer in the family. Blood samples will be taken from the patient, the sibling, and their parents (if possible) and laboratory tests will be performed using those samples. Patients will receive a follow-up evaluation once a year. Patients will not receive the results of the genetic testing and the results will not influence the type and duration of treatment.

NCI HIGH PRIORITY CLINICAL TRIAL— PHASE III RANDOMIZED STUDY OF PROSTATECTOMY VERSUS EXPECTANT MANAGEMENT WITH PALLIATIVE THERAPY IN PATIENTS WITH CLINICALLY LOCALIZED PROSTATE CANCER (PIVOT)

In this randomized Phase III trial, scientists will compare surgery with watchful waiting in men who have stage I or stage II prostate cancer. Watchful waiting until symptoms appear may be effective in patients with prostate cancer. It is not yet known if watchful waiting is more effective than prostatectomy for early prostate cancer.

Patients will be randomly assigned to one of two groups. Within six weeks, patients in group one will undergo surgery to remove lymph nodes in the pelvis, followed within two weeks by surgery to remove the prostate. Patients in group two will be observed until treatment is needed. All patients with disease progression will receive standard therapy. Quality of life will be assessed every six months. Patients will be evaluated every three months for a year and every six months for 15 years.

PHASE I RANDOMFIZED STUDY OF NEOADJUVANT CELECOXIB FOLLOWED BY PROSTATECTOMY IN PATIENTS WITH LOCALIZED PROSTATE CANCER

This is a randomized Phase I trial to determine the effectiveness of celecoxib given before surgery to remove the prostate in patients who have localized prostate cancer. Celecoxib may be an effective treatment for early stage prostate cancer; it is not yet known if celecoxib is more effective than no treatment before surgery for prostate cancer.

Patients will be randomly assigned to one of two groups to receive either celecoxib or a placebo by mouth twice a day for at least four weeks. Patients will then undergo surgery to remove the prostate. All patients will be evaluated within one month and at three months.

PHASE I STUDY OF ACTIVATED AUTOLOGOUS T CELLS (XCELLERATE) IN PATIENTS WITH HORMONE-REFRACTORY PROSTATE CANCER

This Phase I trial will study the effectiveness of T-cell therapy in treating patients who have prostate cancer that has not responded to hormone therapy. Biological therapies use different ways to stimulate the immune system and stop tumor cells from growing. Treating a person's T cells in the laboratory and then reinfusing them may cause a stronger immune response and kill more tumor cells.

Patients' T cells will be collected and treated in the laboratory, and then reinfused into the patients. Patients will be evaluated once a week for four weeks and once a month for three months.

PHASE I STUDY OF DOCETAXEL, ESTRAMUSTINE, MITOXANTRONE, AND PREDNISONE IN PATIENTS WITH ADVANCED PROSTATE CANCER

This is a Phase I trial to study the effectiveness of combination chemotherapy in treating patients who have advanced prostate cancer. Patients will receive oral prednisone twice a day on days 1 through 4, oral estramustine three times a day on days 2 through 6, and infusions of mitoxantrone and docetaxel on day 3. Treatment may be repeated every three weeks for up to six courses. Patients will receive follow-up evaluations every three months.

PHASE I STUDY OF DOCETAXEL, GEMCITABINE, AND FILGRASTIM (G-CSF) IN PATIENTS WITH ADVANCED SOLID TUMORS

This Phase I trial will study the effectiveness of combination chemotherapy plus filgrastim in treating patients who have advanced solid tumors. Colony-stimulating factors such as filgrastim may increase the number of immune cells found in bone marrow or peripheral blood and may help a person's immune system recover from the side effects of chemotherapy.

Patients will receive infusions of docetaxel and gemcitabine on day 1. Beginning on day 2, patients will receive injections of filgrastim once a day until blood counts return to normal. Treatment may be repeated every two weeks for as long as benefit is shown. Patients will be evaluated every two to three weeks during therapy.

PHASE I STUDY OF ESTRAMUSTINE, DOCETAXEL, AND CARBOPLATIN IN PATIENTS WITH HORMONE REFRACTORY PROSTATE CANCER

This Phase I trial will study the effectiveness of estramustine, docetaxel, and carboplatin in treating patients who have prostate cancer that has not responded to hormonal therapy. Patients will receive estramustine by mouth three times a day on days 1 through 5 of week 1. They will also receive infusions of docetaxel once a week during weeks 1 through 3 and an infusion of carboplatin in week 1. Treatment may be repeated every four weeks for up to six courses.

PHASE I STUDY OF GLYCOSYLATED MUC-2-GLOBO H-KLH CONJUGATE VACCINE WITH ADJUVANT GPI-0100 IN PATIENTS WITH BIOCHEMICALLY RELAPSED PROSTATE CANCER

This Phase I trial will study the effectiveness of combining vaccine therapy and biological therapy in treating patients who have relapsed prostate cancer. Biological therapies use different ways to stimulate the immune system and stop cancer cells from growing; combining vaccine therapy with biological therapy may kill more tumor cells.

Patients will receive injections of the vaccine and the biological therapy drug once a week in weeks 1 through 3, 7, 15, and 27. Patients will be evaluated every three months.

PHASE I STUDY OF HIGH-INTENSITY FOCUSED ULTRASOUND USING THE SONABLATE SYSTEM IN PATIENTS WITH LOCALLY RECURRENT PROSTATE CANCER

This Phase I trial will determine the effectiveness of focused ultrasound energy in treating patients who have locally recurrent prostate cancer. Highly focused ultrasound energy may be able to kill cancer cells by heating the tumor without affecting the surrounding tissue.

Patients will receive ultrasound energy to the prostate for approximately two hours through a probe inserted into the rectum. After three months, some patients will receive one additional treatment. Patients will be evaluated regularly over a six-month period.

PHASE I STUDY OF HIGH-INTENSITY FOCUSED ULTRASOUND USING THE SONABLATE SYSTEM IN PATIENTS WITH ORGAN-CONFINED PROSTATE CANCER

In this Phase I trial, scientists will study the effectiveness of focused ultrasound energy in treating patients who have prostate cancer that has not

spread beyond the prostate. Patients will receive ultrasound energy to the prostate for two to three hours through a probe inserted into the rectum. After three months, some patients will receive one additional treatment. Patients will be evaluated regularly over a six-month period.

PHASE I STUDY OF KETOCONAZOLE AND DOCETAXEL IN PATIENTS WITH METASTATIC ANDROGEN-INDEPENDENT PROSTATE CANCER

This Phase I trial will study the effectiveness of combining ketoconazole with docetaxel in treating patients who have metastatic prostate cancer. Androgens can stimulate the growth of prostate cancer cells; drugs such as ketoconazole may stop the adrenal glands from producing androgens. Combining ketoconazole with docetaxel may kill more tumor cells.

Patients will receive an infusion of docetaxel once a week for three weeks. They will also receive ketoconazole by mouth three times a day in weeks 3 and 4. Beginning with course two, patients will receive an infusion of docetaxel once a week for three weeks and ketoconazole by mouth once a day. Treatment may be repeated every four weeks for as long as benefit is shown. Patients will be evaluated once a month.

PHASE I STUDY OF LYCOPENE FOR THE CHEMOPREVENTION OF PROSTATE CANCER

In this Phase I trial, scientists will study the effectiveness of lycopene in preventing prostate cancer. Patients will receive one dose of lycopene by mouth in a mixture of tomato paste, water, and olive oil. Patients will then eat a diet that is low in carotenoids for four weeks. Patients will be evaluated once a week for four weeks.

PHASE I STUDY OF MONOCLONAL ANTIBODY ABX-EGF IN PATIENTS WITH RENAL OR PROSTATE CANCER

This Phase I trial will study the effectiveness of monoclonal antibody therapy in treating patients who have kidney or prostate cancer. Monoclonal antibodies can locate tumor cells and either kill them or deliver tumor-killing substances to them without harming normal cells. Patients will receive an infusion of the monoclonal antibody once a week for four weeks. Patients will be evaluated every two weeks for five weeks.

PHASE I STUDY OF PHOTODYNAMIC THERAPY WITH LUTETIUM TEXAPHYRIN IN PATIENTS WITH LOCALLY RECURRENT PROSTATE ADENOCARCINOMA

This Phase I trial will study the effectiveness of photodynamic therapy with lutetium texaphyrin in treating patients who have locally recurrent prostate cancer. Photodynamic therapy uses light and drugs that make cancer cells more sensitive to light to kill tumor cells, which may be effective treatment for locally recurrent prostate cancer. Photosensitizing drugs such as lutetium texaphyrin are absorbed by cancer cells, and when exposed to light, become active and kill the cancer cells.

Patients will receive an infusion of lutetium texaphyrin followed three to 24 hours later by photodynamic therapy delivered to the prostate through a catheter. Patients will undergo biopsy of the prostate and bladder before and after photodynamic therapy. Patients will receive follow-up evaluations at two weeks, once a month for three months, every three months for two years, every six months for three years, and once a year thereafter.

PHASE I STUDY OF TESTOSTERONE IN PATIENTS WITH PROGRESSIVE ANDROGEN-INDEPENDENT PROSTATE CANCER

This Phase I trial will study the effectiveness of testosterone in treating patients who have progressive prostate cancer that no longer responds to hormone therapy. High doses of testosterone may be effective in killing prostate cancer cells that no longer respond to hormone therapy.

Patients will wear a testosterone patch on the skin for four weeks, changing the patch once a day. Patients will be evaluated on day 1 and at two and four weeks.

PHASE I STUDY OF YTTRIUM Y 90 MONOCLONAL ANTIBODY M170, PACLITAXEL, AND CYCLOSPORINE FOLLOWED BY AUTOLOGOUS PERIPHERAL BLOOD STEM CELL TRANSPLANTATION IN PATIENTS WITH HORMONE-REFRACTORY METASTATIC PROSTATE CANCER

This Phase I trial will study the effectiveness of monoclonal antibody therapy plus chemotherapy followed by peripheral stem cell transplantation in treating patients who have metastatic prostate cancer that has not responded to hormone therapy. Radiolabeled monoclonal antibodies can locate tumor cells and either kill them or deliver tumor-killing substances to them without harming normal cells. Drugs used in chemotherapy use different ways to stop tumor cells from dividing so they stop growing or die. Combining monoclonal antibody therapy and chemotherapy with peripheral stem cell transplantation may be an effective treatment for metastatic prostate cancer.

Peripheral stem cells will be collected. Patients will then receive infusions of radiolabeled and unlabeled monoclonal antibodies on days 4 and 11. Patients will also receive cyclosporine by mouth every 12 hours on days 1 through 29, and will undergo peripheral stem cell transplantation on day 25. They will receive injections of filgrastim beginning on day 25 and continuing until blood counts return to normal. Some patients may receive infusions of paclitaxel on day 13. Patients will be evaluated once a month for three months, every three months for a year, and then every six months for a year.

PHASE I/II RANDOMIZED STUDY OF BMS-247550 WITH OR WITHOUT ESTRAMUSTINE IN PATIENTS WITH PROGRESSIVE ANDROGEN-INDEPENDENT ADENOCARCINOMA OF THE PROSTATE

This randomized Phase I/II trial will study the effectiveness of BMS-247550 with or without estramustine in treating patients who have progressive prostate cancer. It is not yet known which chemotherapy regimen is more effective in treating progressive prostate cancer.

Some patients will receive estramustine by mouth three times a day on days 1 through 5, and an infusion of BMS-247550 on day 2. Other patients will be randomly assigned to one of two groups. Patients in group one will receive infusions of BMS-247550 and estramustine as above. Patients in group two will receive an infusion of BMS-247550 alone. Treatment for all patients may be repeated every three weeks for as long as benefit is shown.

PHASE II NEOADJUVANT STUDY OF ANDROGEN SUPPRESSION AND TRANSPERINEAL ULTRASOUND-GUIDED BRACHYTHERAPY AFTER EXTERNAL BEAM RADIOTHERAPY IN PATIENTS WITH LOCALLY RECURRENT PROSTATE ADENOCARCINOMA

This Phase II trial will study the effectiveness of hormone therapy followed by internal radiation in treating patients who have locally recurrent prostate cancer following external-beam radiation therapy. Androgens can stimulate the growth of prostate cancer cells. Drugs such as goserelin, leuprolide, flutamide, or bicalutamide may stop the adrenal glands from producing androgens. Internal radiation uses radioactive material placed directly into or near a tumor to kill tumor cells. Combining hormone therapy with internal radiation may be effective in treating locally recurrent prostate cancer.

Patients will receive injections of either goserelin or leuprolide no more than once a month for four months, and will also receive flutamide by mouth once a day or bicalutamide by mouth three times a day for four months. Within four weeks after completing hormone therapy, patients will undergo internal radiation therapy. Quality of life will be assessed periodically. Patients will be evaluated every three months for a year, every six months for four years, and once a year for five years.

PHASE II PILOT RANDOMIZED STUDY OF FOWLPOX-PROSTATE-SPECIFIC ANTIGEN VACCINE WITH OR WITHOUT DOCETAXEL IN PATIENTS WITH METASTATIC ANDROGEN-INDEPENDENT PROSTATE CANCER

This randomized Phase II trial will compare the effectiveness of vaccine therapy with or without docetaxel in treating patients who have metastatic prostate cancer. Combining vaccine therapy with chemotherapy may kill more tumor cells.

Patients will receive injections of two different vaccines on day 1 and injections of sargramostim on days 1 through 4. They will then receive an injection of a third vaccine on day 15 and injections of sargramostim on days 15 through 18. Patients will then be randomly assigned to one of two groups. Patients in group one will receive an infusion of docetaxel in weeks 5, 6 and 7, and injections of the vaccine and sargramostim in week 5. Treatment may be repeated beginning in week 8 for one more course. Beginning in week 13, some patients will receive an injection of the vaccine on day 1 of each course and docetaxel once a week for three weeks. Treatment may be repeated every four weeks for as long as benefit is shown. Patients in group two will receive an injection of the vaccine and sargramostim in weeks 5 and 9. After week 13, some patients will stop the vaccine and may receive docetaxel once a week for three weeks. Chemotherapy may be repeated every four weeks for as long as benefit is shown.

PHASE II PILOT STUDY OF A MULTIVALENT CONJUGATE VACCINE WITH ADJUVANT QS21 IN PATIENTS WITH BIOCHEMICALLY RELAPSED PROSTATE CANCER

This Phase II trial will study the effectiveness of combining vaccine therapy and biological therapy in treating patients who have relapsed prostate cancer. Combining vaccine therapy with biological therapy may kill more tumor cells.

Patients will receive injections of the vaccine and the biological therapy drug once a week in weeks 1 through 3, 7, 19, 31, 43, and 55. Patients will be evaluated every three months.

PHASE II PILOT STUDY OF MAGNETIC RESONANCE–GUIDED HIGH-DOSE RATE BRACHYTHERAPY BEFORE AND AFTER EXTERNAL BEAM RADIOTHERAPY IN PATIENTS WITH PROSTATE CANCER

This Phase II trial will evaluate the effectiveness of MRI-guided internal radiation before and after external-beam radiation in treating patients who have prostate cancer. Internal radiation uses radioactive material placed directly into or near a tumor to kill tumor cells. Using magnetic resonance imaging (MRI) to guide the placement of radioactive implants into the tumor may result in more effective radiation therapy.

Patients will undergo external-beam radiation five days a week for five weeks. They will undergo MRI-guided placement of radioactive implants into the prostate once before and once after external-beam radiation. Patients will be evaluated at one month, every three months for six months, every six months for one and a half years, and once a year for three years.

PHASE II PILOT STUDY OF MONOCLONAL ANTIBODY CTLA-4 IN PATIENTS WITH FOLLICULAR OR MANTLE CELL LYMPHOMA, COLON CANCER, OR PROSTATE CANCER REFRACTORY TO VACCINE THERAPY

This Phase II trial will study the effectiveness of monoclonal antibody CTLA-4 in treating patients who have lymphoma, colon cancer, or prostate cancer that has not responded to vaccine therapy. Monoclonal antibodies such as CTLA-4 can locate tumor cells and either kill them or deliver tumor-killing substances to them without harming normal cells.

Patients will receive a 90-minute infusion of monoclonal antibody CTLA-4 every four weeks for up to four courses. Patients will be evaluated every other month.

PHASE II PILOT STUDY OF MONOCLONAL ANTIBODY HUJ591 IN PATIENTS WITH PROGRESSIVE ANDROGEN-INDEPENDENT PROSTATE CANCER

In this Phase II trial, scientists will study the effectiveness of monoclonal antibody therapy in treating patients who have prostate cancer that has not responded to hormone therapy.

Patients will be assigned to one of two groups. Patients in group one will receive an infusion of the monoclonal antibody followed by an infusion of radiolabeled monoclonal antibody. Patients in group two will receive infusions of both monoclonal antibodies at the same time. Treatment in both groups may be repeated every three weeks for up to four courses. Patients will be evaluated for four weeks and then once a month for three months.

PHASE II RANDOMIZED PREVENTION STUDY OF FAT- AND/OR FLAXSEED-MODIFIED DIETS IN PATIENTS WITH NEWLY DIAGNOSED PROSTATE CANCER

This randomized Phase II trial will study the effectiveness of a diet that is low in fat and/or high in flaxseed in slowing or preventing disease progression in patients who have newly diagnosed prostate cancer. A diet that is low in fat and/or high in flaxseed may slow or prevent disease progression of prostate cancer.

Patients will be randomly assigned to one of four groups. Patients in group one will be taught how to add ground flaxseed to their daily diet. Patients in group two will receive instruction on eating a low-fat diet. Patients in group three will receive diet instruction as in both groups one and two. Patients in group four will be contacted once a week, but will not receive diet instruction until after surgery to remove the prostate. Patients will follow the diets for at least three weeks. They will also complete a diet diary until surgery. After surgery, all patients will receive diet counseling.

PHASE II RANDOMIZED STUDY OF BMS-275291 IN PATIENTS WITH HORMONE-REFRACTORY PROSTATE CANCER

This randomized Phase II trial will study the effectiveness of BMS-275291 in treating patients who have prostate cancer that has not responded to hormone therapy. BMS-275291 may halt the growth of prostate cancer by stopping blood flow to the tumor and by blocking the enzymes necessary for tumor cell growth.

Patients will be randomly assigned to one of two groups. Patients in group one will receive oral BMS-275291 once a day. Patients in group two will receive oral BMS-275291 twice a day. Treatment in both groups may continue for as long as benefit is shown. Patients will be evaluated periodically.

PHASE II RANDOMIZED STUDY OF DIETARY SOY IN PATIENTS WITH ELEVATED PSA LEVELS

This randomized Phase II trial will determine the effectiveness of soy protein supplement in preventing prostate cancer in patients who have elevated PSA levels. Soy protein supplement may prevent or delay the development of prostate cancer in patients who have elevated prostate-specific antigen (PSA) levels.

All patients will receive a placebo by mouth once a day for two weeks. Patients will then be randomly assigned to one of two groups. Patients in group one will receive soy protein supplement by mouth once a day for up to a year. Patients in group two will receive a placebo as in group one. Quality of life will be assessed periodically.

PHASE II RANDOMIZED STUDY OF DOCETAXEL AND ESTRAMUSTINE VERSUS BUSULFAN AND THIOTEPA WITH AUTOLOGOUS PERIPHERAL BLOOD STEM CELL TRANSPLANTATION IN PATIENTS WITH HORMONE REFRACTORY METASTATIC PROSTATE CANCER

This randomized Phase II trial will compare combination chemotherapy with or without peripheral stem cell transplantation in treating patients who have metastatic prostate cancer that has not responded to hormone therapy. Combining chemotherapy with peripheral stem cell transplantation may allow the doctor to give higher doses of chemotherapy drugs and kill more tumor cells.

All patients will receive an infusion of docetaxel on day 2, an infusion of cyclophosphamide on day 3, and injections of filgrastim once a day beginning on day 4 and continuing until white blood cells have been collected. Patients will then be randomly assigned to one of two groups. Patients in group one will receive busulfan by mouth every six hours for four days followed by an infusion of thiotepa for two days and then reinfusion of peripheral stem cells. Patients in group two will receive an infusion of docetaxel on day 2 and estramustine by mouth three times a day on days 1 through 5. Treatment may be repeated every three weeks for as long as benefit is shown. All patients will receive injections of filgrastim once a day beginning on day 6 and continuing until blood counts return to normal. Quality of life will be assessed periodically in both groups. Patients will receive follow-up evaluations every three months for a year, every six months for a year, and once a year thereafter.

PHASE II RANDOMIZED STUDY OF DOXERCALCIFEROL IN PATIENTS WITH LOCALIZED PROSTATE CANCER

This randomized Phase II trial will study the effectiveness of giving doxercalciferol before surgery in treating patients who have localized prostate cancer. Patients will be randomly assigned to one of two groups. Patients in group one will receive doxercalciferol once a day for four weeks followed by surgery to remove the prostate gland. Patients in group two will be observed for four weeks followed by surgery as in group one.

PHASE II RANDOMIZED STUDY OF MITOXANTRONE, ESTRAMUSTINE, AND VINORELBINE VERSUS ISOTRETINOIN, INTERFERON ALFA, AND PACLITAXEL IN PATIENTS WITH METASTATIC HORMONE-REFRACTORY PROSTATE CANCER

This randomized Phase II trial will compare the effectiveness of combination chemotherapy with that of chemotherapy plus biological therapy in treating patients who have progressive or metastatic prostate cancer that has not responded to hormone therapy.

Patients will be randomly assigned to one of two groups. Patients in group one will receive infusions of vinorelbine on days 2 and 9 and an infusion of mitoxantrone on day 2. They will also receive estramustine by mouth every 12 hours on days 1 through 5. Treatment may be repeated every three weeks for as long as benefit is shown. Patients in group two will receive isotretinoin by mouth and injections of interferon alfa on days 1 and 2. They will also receive a one-hour infusion of paclitaxel once a week for six weeks. Treatment may be repeated every eight weeks for as long as benefit is shown. Quality of life will be assessed periodically. Patients will be evaluated every three months for two years, every six months for three years, and once a year thereafter.

PHASE II RANDOMIZED STUDY OF RADIOTHERAPY WITH OR WITHOUT VACCINE CONTAINING RECOMBINANT VACCINIA PROSTATE SPECIFIC ANTIGEN (PSA) AND RV-B7.1 PLUS RECOMBINANT FOWLPOX PSA VACCINE IN PATIENTS WITH LOCALIZED PROSTATE CANCER

This randomized Phase II trial will compare the effectiveness of radiation therapy with or without vaccine therapy in treating patients who have prostate cancer. Patients will be randomly assigned to one of two groups. Patients in group one will receive vaccinations every four weeks for 29 weeks. They will also receive sargramostim four days a week and interleukin-2 five days a week every four weeks during the same 29-week period. Beginning in week 13, patients will undergo radiation therapy five days a week. Patients in group two will receive radiation therapy alone five days a week. All patients will receive follow-up evaluations every three months for two years and every six months thereafter.

PHASE II RANDOMIZED STUDY OF RECOMBINANT FOWLPOX PROSTATE-SPECIFIC ANTIGEN (PSA) VACCINE AND RECOMBINANT VACCINIA PSA VACCINE IN PATIENTS WITH ADVANCED ADENOCARCINOMA OF THE PROSTATE

This randomized Phase II trial will determine the effectiveness of vaccine therapy in treating patients who have advanced prostate cancer.

Patients will be randomly assigned to one of two groups. Patients in group one will receive an injection of one vaccine every four weeks for three courses and an injection of a second vaccine every four weeks for two courses. Patients in group two will receive the same vaccines but in reverse order. Treatment may be repeated every six months for as long as benefit is shown. Patients will be evaluated every three months.

PHASE II RANDOMIZED STUDY OF SGN-15 (CBR96-DOXORUBICIN IMMUNOCONJUGATE) COMBINED WITH DOCETAXEL VS DOCETAXEL ALONE IN PATIENTS WITH HORMONE-REFRACTORY PROSTATE CARCINOMA

This randomized Phase II trial will study the effectiveness of docetaxel with or without monoclonal antibody therapy in treating patients who have refractory prostate cancer. Patients will be randomly assigned to one of two groups. Patients in group one will receive an infusion of monoclonal antibody followed by an infusion of docetaxel once a week for six weeks, whereas patients in group two will receive docetaxel alone. Treatment in both groups may be repeated every eight weeks for up to six courses. Quality of life will be assessed periodically.

PHASE II RANDOMIZED STUDY OF TG4010 IN PATIENTS WITH ADENOCARCINOMA OF THE PROSTATE

This randomized Phase II trial will determine the effectiveness of TG4010 in treating patients who have prostate cancer. Vaccines made from a gene-modified virus may make the body build an immune response to kill tumor cells.

Patients will be randomly assigned to one of two groups. Patients in group one will receive an injection of TG4010 once a week for six weeks and then once every three weeks. Patients in group two will receive an injection of TG4010 every three weeks.

Treatment in both groups will continue for as long as benefit is shown. Patients will be evaluated every three months for two years.

PHASE II RANDOMIZED STUDY OF THE EFFECTS OF A LOW FAT, HIGH FIBER DIET ON SERUM FACTORS IN PATIENTS WITH PROSTATE CANCER

This randomized Phase II trial will compare the effectiveness of a low-fat, high-fiber diet with that of a standard diet in treating patients who have prostate cancer. Patients will be randomly assigned to one of two groups. Patients in group one will eat a low-fat, high-fiber diet for three weeks, whereas patients in group two will eat a standard diet.

PHASE II RANDOMIZED STUDY OF TOREMIFENE FOLLOWED BY RADICAL PROSTATECTOMY IN PATIENTS WITH STAGE I OR II ADENOCARCINOMA OF THE PROSTATE

This randomized Phase II trial will study the effectiveness of toremifene followed by radical prostatectomy in treating patients who have stage I or stage II prostate cancer. Androgens can stimulate the growth of prostate cancer cells; hormone therapy using toremifene may fight prostate cancer by reducing the production of androgens.

Patients will be randomly assigned to one of two groups. Patients in group one will receive toremifene by mouth once a day for up to six weeks, and patients in group two will undergo observation only. All patients will then undergo radical prostatectomy.

PHASE II RANDOMIZED STUDY OF VACCINE CONTAINING RECOMBINANT VACCINIA PROSTATE-SPECIFIC ANTIGEN (PSA) ADMIXED WITH RV-B7.1 PLUS RECOMBINANT FOWLPOX-PSA VACCINE, SARGRAMOSTIM (GM-CSF), AND INTERLEUKIN-2 VERSUS NILUTAMIDE ALONE IN PATIENTS WITH HORMONE-REFRACTORY PROSTATE CANCER

This randomized Phase II trial will compare the effectiveness of vaccine therapy plus sargramostim and interleukin-2 with that of nilutamide alone in treating patients who have prostate cancer that has not responded to hormone therapy. Vaccines made from prostate cancer cells may make the body build an immune response to kill tumor cells. Colony-stimulating factors such as sargramostim may increase the number of immune cells found in bone marrow or peripheral blood. Interleukin-2 may stimulate a person's white blood cells to kill prostate cancer cells. Androgens can stimulate the growth of prostate cancer cells. Hormone therapy using nilutamide may fight prostate cancer by reducing the production of androgens. It is not yet known which treatment regimen is more effective for treating prostate cancer.

Patients will be randomly assigned to one of two groups. Patients in group one will receive a vaccination on day 2. Beginning four weeks later, they will receive a vaccination every four weeks for 12 vaccinations and once every 12 weeks thereafter. They will also receive injections of sargramostim on days 1 through 4 and injections of interleukin-2 on days 8 through 12 after each vaccination. Patients in group two will receive nilutamide by mouth once a day. Treatment in both groups may continue for at least six months. After six months of treatment, some patients in both groups may also receive treatment in the opposite group. Patients will be evaluated once a month for six months and every two months thereafter.

PHASE II RANDOMIZED STUDY OF ZOLEDRONATE WITH OR WITHOUT BMS-275291 IN PATIENTS WITH HORMONE-REFRACTORY PROSTATE CANCER

This randomized Phase II trial will compare the effectiveness of zoledronate with or without BMS-275291 in treating patients who have prostate cancer that has not responded to previous hormone therapy. Zoledronate may prevent bone loss and stop the growth of tumor cells in bone. BMS-275291 may stop the growth of tumor cells by blocking the enzymes necessary for cancer cell growth. It is not yet known if zoledronate is more effective with or without BMS-275291 in treating prostate cancer that has not responded to hormone therapy.

Patients will be randomly assigned to one of two groups. Patients in both groups will receive an infusion of zoledronate once every four weeks for as long as benefit is shown. Patients in group one will also receive BMS-275291 by mouth once a day for as long as benefit is shown. All patients will be evaluated periodically.

PHASE II STUDY OF ANDROGEN-SUPPRESSION THERAPY COMBINED WITH EXTERNAL-BEAM RADIOTHERAPY AND BOOST BRACHYTHERAPY IN PATIENTS WITH INTERMEDIATE-RISK LOCALIZED PROSTATE CANCER

This Phase II trial will study the effectiveness of androgen suppression with either leuprolide or goserelin and either flutamide or bicalutamide plus radiation therapy in treating patients who have prostate cancer. Androgens can stimulate the growth of prostate cancer cells, and so androgen suppression may fight prostate cancer by reducing the production of male hormones. Androgen suppression plus radiation therapy may kill more tumor cells.

Patients will receive injections of either leuprolide or goserelin every 12 weeks for 24 weeks. They will also receive either flutamide by mouth three times a day or bicalutamide by mouth once a day for four weeks. Patients will then undergo external-beam radiation five days a week for five weeks. Two weeks after completing this radiation therapy, patients will undergo implant radiation. Patients will be evaluated every three months for two years, and then every six months for four years.

PHASE II STUDY OF ANTINEOPLASTON A10 AND AS2-1 CAPSULES FOR STAGE III OR IV ADENOCARCINOMA OF THE PROSTATE

This Phase II trial will study the effectiveness of antineoplaston therapy in treating patients who have stage III or stage IV prostate cancer. Antineoplastons are naturally-occurring substances found in urine, which may inhibit the growth of cancer cells.

Patients will receive antineoplastons by mouth six to seven times a day. Treatment may continue for as long as benefit is shown. Tumors will be measured every four months for the first two years, every six months for the next two years, and once a year thereafter.

PHASE II STUDY OF ANTINEOPLASTONS A10 AND AS2-1 CAPSULES WITH TOTAL ANDROGEN BLOCKADE IN PATIENTS WITH STAGE III OR IV ADENOCARCINOMA OF THE PROSTATE

This Phase II trial will study the effectiveness of antineoplaston therapy in treating patients who have stage III or stage IV prostate cancer. Patients receive six or seven doses of antineoplastons by mouth each day, and treatment may be repeated for as long as benefit is shown. Patients will continue hormone therapy. Patients will be evaluated every four months for two years, every six months for two years, and then once a year for two years.

PHASE II STUDY OF ANTINEOPLASTONS A10 AND AS2-1 IN PATIENTS WITH METASTATIC, HORMONE-REFRACTORY ADENOCARCINOMA OF THE PROSTATE

This Phase II trial will study the effectiveness of antineoplaston therapy in treating patients who have metastatic prostate cancer that has not responded to hormone therapy. Patients will receive an infusion of antineoplastons six times a day. Treatment may continue for as long as benefit is shown. Tumors will be measured every two months for a year and every three months for a year.

PHASE II STUDY OF ANTINEOPLASTONS A10 AND AS2-1 IN PATIENTS WITH REFRACTORY STAGE IV ADENOCARCINOMA OF THE PROSTATE

This Phase II trial will study the effectiveness of antineoplaston therapy in treating patients who have refractory stage IV prostate cancer. Patients will receive injections of antineoplastons six times a day, and treatment may continue for as long as benefit is shown. Tumors will be measured every two months during the first year and every three months during the second year.

PHASE II STUDY OF ARSENIC TRIOXIDE IN PATIENTS WITH METASTATIC HORMONE-REFRACTORY PROSTATE CANCER

This Phase II trial will study the effectiveness of arsenic trioxide in treating patients who have stage IV prostate cancer that has not responded to hormone therapy. Patients will receive infusions of arsenic trioxide five days a week for two weeks, and treatment will continue twice a week for at least 14 more weeks. Patients will periodically complete a pain assessment questionnaire.

PHASE II STUDY OF BMS-247550 IN PATIENTS WITH HORMONE-REFRACTORY PROSTATE CANCER

This Phase II trial will study the effectiveness of BMS-247550 in treating patients who have prostate cancer that has not responded to hormone therapy.

Patients will receive an infusion of BMS-247550 every three weeks for as long as benefit is shown. Patients will be evaluated every three months for one year and then every six months for two years.

PHASE II STUDY OF DHA-PACLITAXEL IN PATIENTS WITH METASTATIC HORMONE-REFRACTORY PROSTATE CANCER

This Phase II trial will study the effectiveness of DHA-paclitaxel in treating patients who have metastatic prostate cancer that has not responded to hormone therapy. Patients will receive an infusion of DHA-paclitaxel once every three weeks for as long as benefit is shown. Quality of life will be assessed periodically, and patients will be evaluated every three months.

PHASE II STUDY OF DOCETAXEL PLUS ESTRAMUSTINE IN COMBINATION WITH ANDROGEN DEPRIVATION THERAPY IN PATIENTS WITH PSA ELEVATION FOLLOWING RADIOTHERAPY OR RADICAL PROSTATECTOMY FOR EARLY PROSTATE CANCER

This Phase II trial will study the effectiveness of docetaxel and estramustine plus hormone therapy in treating patients who have previously undergone radiation therapy or surgical removal of the prostate for stage I prostate cancer. Patients will receive estramustine by mouth three times a day on days 1 through 5, and an infusion of docetaxel on day 2. Treatment may be repeated every three weeks for four courses. Patients will then receive bicalutamide by mouth once a day and injections of leuprolide once every three months for 15 months. Patients will receive follow-up evaluations every three months for two years, every four months for a year, and every six months thereafter.

PHASE II STUDY OF DOCETAXEL, ESTRAMUSTINE, AND EXISULIND IN PATIENTS WITH HORMONE-REFRACTORY METASTATIC PROSTATE CANCER

This Phase II trial will study the effectiveness of combining estramustine with exisulind and docetaxel in treating patients who have metastatic prostate cancer that has not responded to hormone therapy. Patients will receive extramustine by mouth three times a day for five days and a one-hour infusion of docetaxel on day 2. Patients will also receive exisulind by mouth twice a day for three weeks. Treatment may be repeated every three weeks for as long as benefit is shown. Patients will be evaluated every three months for two years.

PHASE II STUDY OF DOCETAXEL, ESTRAMUSTINE, AND THALIDOMIDE IN PATIENTS WITH HORMONE-REFRACTORY PROSTATE CANCER

This Phase II trial will study the effectiveness of combining docetaxel and estramustine with thalidomide in treating patients who have prostate cancer previously treated with hormone therapy. Thalidomide may stop the growth of prostate cancer by stopping blood flow to the tumor. Combining chemotherapy with thalidomide may kill more tumor cells than using chemotherapy alone.

Patients will receive estramustine by mouth for three days and a one-hour infusion of docetaxel on day 2. This treatment will continue for three weeks. Treatment may be repeated every four weeks for at least six courses. Patients will also receive thalidomide by mouth once a day for up to a year, and will be evaluated once a month.

PHASE II STUDY OF EARLY ESTRAMUSTINE, ETOPOSIDE, AND PACLITAXEL WITH COMBINED ANDROGEN BLOCKADE THERAPY IN PATIENTS WITH HIGH-RISK METASTATIC ADENOCARCINOMA OF THE PROSTATE

This Phase II trial will study the effectiveness of combination chemotherapy plus hormone therapy in treating patients who have metastatic prostate cancer. Androgens can stimulate the growth of prostate cancer cells; drugs such as goserelin, leuprolide, flutamide, or bicalutamide may stop the adrenal glands from producing androgens. Combining chemotherapy with hormone therapy may kill more tumor cells.

Patients will receive an injection of either goserelin or leuprolide once a month or once every three to four months. Patients will also receive bicalutamide, flutamide, or nilutamide by mouth once a day. Treatment may continue for as long as benefit is shown. Beginning two to four weeks after the start of the hormone therapy, patients will receive estramustine by mouth three times a day for three weeks, an infusion of paclitaxel on day 2, and etoposide by

mouth once a day for two weeks. Treatment may be repeated every three weeks for up to four courses. Patients will be evaluated every six months for two years and once a year for three years.

PHASE II STUDY OF EPOTHILONE B IN PATIENTS WITH HORMONE- AND CHEMOTHERAPY-REFRACTORY PROSTATE CANCER

This Phase II trial will study the effectiveness of epothilone B in treating patients with prostate cancer that has not responded to hormone therapy and chemotherapy. Patients will receive an infusion of epothilone B once a week for three weeks. Treatment may be repeated every four weeks for as long as benefit is shown, and quality of life will be assessed periodically. Patients will be evaluated every three months for two years and every six months for three years.

PHASE II STUDY OF GLYCOSYLATED MUC-2-GLOBO H-KLH CONJUGATE VACCINE WITH ADJUVANT QS21 IN PATIENTS WITH PROSTATE CANCER

This is a Phase II trial to study the effectiveness of combining vaccine therapy with QS21 in treating patients who have prostate cancer. Vaccines may make the body build an immune response to kill tumor cells. Biological therapies such as QS21 use different ways to stimulate the immune system and stop cancer cells from growing. Combining vaccine therapy with QS21 may kill more tumor cells.

Patients will receive injections of the vaccine combined with QS21 once a week in weeks 1 through 3, 7, 15, and 27. Some patients may receive a seventh vaccination after week 50. Patients will be evaluated every three months for a year.

PHASE II STUDY OF HIGH-DOSE THREE-DIMENSIONAL CONFORMAL RADIOTHERAPY (3D-CRT) IN PATIENTS WITH INTERMEDIATE PROGNOSTIC RISK ADENOCARCINOMA OF THE PROSTATE

This Phase II trial will study the effectiveness of radiation therapy that has been planned with a computer in treating patients who have prostate cancer. Computer systems that allow doctors to create a three-dimensional picture of the tumor in order to plan treatment may result in more effective radiation therapy.

Patients will receive high-dose radiation therapy four to five days a week for at least nine weeks. Patients will be evaluated at least once a week during treatment, at two and four months after treatment, and then every six months for three years.

PHASE II STUDY OF IMMUNIZATION WITH PROSTATE-SPECIFIC MEMBRANE ANTIGEN–PULSED AUTOLOGOUS PERIPHERAL BLOOD MONONUCLEAR CELLS AND INTERLEUKIN-12 IN PATIENTS WITH METASTATIC HORMONE-REFRACTORY PROSTATE CANCER

This Phase II trial will study the effectiveness of vaccine therapy combined with interleukin-12 in treating patients who have metastatic prostate cancer that has not responded to hormone therapy. Interleukin-12 may kill cancer cells by stopping blood flow to the tumor and by stimulating a person's white blood cells to kill cancer cells. Combining vaccine therapy with interleukin-12 may kill more tumor cells.

Patients will receive an injection of the vaccine on day 1, and an injection of interleukin-12 on days 1, 3, and 5. Treatment may be repeated every three weeks for up to nine courses. Patients will be evaluated every three months.

PHASE II STUDY OF MEN-10755 IN PATIENTS WITH PROGRESSIVE HORMONE-REFRACTORY ADENOCARCINOMA OF THE PROSTATE

This Phase II trial will study the effectiveness of MEN-10755 in treating patients who have progressive prostate cancer that has not responded to hormone therapy. Patients will receive an infusion of MEN-10755 every three weeks for at least four courses. Patients will be evaluated every six weeks.

PHASE II STUDY OF MITOXANTRONE IN COMBINATION WITH VINORELBINE AS FIRST LINE THERAPY IN PATIENTS WITH METASTATIC HORMONE REFRACTORY ADENOCARCINOMA OF THE PROSTATE

This Phase II trial will study the effectiveness of combination chemotherapy in treating patients who have metastatic prostate cancer that has not responded to hormone therapy. Patients will receive infusions of vinorelbine on days 1 and 8 and an infusion of mitoxantrone on day 8. Treatment may be repeated every three weeks for up to nine courses. Quality of life will be assessed periodically. Patients will receive follow-up evaluations every three months.

PHASE II STUDY OF NEOADJUVANT DOCETAXEL AND MITOXANTRONE FOLLOWED BY PROSTATECTOMY IN PATIENTS WITH HIGH-RISK LOCALIZED PROSTATE CANCER

This Phase I/II trial will study the effectiveness of combination chemotherapy followed by surgery in treating patients who have localized prostate cancer. Combining more than one drug and giving chemotherapy before surgery may shrink the tumor so that it can be removed during surgery.

Patients will receive docetaxel and mitoxantrone once a week for three weeks. Treatment may be repeated for up to four courses. Following chemotherapy, patients will undergo surgery to remove the prostate.

PHASE II STUDY OF NEOADJUVANT PACLITAXEL, ESTRAMUSTINE, CARBOPLATIN, AND ANDROGEN ABLATION FOLLOWED BY RADIOTHERAPY IN PATIENTS WITH POOR-PROGNOSIS LOCALLY ADVANCED PROSTATE CANCER

This Phase II trial will study the effectiveness of combining chemotherapy, hormone therapy, and radiation therapy in treating patients who have locally advanced prostate cancer. Patients will receive a one-hour infusion of paclitaxel once a week and a one-hour infusion of carboplatin once a month. They will receive estramustine by mouth three times a day, five days a week. Treatment may be repeated every four weeks for six courses. Patients will also receive an injection of either goserelin or leuprolide once a month for six courses. After completing chemotherapy, patients will undergo radiation therapy once a day for eight weeks. Patients will be evaluated every three months for two years and then every six months for four years.

PHASE II STUDY OF NONMYELOBLATIVE ALLOGENEIC PERIPHERAL BLOOD STEM CELL TRANSPLANTATION AND DONOR LYMPHOCYTE INFUSIONS IN PATIENTS WITH REFRACTORY METASTATIC SOLID TUMORS

This Phase II trial will study the effectiveness of peripheral stem cell transplantation and donor white blood cell transfusions in treating patients who have refractory metastatic solid tumors. Peripheral stem cell transplantation may be able to replace immune cells that were destroyed by chemotherapy used to kill tumor cells. Sometimes the transplanted cells are rejected by the body's normal tissues; antithymocyte globulin and cyclosporine may prevent this from happening.

Patients will receive infusions of cyclophosphamide and fludarabine for one week. Some patients may also receive infusions of antithymocyte globulin for four days. Patients will then undergo transplantation of donated peripheral stem cells. Patients will receive cyclosporine by continuous infusion or by mouth twice a day for 15 weeks. Some patients may then receive transfusions of donated white blood cells every four weeks. Patients will receive follow-up evaluations every other month for a year, every three months for two years, and every six months for two years.

PHASE II STUDY OF PACLITAXEL AND CARBOPLATIN IN PATIENTS WITH METASTATIC HORMONE-REFRACTORY PROSTATE CANCER

This Phase II trial will study the effectiveness of combining paclitaxel with carboplatin in treating patients who have metastatic prostate cancer that has not responded to hormone therapy.

Patients will receive an infusion of paclitaxel once a week for three weeks, and an infusion of carboplatin in week 1. Treatment may be repeated every four weeks for as long as benefit is shown. Patients will be evaluated every four weeks for 12 weeks and every two months thereafter.

PHASE II STUDY OF PATIENT POSITIONING USING MULTIPLE CT SCANS IN PATIENTS WITH PROSTATE CANCER UNDERGOING EXTERNAL BEAM RADIOTHERAPY

This Phase I trial will study the effectiveness of multiple CT scans in guiding the treatment of patients who have prostate cancer and are undergoing radiation therapy. Multiple CT scans may improve the accuracy of radiation therapy for prostate cancer. Patients will undergo radiation therapy for nine weeks, and will undergo a CT scan immediately before receiving radiation therapy on days 3 through 8, and once a week thereafter. On three different days, patients also will undergo a CT scan immediately after radiation therapy. The patient's positioning for radiation therapy may be adjusted on the basis of the results of the CT scans.

PHASE II STUDY OF RADICAL PROSTATECTOMY IN PATIENTS WITH LOCALLY ADVANCED ADENOCARCINOMA OF THE PROSTATE

This Phase II trial will study the effectiveness of radical prostatectomy in treating patients who have locally advanced prostate cancer. Patients will undergo surgery to remove lymph nodes in the pelvis and will then undergo a retropubic prostatectomy. Some patients may receive further treatment. Patients will be evaluated every three months for a year, every four months for two years, and every six months for two years.

PHASE II STUDY OF THE ROLE OF SALVAGE PROSTATECTOMY AFTER RADIATION FAILURE IN PATIENTS WITH PROSTATE CANCER

This Phase II trial will study the effectiveness of prostatectomy in treating patients who have recurrent or persistent prostate cancer that has not responded to radiation therapy. Prostatectomy may be an effective treatment for prostate cancer that has not responded to radiation therapy. Patients' pelvic lymph nodes will be examined for cancer cells, and patients may then undergo prostatectomy. Some patients may also receive hormone therapy. Quality of life will be assessed before surgery and every three to six months after surgery for two years. Patients will be evaluated at least every three months for two years, every six months for two years, and once a year thereafter.

PHASE II STUDY OF TOPICAL AMIFOSTINE FOR RECTAL PROTECTION DURING RADIOTHERAPY IN PATIENTS WITH PROSTATE CANCER

This Phase II trial will study the effectiveness of topical amifostine in protecting the rectum in patients who are undergoing radiation therapy for prostate cancer. Applying topical amifostine to the rectum before undergoing radiation therapy may protect healthy tissue and decrease the side effects of radiation therapy.

Patients will receive amifostine inserted into the rectum before undergoing radiation therapy five days a week for seven to eight weeks. Quality of life will be assessed periodically, and patients will be evaluated at one month, every three months for six months, every six months for one and a half years, and once a year for three years.

PHASE II/III DIAGNOSTIC STUDY OF C11-METHIONINE AND 2-F18-FLUORO-2-DEOXY-D-GLUCOSE (FDG) POSITRON EMISSION TOMOGRAPHY (PET) IMAGING IN PATIENTS WITH PROGRESSIVE PROSTATE CANCER

This diagnostic trial will study the effectiveness of PET scans in treating patients with metastatic prostate cancer. New imaging procedures, such as PET scans, may improve the ability to detect new or recurrent prostate cancer.

Patients will fast for six hours and then receive an intravenous infusion of a radiolabeled amino acid, followed by PET scans for one hour. Patients will next receive an intravenous infusion of a sugar molecule followed by PET scans for one hour.

PHASE IIB RANDOMIZED CHEMOPREVENTION STUDY OF EFLORNITHINE (DFMO) IN MEN AT HIGH GENETIC RISK FOR PROSTATE CANCER

This randomized Phase II trial will try to determine the effectiveness of eflornithine in preventing prostate cancer in men who are at high risk of developing the disease. All patients will receive a placebo by mouth once a day for four weeks. Patients will then be randomly assigned to one of two groups. Patients in group one will receive a placebo once a day, and patients in group two will receive eflornithine by mouth once a day. Treatment may continue for up to one year.

PHASE III EXTENSION STUDY OF ATRASENTAN IN PATIENTS WITH HORMONE-REFRACTORY PROSTATE CANCER

This Phase III trial will determine the effectiveness of atrasentan in treating patients who have prostate cancer that has not responded to hormone therapy. Patients will receive atrasentan by mouth once a day for three years. Patients will be evaluated at one month and every three months for two years.

PHASE III RANDOMIZED ADJUVANT STUDY OF RADIOTHERAPY WITH HORMONAL THERAPY VERSUS RADIOTHERAPY ALONE VERSUS HORMONAL THERAPY ALONE IN PATIENTS WITH HIGH-RISK STAGE II OR III PROSTATE CANCER

This randomized Phase III trial will compare the effectiveness of radiation therapy plus hormone therapy to that of radiation therapy alone or hormone therapy alone in treating patients who have stage III prostate cancer. Combining radiation therapy with hormone therapy may be an effective treatment for stage III prostate cancer. It is not yet known if radiation therapy combined with hormone therapy is more effective than either radiation therapy alone or hormone therapy alone in treating stage III prostate cancer.

Patients will be randomly assigned to one of three groups. Patients in group one will receive radiation therapy five days a week for seven weeks. At the same time, they will also receive injections of either goserelin or leuprolide every one to four months for two years, and either flutamide by mouth three times a day or bicalutamide once a day for a month. Patients in group two will receive radiation therapy alone as in group one. Patients in group three will receive hormone therapy alone as in group one. All patients will be evaluated every three months for a year, every six months for four years, and once a year thereafter.

PHASE III RANDOMIZED STUDY OF ADJUVANT ANDROGEN DEPRIVATION THERAPY WITH OR WITHOUT MITOXANTRONE AND PREDNISONE AFTER RADICAL PROSTATECTOMY IN PATIENTS WITH HIGH-RISK ADENOCARCINOMA OF THE PROSTATE

This randomized Phase III trial will compare the effectiveness of hormone therapy with or without mitoxantrone and prednisone in treating patients who have undergone radical prostatectomy for prostate cancer. It is not yet known whether hormone therapy plus mitoxantrone and prednisone is more effective than hormone therapy alone for prostate cancer.

Patients will be randomly assigned to one of two groups. Patients in group one will receive an injection of goserelin once every three months and bicalutamide by mouth once a day for two years.

Patients in group two will receive goserelin and bicalutamide as in group one plus an infusion of mitoxantrone on day 1 and prednisone by mouth twice a day for three weeks. Treatment may be repeated every three weeks for six courses. Some patients may also receive radiation therapy. Patients will be evaluated every six months for two years and then once a year for up to 13 years.

PHASE III RANDOMIZED STUDY OF ANDROGEN BLOCKADE WITH CONCURRENT CHEMOTHERAPY VERSUS DELAYED CHEMOTHERAPY IN PATIENTS WITH HIGH-RISK HORMONE-NAIVE PROSTATE CANCER

This randomized Phase III trial will compare the effectiveness of chemotherapy given at the same time as hormone therapy with that of chemotherapy given after hormone therapy in treating patients who have prostate cancer. Drugs such as goserelin, leuprolide, flutamide, or bicalutamide may stop the adrenal glands from producing androgens, which can stimulate the growth of prostate cancer cells. It is not yet known if chemotherapy given at the same time as hormone therapy is more effective than chemotherapy given after hormone therapy in treating prostate cancer.

Patients will be randomly assigned to one of two groups. Patients in group one will receive injections of either leuprolide or goserelin once every one to three months. They will also receive either flutamide or bicalutamide by mouth once a day for at least a month. Within two weeks of starting hormone therapy, patients will receive one of five different chemotherapy regimens for approximately six months. Patients in group two will receive hormone therapy as in group one for as long as benefit is shown. Some patients may then receive one of the chemotherapy regimens as in group one. All patients will be evaluated every three months for two years, every six months for three years, and once a year thereafter.

PHASE III RANDOMIZED STUDY OF ANDROGEN SUPPRESSION AND RADIOTHERAPY WITH OR WITHOUT SUBSEQUENT PACLITAXEL, ESTRAMUSTINE, AND ETOPOSIDE IN PATIENTS WITH LOCALIZED HIGH-RISK PROSTATE CANCER

This randomized Phase III trial will compare the effectiveness of hormone therapy plus radiation therapy with or without combination chemotherapy in treating patients who have prostate cancer. It is not yet known whether hormone therapy plus radiation therapy is more effective with or without combination chemotherapy for prostate cancer.

Patients will receive hormone therapy for four months. Eight weeks after beginning hormone therapy, patients will undergo radiation therapy five days a week for seven to eight weeks. Patients will then be randomly assigned to one of two groups. Patients in group one will continue to receive hormone therapy for about 20 more months after completing radiation therapy. Patients in group two will receive treatment as in group one plus combination chemotherapy every three weeks for four courses. Patients will be evaluated every three months for two years, every six months for three years, and once a year thereafter.

PHASE III RANDOMIZED STUDY OF ATRASENTAN IN PATIENTS WITH NONMETASTATIC HORMONE-REFRACTORY PROSTATE CANCER

This randomized Phase III trial will study the effectiveness of atrasentan in treating patients who have nonmetastatic prostate cancer that has not responded to hormone therapy. Patients will be randomly assigned to one of two groups. Patients in group one will receive atrasentan by mouth once a day; patients in group two will receive a placebo by mouth once a day. Treatment in both groups may continue for as long as benefit is shown.

PHASE III RANDOMIZED STUDY OF CALCIUM AND CHOLECALCIFEROL WITH OR WITHOUT CONJUGATED ESTROGENS AND WITH OR WITHOUT RISEDRONATE FOR THE PREVENTION OF OSTEOPOROSIS IN PATIENTS WITH PROSTATE CANCER RECEIVING ANDROGEN ABLATION THERAPY

This randomized Phase III trial will compare the effectiveness of two forms of calcium with or without estrogen and/or risedronate in preventing osteoporosis in patients with prostate cancer who are receiving androgen ablation therapy. Preventing bone loss in patients who are undergoing androgen ablation for prostate cancer may decrease the risk of fractures and may help patients live more comfortably. It is not yet known whether calcium is more effective with or without estrogen and/or risedronate in preventing osteoporosis.

Patients will be randomly assigned to one of four groups. Patients in group one will receive two forms of calcium by mouth, a risedronate placebo by mouth, and an estrogen placebo by mouth. Patients in group two will receive two forms of calcium by mouth, risedronate by mouth, and an estrogen placebo by mouth. Patients in group three will receive two forms of calcium by mouth, estrogen by mouth, and a risedronate placebo by mouth. Patients in group four will receive two forms of calcium by mouth, estrogen by mouth, and risedronate by mouth. Treatment in all groups will be repeated once a day for two years, during which quality of life and bone mineral density will be assessed periodically.

PHASE III RANDOMIZED STUDY OF CONSOLIDATION THERAPY WITH OR WITHOUT STRONTIUM CHLORIDE SR 89 AFTER INDUCTION CHEMOTHERAPY IN PATIENTS WITH ANDROGEN-INDEPENDENT PROSTATE CANCER

This randomized Phase III trial will compare the effectiveness of chemotherapy with or without strontium-89 in treating patients who have prostate cancer that has spread to the bone. Radioactive substances such as strontium-89 may relieve bone pain associated with prostate cancer.

Patients will receive one of two chemotherapy regimens for six weeks. Treatment may be repeated every eight weeks for up to two courses. Some patients will then be randomly assigned to one of two groups. Patients in group one will receive a 24-hour continuous infusion of doxorubicin once a week for six weeks plus an infusion of strontium-89 at the beginning of chemotherapy. Patients in group two will receive doxorubicin as in group one. Patients will be evaluated every three months.

PHASE III RANDOMIZED STUDY OF CYPROTERONE ACETATE IN PATIENTS WITH HOT FLASHES FOLLOWING SURGICAL OR CHEMICAL CASTRATION FOR PROSTATE CANCER

This randomized Phase III trial will determine the effectiveness of cyproterone acetate in treating patients who have hot flashes following surgical or chemical castration for prostate cancer. Cyproterone acetate may be effective treatment for hot flashes following surgical or chemical castration for prostate cancer, but it is not yet known which regimen of cyproterone acetate is more effective for hot flashes.

Patients will be randomly assigned to receive one of two doses of cyproterone acetate or a placebo by mouth for 12 weeks. Patients in both groups will then receive cyproterone acetate for six to nine months. Quality of life will be assessed.

PHASE III RANDOMIZED STUDY OF DENDRITIC CELL–RECOMBINANT PROSTATE-SPECIFIC MEMBRANE ANTIGEN VACCINE (DCVAX-RPSMA) IN PATIENTS WITH METASTATIC, HORMONE-REFRACTORY ADENOCARCINOMA OF THE PROSTATE

This randomized Phase III trial will study the effectiveness of vaccine therapy in treating patients who have metastatic prostate cancer that has not responded to hormone therapy.

White blood cells will be collected from patients to make the vaccine. Patients will then be randomly assigned to one of two groups to receive injections of either the vaccine or a placebo in weeks 1, 5, 9, 13, 21, and 39. Patients will be evaluated periodically for a year and every six months for two years.

PHASE III RANDOMIZED STUDY OF DOCETAXEL AND ESTRAMUSTINE VERSUS MITOXANTRONE AND PREDNISONE IN PATIENTS WITH HORMONE-REFRACTORY, METASTATIC ADENOCARCINOMA OF THE PROSTATE

This randomized Phase III trial will compare the effectiveness of estramustine plus docetaxel with that of mitoxantrone plus prednisone in treating patients who have stage IV prostate cancer that has not responded to hormone therapy. It is not yet known whether estramustine plus docetaxel is more effective than mitoxantrone plus prednisone for prostate cancer.

Patients will be randomly assigned to one of two groups. Patients in group one will receive estramustine by mouth three times a day for five days plus a one-hour infusion of docetaxel on day 2. Patients in group two will receive an infusion of mitoxantrone on day 1 plus prednisone by mouth two times a day for three weeks. Treatment in both groups may be repeated every three weeks for up to 12 courses. Quality of life will be assessed periodically before, during, and after treatment. Patients will receive follow-up evaluations every six months for two years and then at year 3.

PHASE III RANDOMIZED STUDY OF GABAPENTIN FOR THE MANAGEMENT OF HOT FLASHES IN PATIENTS WITH PROSTATE CANCER

This randomized Phase III trial will compare different regimens of gabapentin in treating men who have prostate cancer. Gabapentin may be effective in relieving hot flashes in men who have prostate cancer. It is not yet known which regimen of gabapentin is most effective in treating hot flashes.

Patients will be randomly assigned to one of four groups. Patients in group one will receive gabapentin by mouth once a day for four weeks. Patients in group two will receive gabapentin by mouth once a day for a week and twice a day for three weeks. Patients in group three will receive gabapentin by mouth once a day for a week, twice a day for a week, and three times a day for two weeks. Patients in group four will receive a placebo by mouth as in either group one, group two, or group three. Treatment may be repeated for an additional eight weeks. Quality of life will be assessed periodically. Patients will be evaluated at six months and once a year for two years.

PHASE III RANDOMIZED STUDY OF HIGH-VERSUS STANDARD-DOSE THREE-DIMENSIONAL CONFORMAL RADIOTHERAPY IN PATIENTS WITH STAGE I OR II ADENOCARCINOMA OF THE PROSTATE

This randomized Phase III trial will compare the effectiveness of two different doses of specialized radiation therapy in treating patients who have stage I or stage II prostate cancer. Specialized radiation therapy that delivers a high dose of radiation directly to the tumor may kill more tumor cells and cause less damage to normal tissue. It is not yet known which dose of radiation therapy is more effective in treating stage I or stage II prostate cancer.

Patients will be randomly assigned to one of two groups. Patients in group one will undergo standard-dose specialized radiation therapy five days a week for approximately eight weeks. Patients in group two will undergo high-dose specialized radiation therapy five days a week for approximately nine weeks. Quality of life will be assessed periodically. Patients will be evaluated every three months for two years, every six months for three years, and once a year thereafter.

PHASE III RANDOMIZED STUDY OF *HYPERICUM PERFORATUM* (ST. JOHN'S WORT) COMBINED WITH DOCETAXEL IN PATIENTS WITH UNRESECTABLE SOLID TUMORS

This randomized Phase III trial will compare the effectiveness of docetaxel with or without St. John's wort in treating patients who have solid tumors that cannot be removed by surgery. St. John's wort may interfere with the effectiveness of chemotherapy. It is not yet known if chemotherapy is more effective with or without St. John's wort in treating solid tumors.

Patients who have not previously received St. John's wort will be randomly assigned to one of two groups. Patients in group one will receive a placebo by mouth three times a day for two weeks followed by a one-hour infusion of docetaxel on day 15. Patients in group two will receive St. John's wort by mouth three times a day for two weeks followed by docetaxel as in group one. Patients who have previously received St. John's wort will receive their usual regimen for two weeks followed by docetaxel as in group one. Treatment in all groups may be repeated every three weeks for two courses. Patients will be evaluated periodically.

PHASE III RANDOMIZED STUDY OF INITIAL BICALUTAMIDE VERSUS OBSERVATION FOLLOWED BY BICALUTAMIDE WITH EITHER GOSERELIN OR BILATERAL ORCHIECTOMY IN PATIENTS WITH PROSTATE CANCER

This randomized Phase III trial will compare the effectiveness of bicalutamide with that of observation followed by bicalutamide plus either goserelin or orchiectomy for patients who have prostate cancer. Testosterone can stimulate the growth of cancer cells. Bicalutamide and goserelin may fight prostate cancer by reducing the production of testosterone. It is not yet known which hormone therapy regimen is most effective for prostate cancer.

Patients will be randomly assigned to one of two groups. Patients in group one will receive bicalutamide by mouth once a day. At the first symptom of disease progression, patients will also receive either an injection of goserelin every four or 12 weeks or will undergo bilateral orchiectomy. Some patients will then stop taking bicalutamide. Patients in group two will be observed, and at the first symptom of disease progression will begin taking bicalutamide and will either receive goserelin or undergo bilateral orchiectomy as in group one. Some patients in group two will also stop taking the bicalutamide as in group one. Quality of life will be assessed in both groups periodically. Patients will be evaluated once a year.

PHASE III RANDOMIZED STUDY OF INTERMITTENT VERSUS CONTINUOUS ANDROGEN SUPPRESSION IN PATIENTS WITH PROSTATE-SPECIFIC ANTIGEN PROGRESSION IN THE CLINICAL ABSENCE OF DISTANT METASTASES AFTER PRIOR RADIOTHERAPY FOR PROSTATE CANCER

This randomized Phase III trial will compare the effectiveness of intermittent or continuous hormone therapy in treating patients with rising PSA levels following radiation therapy for prostate cancer. It is not yet known which androgen suppression regimen is more effective for prostate cancer.

Patients will be randomly assigned to one of two groups. Patients in group one will receive a luteinizing hormone–releasing hormone (LHRH) analog implant injected under the skin every one to four months and an antiandrogen by mouth one to three times a day for eight months. When PSA levels return to normal, therapy will stop. If PSA levels rise again, treatment will continue for eight more months. Treatment may be repeated for as long as benefit is shown. Patients in group two will receive LHRH analog and an antiandrogen without interruptions with or without surgery to remove the testicles. Quality of life will be assessed periodically. Patients will be evaluated once a year.

PHASE III RANDOMIZED STUDY OF INTERMITTENT VERSUS CONTINUOUS COMBINED ANDROGEN-DEPRIVATION THERAPY COMPRISING BICALUTAMIDE AND GOSERELIN IN PATIENTS WITH METASTATIC STAGE IV PROSTATE CANCER RESPONSIVE TO SUCH THERAPY

This randomized Phase III trial will compare the effectiveness of two hormone therapies in treating

men who have stage IV prostate cancer. Testosterone can stimulate the growth of prostate cancer cells, and hormone therapy may be effective treatment for prostate cancer. It is not yet known which regimen of hormone therapy is most effective for stage IV prostate cancer.

Patients will receive an injection of goserelin once a month and bicalutamide by mouth once a day for seven months. Patients will then be randomly assigned to one of two groups. Patients in group one will continue to receive the same hormone therapy for as long as benefit is shown. Patients in group two will receive hormone therapy periodically. Quality of life will be assessed before treatment, and at eight, 11, 17, and 23 months, and patients will be evaluated every six months.

PHASE III RANDOMIZED STUDY OF NEOADJUVANT TOTAL ANDROGEN SUPPRESSION AND RADIOTHERAPY IN PATIENTS WITH INTERMEDIATE-RISK ADENOCARCINOMA OF THE PROSTATE

This randomized Phase III trial will compare the effectiveness of two different regimens of hormone therapy and radiation therapy in treating patients who have prostate cancer. It is not yet known which regimen of hormone therapy and radiation therapy is more effective for prostate cancer.

Patients will be randomly assigned to one of two groups. Patients in group one will receive goserelin or leuprolide every one to three months and bicalutamide or flutamide by mouth once a day for 16 weeks. Beginning in week 9, patients will also receive radiation therapy five days a week for eight weeks. Patients in group two will receive hormone therapy as in group one for 36 weeks. Beginning in week 29, they will receive radiation therapy as in group one. Patients will receive follow-up evaluations every three months for a year, every six months for four years, and once a year thereafter.

PHASE III RANDOMIZED STUDY OF OCTREOTIDE FOR PREVENTION OF ACUTE DIARRHEA IN PATIENTS RECEIVING RADIOTHERAPY TO THE PELVIS

This is a randomized Phase III trial designed to determine the effectiveness of octreotide in preventing diarrhea in patients who are undergoing radiation therapy to the pelvis. Octreotide may be effective in preventing or controlling diarrhea in patients who are undergoing radiation therapy to the pelvis. It is not yet known whether octreotide is effective for diarrhea.

No more than four days after beginning radiation therapy, patients will be randomly assigned to one of two groups. Patients in group one will receive an injection of short-acting octreotide on day 1 and an injection of long-acting octreotide on days 2 and 29. Patients in group two will receive an injection of a placebo as in group one. Treatment in both groups may continue for as long as benefit is shown. Patients will complete questionnaires periodically. They will be evaluated once a week for four weeks, at one year, and at two years.

PHASE III RANDOMIZED STUDY OF ORAL THALIDOMIDE VERSUS PLACEBO IN PATIENTS WITH ANDROGEN DEPENDENT STAGE IV NONMETASTATIC PROSTATE CANCER FOLLOWING LIMITED HORMONAL ABLATION

This randomized Phase III trial will determine the effectiveness of leuprolide or goserelin plus thalidomide in treating patients who have nonmetastatic stage IV prostate cancer. Thalidomide may stop the growth of prostate cancer by stopping blood flow to the tumor. It is not yet known whether leuprolide or goserelin plus thalidomide is more effective than leuprolide or goserelin alone for prostate cancer.

Patients who have a rising PSA level will be randomly assigned to receive injections of either leuprolide or goserelin once a month, followed by either thalidomide or a placebo by mouth once a day until disease progression. Patients will then receive an additional six months of leuprolide or goserelin. Patients who have received the placebo will then receive thalidomide, and patients who had received thalidomide will then receive a placebo. Treatment will continue for as long as benefit is shown. Patients will be evaluated once a month.

PHASE III RANDOMIZED STUDY OF POSTOPERATIVE EXTERNAL RADIOTHERAPY VS NO IMMEDIATE FURTHER TREATMENT IN PATIENTS WITH PT3 PN0 PROSTATIC ADENOCARCINOMA

This randomized Phase III trial will compare radiation therapy with no further treatment in treating patients with stage III prostate cancer following radical prostatectomy.

Patients will be randomized to one of two groups. Patient in the first group will receive radiation therapy five days a week for five weeks, followed by additional radiation therapy for one to one and a half weeks. Those in the second group will undergo observation, except patients in relapse will receive radiation therapy. Patients will receive follow-up evaluation every three months during the first year after surgery, every six months until year five, and once a year thereafter.

PHASE III RANDOMIZED STUDY OF RADICAL PROSTATECTOMY VERSUS BRACHYTHERAPY IN PATIENTS WITH STAGE II PROSTATE CANCER

This is a randomized Phase III trial to compare the effectiveness of surgery with that of internal radiation in treating patients who have stage II prostate cancer. Internal radiation uses radioactive material placed directly into or near a tumor to kill tumor cells. It is not yet known whether surgery is more effective than internal radiation in treating prostate cancer.

Patients will be randomly assigned to one of two groups. Patients in group one will undergo surgery to remove the prostate. Patients in group two will undergo internal radiation. Patients will be evaluated every six months for five years and once a year thereafter.

PHASE III RANDOMIZED STUDY OF RADIOTHERAPY TO THE PROSTATE WITH OR WITHOUT RADIOTHERAPY TO THE PELVIS IN PATIENTS WITH STAGE I, II, OR III ADENOCARCINOMA OF THE PROSTATE

This randomized Phase III trial will compare the effectiveness of radiation therapy to the prostate with or without radiation to the pelvis in treating patients with stage I, stage II, or stage III prostate cancer.

Patients will be randomized to receive either radiation therapy to the prostate and pelvis or radiation therapy only to the prostate. Treatment for both groups will be given five days a week for seven weeks. Quality of life will be assessed before therapy, 12 months after therapy, and then once a year. Patients will be evaluated at two and six months and every six months thereafter.

PHASE III RANDOMIZED STUDY OF RADIOTHERAPY WITH OR WITHOUT ADJUVANT BICALUTAMIDE AND GOSERELIN IN PATIENTS WITH LOCALIZED PROSTATE CANCER

This randomized Phase III trial will compare the effectiveness of radiation therapy with or without bicalutamide and goserelin in treating patients who have localized prostate cancer. Bicalutamide and goserelin may fight prostate cancer by reducing the production of testosterone. It is not yet known if radiation therapy is more effective with or without bicalutamide and goserelin in treating prostate cancer.

Patients will be randomly assigned to one of two groups. Patients in group one will receive bicalutamide by mouth once a day for 30 days. They will also receive an injection of goserelin in week 2 and again three months later. Beginning in week 2, patients will undergo radiation therapy five days a week for up to seven and a half weeks. Patients in group two will undergo radiation therapy as in group one. Quality of life will be assessed periodically. Patients will be evaluated every six months for five years and once a year thereafter.

PHASE III RANDOMIZED STUDY OF RADIOTHERAPY WITH OR WITHOUT BICALUTAMIDE IN PATIENTS WITH PSA ELEVATION FOLLOWING RADICAL PROSTATECTOMY FOR CARCINOMA OF THE PROSTATE

This randomized Phase III trial will compare the effectiveness of radiation therapy with or without bicalutamide in treating patients who have stage II, stage III, or recurrent prostate cancer and elevated PSA levels following radical prostatectomy.

Patients will be randomly assigned to one of two groups. Patients in group one will receive radiation therapy for 7.2 weeks plus bicalutamide by mouth daily for two years. Patients in group two will receive radiation therapy for 7.2 weeks plus a placebo by mouth daily for two years. Patients will receive follow-up evaluations every three months for two years, every six months for three years, and once a year thereafter.

PHASE III RANDOMIZED STUDY OF SECOND-LINE HORMONAL THERAPY (KETOCONAZOLE AND HYDROCORTISONE) VERSUS COMBINATION CHEMOTHERAPY (DOCETAXEL AND ESTRAMUSTINE) IN ASYMPTOMATIC PATIENTS WITH PROSTATE CANCER AND A RISING PSA AFTER ANDROGEN SUPPRESSION

This randomized Phase III trial will compare the effectiveness of hormone therapy with that of combination chemotherapy in treating patients who have prostate cancer that has been previously treated with androgen suppression.

Patients will be randomly assigned to one of two groups. Patients in group one will receive ketoconazole by mouth three times a day and hydrocortisone by mouth twice a day for as long as benefit is shown. Patients in group two will receive estramustine by mouth three times a day on days 1 through 5. On day 2 they will receive a one-hour infusion of docetaxel. Treatment may be repeated every three weeks for up to six courses. Quality of life will be assessed periodically. Patients will be evaluated every three months for two years, every six months for five years, and once a year for five years.

PHASE III RANDOMIZED STUDY OF SELENIUM AND VITAMIN E FOR THE PREVENTION OF PROSTATE CANCER (SELECT TRIAL)

This randomized Phase III trial will determine the effectiveness of selenium and vitamin E, either alone or together, in preventing prostate cancer. It is not yet known which regimen of selenium and/or vitamin E may be more effective in preventing prostate cancer.

Patients will be randomly assigned to one of four groups. Patients in group one will receive two different placebos by mouth once a day. Patients in group two will receive selenium and a placebo by mouth once a day. Those in group three will receive vitamin E and a placebo by mouth once a day, and patients in group four will receive selenium and vitamin E by mouth once a day. Treatment may continue for seven to 12 years. Quality of life will be assessed periodically. Patients will be evaluated periodically.

PHASE III RANDOMIZED STUDY OF TOTAL ANDROGEN BLOCKADE WITH OR WITHOUT PELVIC IRRADIATION IN PATIENTS WITH LOCALLY ADVANCED ADENOCARCINOMA OF THE PROSTATE

This randomized Phase III trial will compare the effectiveness of hormone therapy alone, hormone therapy plus bilateral orchiectomy, or hormone therapy plus radiation therapy in treating patients who have stage III or stage IV prostate cancer.

Patients will be randomly assigned to one of two groups. Patients in group one will receive hormone therapy with or without surgery. Patients in group two will receive hormone therapy as in group one plus radiation therapy. Hormone therapy will be repeated every four to eight weeks for as long as benefit is shown. Patients will receive radiation therapy five days a week for approximately seven weeks. Quality of life will be assessed periodically. Patients will be evaluated at one, two and six months and every six months thereafter.

PHASE III RANDOMIZED STUDY OF ZOLEDRONATE AND ESTRADIOL FOR THE PREVENTION OF BONE LOSS IN PATIENTS WITH PROSTATE CANCER UNDERGOING HORMONAL BLOCKADE THERAPY

This randomized Phase III trial will compare the effectiveness of zoledronate and estradiol alone to that of zoledronate combined with estradiol in preventing bone loss in patients who are receiving hormone therapy for prostate cancer. It is not yet known whether zoledronate and estradiol are more effective alone or in combination in preventing bone loss in patients who are receiving hormone therapy for prostate cancer.

Patients will be randomly assigned to one of four groups. Patients in group one will receive an infusion of zoledronate and estradiol by skin patch. Patients in group two will receive an infusion of zoledronate and a placebo by skin patch. Patients in group three will receive an infusion of a placebo and estradiol by skin patch. Patients in group four will receive an infusion of a placebo and a placebo by skin patch. Treatment in all groups may be repeated every three months for four courses, and all patients will also receive calcium and vitamin D

by mouth once a day. Quality of life will be assessed periodically.

PHASE III STUDY OF CHEMO/HORMONAL THERAPY VS ANDROGEN ABLATION ALONE AS INITIAL THERAPY IN PATIENTS WITH UNRESECTABLE/METASTATIC ADENOCARCINOMA OF THE PROSTATE

This randomized Phase III trial will compare the effectiveness of chemotherapy plus hormone therapy versus androgen suppression alone as initial therapy in patients with prostate cancer that is metastatic or that cannot be removed surgically.

Patients will be randomized to one of two groups. Patients in group one will undergo medical or surgical castration followed by antiandrogen therapy. Patients in group two will have a catheter placed and will receive three eight-week courses of chemotherapy plus hormone therapy followed by total androgen ablation.

PHASE III STUDY OF LONG TERM ADJUVANT HORMONAL TREATMENT WITH LHRH ANALOG (TRIPTORELIN) VERSUS NO FURTHER TREATMENT IN PATIENTS WITH LOCALLY ADVANCED PROSTATIC CARCINOMA TREATED BY EXTERNAL IRRADIATION AND A SIX MONTH COMBINED ANDROGEN BLOCKAGE

This randomized Phase III trial will compare the effectiveness of long-term hormone therapy and triptorelin with no further treatment in treating patients who have advanced prostate cancer previously treated with radiation therapy and six months of androgen suppression. Hormone therapy using triptorelin may fight prostate cancer by reducing the production of androgens.

Patients will receive radiation therapy for seven weeks, followed by treatment with flutamide or bicalutamide. Patients will then be randomly assigned to one of two groups. Patients in group one will receive no further treatment. Patients in group two will receive injections of triptorelin every three months for two and a half years. Patients in group two will receive triptorelin for an additional 30 months without continued flutamide or bicalutamide. Patients will receive follow-up evaluations every six months during the first five years after treatment and then once a year thereafter.

PILOT STUDY OF MARIJUANA IN COMBINATION WITH MORPHINE FOR THE TREATMENT OF PERSISTENT PAIN SECONDARY TO BONE METASTASES IN PATIENTS WITH BREAST OR PROSTATE CANCER

This clinical trial will study the effectiveness of combining morphine with marijuana in treating pain caused by bone metastases in patients who have breast or prostate cancer. Morphine helps to relieve the pain associated with bone metastases. Marijuana may be effective in controlling pain and nausea and vomiting. Combining morphine with marijuana may provide more pain relief and may help to reduce or prevent nausea and vomiting in patients treated with opioids.

Patients will smoke one marijuana cigarette three times a day for a week, and receive morphine by mouth. Patients will complete questionnaires and undergo assessments of pain, nausea, and vomiting periodically.

RANDOMIZED HOME-BASED STUDY OF A DIET- AND EXERCISE-BASED COUNSELING PROGRAM VERSUS A STANDARD COUNSELING PROGRAM FOR PATIENTS WITH EARLY-STAGE BREAST OR PROSTATE CANCER

This randomized clinical trial will compare the effectiveness of a diet- and exercise-based counseling program with that of a standard counseling program in patients who have early-stage prostate cancer or breast cancer. An individualized, computer-designed health program may promote changes in diet and physical activity and may improve quality of life in prostate or breast cancer survivors.

Patients will be randomly assigned to one of two groups. Patients in group one will participate for 10 months in a computer-designed correspondence course that includes a personalized diet, exercise, and other health information. Patients in group two will receive standard reading materials about diet, exercise, cancer, and other health issues. Some patients may undergo collection of blood samples and have height and weight measured periodically. Some patients may also be asked to wear a device for a week that measures walking distance. In both groups, diet and exercise behavior, quality of life, and other health issues will be evaluated by telephone interview periodically during and after the study.

RANDOMIZED PILOT STUDY OF ISOFLAVONES VERSUS LYCOPENE PRIOR TO RADICAL PROSTATECTOMY IN PATIENTS WITH LOCALIZED PROSTATE CANCER

This randomized clinical trial will compare the effectiveness of isoflavones with that of lycopene before surgery in treating patients who have stage I or stage II prostate cancer. Chemoprevention therapy is the use of certain substances to try to prevent the development or recurrence of cancer. Eating a diet rich in isoflavones, compounds found in soy foods, or lycopene, a substance found in tomatoes, may prevent the development of cancer.

Patients will be randomly assigned to one of seven groups. Patients in groups one, two, and three will receive one of three doses of isoflavones by mouth twice a day plus a multivitamin once a day. Patients in groups four, five, and six will receive one of three doses of lycopene by mouth twice a day plus a multivitamin once a day. Patients in group seven will receive a multivitamin alone once a day. Treatment may continue for up to six weeks.

RANDOMIZED PILOT STUDY TO EVALUATE EDUCATIONAL INTERVENTION AND BEHAVIORAL SKILLS TRAINING FOR PAIN CONTROL IN PATIENTS WITH RECURRENT OR METASTATIC BREAST OR PROSTATE CANCER

This randomized pilot study will evaluate whether an outpatient educational and behavioral skills training program will improve pain control in patients who have metastatic or recurrent prostate cancer. An outpatient educational and behavioral skills training program may help patients with metastatic prostate cancer live longer and more comfortably.

Patients will be randomized to one of two groups. Patients in group one will receive standard pain management, but patients in group two will receive standard pain management plus educational intervention and behavior-skills training. Patients in group two will view and discuss pain management videos, listen to relaxation audio-tapes, and receive a schedule of practice relaxation sessions. Patients in group two will receive a follow-up phone call to review their pain status. Patients in both groups will undergo pain and psychological assessments on days 1 and 15.

RANDOMIZED STUDY OF HEALTH PROMOTION IN PATIENTS WHO ARE PROSTATE OR BREAST CANCER SURVIVORS

This randomized clinical trial will compare the effectiveness of an individualized, computer-designed program with that of a standard program in promoting health in patients who have early-stage breast cancer or prostate cancer. Telephone counseling by a nutritionist and a personal trainer may improve physical function and quality of life in patients who have early-stage breast cancer or prostate cancer.

Patients will be randomly assigned to one of two groups. Patients in group one will receive telephone counseling about diet and exercise. Patients in group two will receive telephone counseling about general health topics such as sun exposure, cancer screening, and falls prevention. Counseling in both groups will continue every two weeks for six months. All patients will be evaluated at six months.

RANDOMIZED STUDY OF HEALTH-RELATED QUALITY OF LIFE IN PATIENTS WITH STAGE II PROSTATE CANCER TREATED WITH RADICAL PROSTATECTOMY OR BRACHYTHERAPY

This randomized clinical trial will study quality of life in patients undergoing surgery or brachytherapy for stage II prostate cancer. Quality of life assessment in patients undergoing prostate cancer treatment may help determine the intermediate-term and long-term effects of surgery and brachytherapy.

Patients will be randomly assigned to undergo either radical prostatectomy or brachytherapy. Patients in both groups will complete quality-of-life questionnaires before, during, and for 10 years after treatment.

RANDOMIZED STUDY OF ISOFLAVONES IN REDUCING RISK FACTORS IN PATIENTS WITH PROSTATE CANCER

This randomized clinical trial is studying the effectiveness of isoflavones in preventing prostate cancer. Soy isoflavones may reduce the risk of some types of cancer. It is not yet known if isoflavones are effective in preventing prostate cancer.

Patients will be randomly assigned to one of two groups. Patients in group one will receive isoflavones by mouth twice a day and a multivitamin once a day for 12 weeks. Patients in group two will receive a placebo and a multivitamin as in group one.

RANDOMIZED STUDY OF SELENIUM AS CHEMOPREVENTION OF PROSTATE CANCER IN PATIENTS WITH HIGH-GRADE PROSTATIC INTRAEPITHELIAL NEOPLASIA

This randomized clinical trial will study the effectiveness of selenium in preventing prostate cancer in patients who have neoplasia of the prostate.

Patients will be randomly assigned to one of two groups. Patients in group one will receive selenium by mouth once a day for up to three years. Patients in group two will receive a placebo by mouth once a day for up to three years. Patients will be evaluated every six months for two years and once a year for eight years.

STUDY OF ANDROGEN ABLATION AND BONE RESORPTION IN PATIENTS WITH OR WITHOUT BONE METASTASES SECONDARY TO PROSTATE CANCER

This clinical trial will determine the effect of androgen suppression on bone loss in patients who have prostate cancer. Assessing the effect of androgen suppression on bone loss in prostate cancer patients may improve the ability to plan treatment, may decrease the risk of fractures and bony pain, and may help patients live more comfortably.

Patients will undergo blood work and 24-hour urine collection. The blood work and urine collection will be repeated six to eight weeks later. Some patients will undergo an X ray scan.

STUDY OF THE EORTC QLQ-C30 AND PROSTATE CANCER–SPECIFIC QLQ-PR25 QUESTIONNAIRES TO ASSESS QUALITY OF LIFE OF PATIENTS WITH STAGE I–IV PROSTATE CANCER

This clinical trial will study the effectiveness of two questionnaires in assessing quality of life of patients who have prostate cancer. Quality of life assessment in patients undergoing prostate cancer treatment may help determine the intermediate and long-term effects of the treatment on these patients.

Patients will complete two questionnaires before therapy and three months after the start of therapy. Some patients will also complete questionnaires at six months after the start of therapy.

SUPPORTIVE-EXPRESSIVE GROUP THERAPY FOR MEN WITH STAGE I/II PROSTATE CANCER

This randomized clinical trial will study the effect of group therapy compared with written educational materials on the quality of life of men with stage I or stage II prostate cancer.

Patients will be randomized to one of two groups. One group will attend 12 weekly 90-minute group therapy meetings where they will have an opportunity to express their thoughts, feelings and emotions; set goals; and participate in stress reduction exercises. The other group will receive a packet of educational booklets about coping with prostate cancer. Both groups will fill out quality-of-life questionnaires every three to six months for two years.

GLOSSARY

antigen   A protein marker on the surface of a cell that identifies the cell.

androgen   A hormone that promotes the development and maintenance of male sex characteristics. Testosterone is the primary androgen.

antegrade ejaculation   Normal forward ejaculation.

azoospermia   Semen containing no sperm, either because the testicles cannot make sperm, there is a blockage in the reproductive tract, or the patient has had a vasectomy.

biopsy   Removal of a small tissue sample for microscopic examination.

capsule   The layer of cells around an organ such as the prostate.

carcinoma   Cancer that begins in the tissues that line or cover an organ.

central nervous system   Brain and spinal cord. Extragonadal germ cell tumors can arise in the central nervous system, often in the pineal gland. Metastatic germ cell tumors can also spread to the central nervous system.

clinical trial   A research study designed to answer specific questions about a particular disease.

differentiation   The degree to which a tumor resembles normal tissue. Typically, the closer the resemblance, the better the prognosis. Well-differentiated tumors are very similar to normal tissue.

ejaculate   The semen and sperm expelled during ejaculation.

epididymis   A soft, tubelike structure behind the testicle that collects and carries sperm; inside it, the developing sperm complete their maturation. The mature sperm leave the epididymis through the vas deferens, where they may live for several weeks.

epididymitis   Inflammation of the epididymis. This common problem is usually caused by infection.

external urethral sphincter muscle   A voluntary and involuntary ringlike band of muscle fibers that a person can voluntarily contract to stop urination.

false negative   A negative result of a test that occurs when in reality the test result is positive.

false positive   A positive result of a test that occurs when in reality the test result is negative.

funiculitis   Inflammation of the spermatic cord.

germ cell   The testicular cell that divides to produce the immature sperm cells. A man's germ cells remain intact throughout his reproductive life. Most (95 percent) testicular tumors are germ cell tumors.

gonad   The gland that makes reproductive cells and sex hormones. This includes the testicles, which make sperm and testosterone.

lymph   A nearly colorless fluid that bathes body tissues and contains cells that help the body fight infection.

lymph nodes   Small bean-shaped structures located throughout the body along the channels of the lymphatic system (also called lymph glands). Nodes filter circulating lymph and trap bacteria or cancer cells that may travel through the lymphatic system.

metastasis   The spread of cancer cells to distant areas of the body via the lymph system or bloodstream.

natural killer cells (NK cells)   White blood cells that can kill tumor cells and infected body cells. NK cells kill on contact, binding to the target cell and releasing toxic chemicals. Normal cells are not affected by NK cells, which play a major role in cancer prevention by destroying abnormal cells to prevent them from becoming dangerous.

oligospermia   Low production of sperm.

perineum   The tissue located between the anus and scrotum.

peripheral neuropathy A condition of the nervous system that usually begins in the hands or feet, causing numbness, tingling, burning, and weakness. It is sometimes caused by certain chemotherapy drugs, such as cisplatin.

recurrence The return of cancer after treatment, which may occur either at the original site of the disease or at another location (metastasis).

rete testis A network of tubules that basically connects the seminiferous tubules in the testis to the epididymis.

retroperitoneum The back of the abdomen, where the kidneys lie and the great blood vessels run.

tunica albuginea A white fibrous tissue that encapsulates the testis.

tunica vaginalis A double-layered pouch that covers each testis, composed of a membrane that provides lubrication.

vas deferens A small thin cord that carries mature sperm from the testicle and epididymis to the ejaculatory ducts near the prostate gland in the urethra.

BIBLIOGRAPHY

The Alpha-Tocopherol, Beta Carotene Cancer Prevention Study Group. "The Effect of Vitamin E and Beta Carotene on the Incidence of Lung Cancer and Other Cancers in Male Smokers." *New England Journal of Medicine* 330 (1994): 1,029–1,035.

Adlercreutz, H. "Evolution, Nutrition, Intestinal Microflora, and Prevention of Cancer: A Hypothesis." *Proceedings of the Society for Experimental Biology and Medicine* 217 (1998): 241–246.

Albertsen, P. C. "The Positive Yield of Imaging Studies in the Evaluation of Men with Newly Diagnosed Prostate Cancer: A Population Based Analysis." *Journal of Urology* 163 (2000): 1,138–1,143.

Altman, Roberta, and Michael J. Sarg, *The Cancer Dictionary.* New York: Facts On File, 2000.

Amagase, H., et al. "Intake of Garlic and Its Bioactive Components." *Journal of Nutrition* 131 (2001): 9,55S–9,26S.

American Cancer Society. "American Cancer Society Updates Prostate Cancer Screening Guidelines." Available at: http://www.cancer.org.

———. "Unproven Methods of Cancer Management: Laetrile." *CA: A Cancer Journal for Clinicians* 41, no. 3 (1991): 187–192.

Anderson, J. J. B., and S. C. Garner. "Phytoestrogens and Human Function." *Nutrition Today* 32 (1997): 39.

Armstrong, C., C. Stern, and B. Corn. "Memory Performance Used to Detect Radiation Effects on Cognitive Functioning." *Applied Neuropsychology,* 8 (2001): 129–139.

Bal, D. G., and S. B. Forester. "Dietary Strategies for Cancer Prevention." *Cancer* 72 (1992): 1,005–1,010.

Beecher, C. W. W. "Cancer Preventive Properties of Varieties of *Brassica oleracea:* A Review." *American Journal of Clinical Nutrition* 59 (1994): 166S–1170S.

Brawley, O. W., K. Knopf, and I. Thompson. "The Epidemiology of Prostate Cancer. Part II. The Risk Factors." *Seminars in Urologic Oncology* 16, no. 4 (1998): 193–201.

Bruera, E. "Current Pharmacological Management of Anorexia in Cancer Patients." *Oncology* 6, no. 1 (1992): 125–130.

Browne, R. F., et al. "Technical Report. Intra–operative Ultrasound-guided Needle Localization for Impalpable Testicular Lesions." *Clinical Radiology* 58, no. 7 (July 2003): 566–569.

Byers, T., and N. Guerrero. "Epidemiologic Evidence for Vitamin C and Vitamin E in Cancer Prevention." *American Journal of Clinical Nutrition* 62 (1995): 1,385S–1,392S.

Chaudhary, U. B., and J. R. Haldas. "Long-term Complications of Chemotherapy for Germ Cell Tumours." *Drugs* 63, no. 15 (2003): 1,565–1,577.

Clegg, L. X., et al. "Comparison of Self-Reported Initial Treatment with Medical Records: Results from the Prostate Cancer Outcomes Study." *American Journal of Epidemiology* 154 (2001): 582–587.

Coley, C. M., et al. "Early Detection of Prostate Cancer. Part II. Estimating the Risks, Benefits, and Costs." *Annals of Internal Medicine* 126 (1997): 468–479.

Culkin, D. J., and T. M. Beer. "Advanced Penile Carcinoma." *Journal of Urology* 170, no. 2 (pt. 1) (August 2003): 359–365.

Dearnaley, D. P., et al. "A double-blind, Placebo-controlled, Randomized Trial of Oral Sodium Clodronate for Metastatic Prostate Cancer (MRC PR05 Trial)." *Journal of the National Cancer Institute* 95, no. 17 (September 3, 2003): 1,300–1,311.

Dibble, S. L., et al. "Acupressure for Nausea: Results of a Pilot Study." *Oncology Nursing Forum* 27, no. 1 (February 2000): 41–47.

Donohue, J. P. "Evolution of Retroperitoneal Lymphadenectomy (RPLND) in the Management of

Nonseminomatous Testicular Cancer (NSGCT)." *Urological Oncology* 21, no. 2 (March–April 2003): 129–132.

Downing, S. R., P. J. Russell, and P. Jackson. "Alterations of p53 Are Common in Early Stage Prostate Cancer." *Canadian Journal of Urology* 10, no. 4 (August 2003): 1,924–1,933.

Duyff, R. L. *The American Dietetic Association's Complete Food and Nutrition Guide.* Minneapolis, Minn.: Chronimed, 1996.

Dufresne, C. J., and E. R. Farnworth. "A Review of Latest Research Findings on the Health Promotion Properties of Tea." *Journal of Nutritional Biochemistry* 12, no. 7 (2001): 404–421.

Ellison, N. M., D. P. Byar, and G. R. Newell. "Special Report on Laetrile: The NCI Laetrile Review: Results of the National Cancer Institute's Retrospective Laetrile Analysis." *New England Journal of Medicine* 299, no. 10 (1978): 549–552.

Fleischauer, A. T., and L. Arab. "Garlic and Cancer: A Critical Review of the Epidemiologic Literature." *Journal of Nutrition* 131 (2001): 1,032S–1,040S.

Fossa, S. D., et al. "Optimal Planning Target Volume for Stage I Testicular Seminoma: A Medical Research Council Randomized Trial, Medical Research Council Testicular Tumor Working Group." *Journal of Clinical Oncology* 17 (1999): 1,146.

Friedenreich, C. M., and K. S. Courneya. "Exercise as Rehabilitation for Cancer Patients." *Clinical Journal of Sport Medicine* 6 (1996): 237–244.

Frydenberg, M., P. D. Stricker, and K. W. Kaye. "Prostate Cancer Diagnosis and Management." *The Lancet* 349 (1997): 1,681–1,687.

Gann, P. H., et al. "Prospective Study of Sex Hormone Levels and Risk of Prostate Cancer." *Journal of the National Cancer Institute* 88 (1996): 1,118–1,126.

Gann, P. H., et al. "Prospective Study of Plasma Fatty Acids and Risk of Prostate Cancer." *Journal of the National Institute of Cancer* 86 (1994): 281–286.

Gann, P. H., et al. "Lower Prostate Cancer Risk in Men with Elevated Plasma Lycopene Levels: Results of a Prospective Analysis." *Cancer Research* 59 (1999): 1,225–1,230.

Garner, M. J., et al. Canadian Cancer Registries Epidemiology Research Group. "Dietary Risk Factors for Testicular Carcinoma." *International Journal of Cancer* 106, no. 6 (October 2003): 934–941.

Gill, W. B., G. F. B. Schumacher, and M. Bibbo. "Structural and Functional Abnormalities in the Sex Organs of Male Offspring of Mothers Treated with Diethylstilbestrol (DES)." *Journal of Reproductive Medicine* 16 (1976): 147–153.

Gilliland, F. D., et al. "Predicting Extracapsular Extension of Prostate Cancer in Men Treated with Radical Prostatectomy: Results from the Population-Based Prostate Cancer Outcomes Study." *Journal of Urology* 162 (1999): 1,341–1,345.

Giovannucci, E. "Selenium and Risk of Prostate Cancer." *Lancet* 352 (1998): 755–756.

Goldbohm, R. A., et al., "Consumption of Black Tea and Cancer Risk: A Prospective Cohort Study." *Journal of the National Cancer Institute* 88, no. 2 (1996): 93–100.

Gray, S., and O. I. Olopade. "Direct-to-consumer Marketing of Genetic Tests for Cancer: Buyer Beware." *Journal of Clinical Oncology* 21 (2003): 3,191–3,193.

Greenlee, R. T., et al. "Cancer Statistics, 2001." *CA: A Cancer Journal for Clinicians* 56 (2001): 15–36.

Greenwald, P. "The Potential of Dietary Modification to Prevent Cancer." *Preventive Medicine* 25 (1996): 41–43.

Griffiths, K., et al. "Possible Relationship between Dietary Factors and Pathogenesis of Prostate Cancer." *International Journal of Urology* 5 (1998): 195–213.

Hamilton, A. S., et al. "Health Outcomes after External-Beam Radiation Therapy for Clinically Localized Prostate Cancer: Results from the Prostate Cancer Outcomes Study." *Journal of Clinical Oncology* 19, no. 9 (2001): 2,517–2,526.

Hammar, M., et al. "Acupuncture Treatment of Vasomotor Symptoms in Men with Prostatic Carcinoma: A Pilot Study." *Journal of Urology* 161 (1999): 853–856.

Harlan, L. C., et al. "Factors Associated with Initial Therapy for Clinically Localized Prostate Cancer: Prostate Cancer Outcomes Study." *Journal of the National Institute of Cancer* 93, no. 24 (December 2001): 1,864–1,871.

Hoffman, R. M., et al. "Factors Associated with Racial and Ethnic Differences in Presenting with

Advanced Stage Prostate Cancer: Results from The Prostate Cancer Outcomes Study." *Journal of the National Institute of Cancer* 93, no. 5 (2001): 388–395.

Hoffman, R. M., et al. "Patient Satisfaction with Treatment Decisions for Clinically Localized Prostate Carcinoma: Results from the Prostate Cancer Outcomes Study." *Cancer* 97, no. 7 (April 1, 2003): 1,653–1,662.

Holm, M., et al. "Increased Risk of Carcinoma in Situ in Patients with Testicular Germ Cell Cancer with Ultrasonic Microlithiasis in the Contralateral Testicle." *Journal of Urology* 170, no. 4 (pt. 1) (October 2003): 1,163–1,167.

Kamradt, J. M., and K. J. Pienta. "The Effect of Hydrazine Sulfate on Prostate Cancer Growth." *Oncology Reports* 5 (1998): 919–921.

Kaegi, E. "Unconventional Therapies for Cancer." *Canadian Medical Association Journal* 158, no. 9 (1998): 1,157–1,159.

Kattlove, H., and R. J. Winn. "Ongoing Care of Patients after Primary Treatment for Their Cancer." *CA: A Cancer Journal for Clinicians* 53 (2003): 172–196.

Kolonel, L. N. "Nutrition and Prostate Cancer." *Cancer Causes Control* 7 (1996): 83–94.

Kramer, B. S., et al. "A National Cancer Institute Sponsored Screening Trial for Prostatic, Lung, Colorectal, and Ovarian Cancers." *Cancer* 71 (suppl. 2) (1993): 589–593.

Legler, J., et al. "Validation Study of Retrospective Recall of Disease-targeted Function: Results from the Prostate Cancer Outcomes Study." *Medical Care* 38, no. 8 (2000): 847–857.

Lerner, I. J. "Laetrile: A Lesson in Cancer Quackery." *CA: A Cancer Journal for Clinicians* 31, no. 2 (1981): 91–95.

Lesko, S. M., et al. "Vasectomy and Prostate Cancer." *Journal of Urology* 161, no. 6 (1999): 1,848–1,852.

Lightfoot, N., et al. "Prostate Cancer Risk: Medical History, Sexual, and Hormonal Factors." *Annals of Epidemiology* 10, no. 7 (2000): 470.

Lindegaard, J. C., et al. "A Retrospective Analysis of 82 Cases of Cancer of the Penis." *British Journal of Urology* 77, no. 6 (1996): 883–890.

Long, A. P., et. al. "Management of Clinically Node Negative Penile Carcinoma: Improved Survival after the Introduction of Dynamic Sentinel Node Biopsy." *Journal of Urology* 170, no. 3 (September 2003): 783–786.

Lynch, D. F., and P. F. Schellhammer. "Tumors of the Penis." In *Campbell's Urology* 7th ed., edited by P. C. Clark, et al. 2,453–2,478. Philadelphia: W.B. Saunders, 1998.

Lynch, H. T., J. A. Ens, and J. F. Lynch. "The Lynch Syndrome II and Urological Malignancies." *Journal of Urology* 143, no. 1 (January 1990): 24–28.

Mandoky, L., et al. "Expression of HER-2/neu in Testicular Tumors." *Anticancer Research* 23, no. 4 (July/August 2003): 3,447–3,451.

Masters, J.R., and B. Koberle. "Curing Metastatic Cancer: Lessons from Testicular Germ-cell Tumors." *National Review of Cancer* 3, no. 7 (July 2003): 517–525.

McLean, M., et al. "The Results of Primary Radiation Therapy in the Management of Squamous Cell Carcinoma of the Penis." *International Journal of Radiation Oncology Biological Physics* 25, no. 4 (1993): 623–628.

Mcleod, D. G., and G. J. Kolvenbag. "Defining the Role of Antiandrogens in the Treatment of Prostate Cancer." *Urology* 47 (suppl. 1A)(1996): 85–89.

Milner, J. A. "Mechanisms by Which Garlic and Allyl Sulfur Compounds Suppress Carcinogen Bioactivation: Garlic and Carcinogenesis." *Advances in Experimental Medicine and Biology* 492 (2001): 69–81.

———. "A Historical Perspective on Garlic and Cancer." *Journal of Nutrition* 131 (2001): 1,027S–1,031S.

Mosharafa, A. A., et al. "Does Retroperitoneal Lymph Node Dissection Have a Curative Role for Patients with Sex Cord–stromal Testicular Tumors?" *Cancer* 98, no. 4 (August 2003): 753–757.

Pais, V., et al. "Estrogen Receptor-beta Expression in Human Testicular Germ cell Tumors." *Clinical Cancer Research* 9, no. 12 (2003): 4,475–4,482.

Parnes, H. L., and J. Aisner. "Protein Calorie Malnutrition and Cancer Therapy." *Drug Safety* 7, no. 6 (1992): 404–416.

Patterson, H., et al. "Combination Carboplatin and Radiotherapy in the Management of Stage II Testicular Seminoma: Comparison with Radiotheraphy Treatment Alone." *Radiotherapy Oncology* 59 (2001): 5–11.

Penson, D. F., et al. "General Quality of Life Two Years Following Treatment for Prostate Cancer: What Influences Outcomes? Results from the Prostate Cancer Outcomes Study." *Journal of Clinical Oncology* 21 (2003): 1,147–1,154.

Perry, B. B., et al. "Adenocarcinoma of the Rete Testis Presenting in an Undescended Testicle." *Journal of Urology* 170, no. 4 (pt. 1)(October 2003): 1,304.

Polsky, E. G., et al. "Primary Malignant Mesothelioma of the Penis: Case Report and Review of the Literature." Urology 62, no. 3 (September 2003): 551.

Potosky, A. L., et al. "Prostate Cancer Practice Patterns and Quality of Life: The Prostate Cancer Outcomes Study." *Journal of the National Cancer Institute* 91 (1999): 1,719–1,724.

Potosky, A. L., et. al. "Health Outcomes after Radical Prostatectomy or Radiotherapy for Clinically Localized Prostate Cancer: Results from the Prostate Cancer Outcomes Study (PCOS)." *Journal of the National Institute of Cancer* 92 (2000): 1,582–1,592.

Potosky, A. L., et al. "Quality of Life Following Localized Prostate Cancer Treated Initially with Androgen Deprivation Therapy or No Therapy." *Journal of the National Institute of Cancer* 94, no. 6 (March 20, 2002): 430–437.

Potosky, A. L., et al. "Quality-of-Life Outcomes after Primary Androgen Deprivation Therapy: Results from the Prostate Cancer Outcomes Study." *Journal of Clinical Oncology* 19 (2001): 3,750–3,757.

Rentinck, M. E., et al. "Chemotherapy for Metastatic Seminoma in Elderly Patients." *Anticancer Research* 23, no. 3C (May–June 2003): 3,093–3,096.

Reyes, A., et al. "Neuroendocrine Carcinomas (Carcinoid Tumor) of the Testis: A Clinicopathologic and Immunohistochemical Study of Ten Cases." *American Journal of Clinical Pathology* 120, no. 2 (August 2003): 182–187.

Roukos, D. H., A. M. Kappas, and E. Tsianos. "Role of Surgery in the Prophylaxis of Hereditary Cancer Syndromes." *Annals of Surgical Oncology* 9 (2002): 607–609.

Schellhammer, P. F., et al. "Clinical Benefits of Bicalutamide Compared with Flutamide Capsules in combined Androgen Blockade for Patients with Advanced Prostatic Carcinoma: Final Report of a Double-Blind, Randomized, Multicenter Trial." *Urology* 50 (1997): 330–336.

Scholz, M., and W. Holtjl. "Stage I Testicular Cancer." *Current Opinions in Urology* 13, no. 6 (November 2003): 473–476.

Schwingl, P. J., and H. A. Guess. "Safety and Effectiveness of Vasectomy." *Fertility and Sterility* 73, no. 5 (2000): 923–936.

Serra-Majem, L., et al. "Changes in Diet and Mortality from Selected Cancers in Southern Mediterranean Countries." *European Journal of Clinical Nutrition* 47 (1993): S25–S34.

Sigurdsson, S., et al. "BRCA2 Mutation in Icelandic Prostate Cancer Patients." *Journal of Molecular Medicine* 75 (1997): 758–761.

Stancik, I., and W. Holtl. "Penile Cancer: Review of the Recent Literature." *Current Opinions in Urology* 13, no. 6 (November 2003): 467–472.

Stanford, J. L., et al. "Vasectomy and Risk of Prostate Cancer." *Cancer Epidemiology, Biomarkers & Prevention* 8, no. 10 (1999): 881–886.

Struewing, J. P., et al. "The Risk of Cancer Associated with Specific Mutations of *BRCA1* and *BRCA2* among Ashkenazi Jews." *New England Journal of Medicine* 336 (1997): 1401–1408.

Taksey, J., N. K. Bissada, and U. B. Chaudhary. "Fertility after Chemotherapy for Testicular Cancer." *Archives of Andrology* 49, no. 5 (September–October 2003): 389–395.

Tamboli, C. P. "Long-term Survivors of Testicular Cancer." *Journal of Clinical Oncology* 21, no. 20 (October 15, 2003): 3888.

Teeley, P., and P. Bashe. *The Complete Cancer Survival Guide*. New York: Doubleday, 2000.

Theodorescu, D., et al. "Outcomes of Initial Surveillance of Invasive Squamous Cell Carcinoma of the Penis and Negative Nodes." *Journal of Urology* 155, no. 5 (1996): 1626–1631.

Vogelzang, N. J., et al., eds. *Comprehensive Textbook of Genitourinary Oncology,* 2d ed. Philadelphia: Lippincott Williams & Wilkins, 2000.

INDEX